THE ADIPOCYTE AND OBESITY:
CELLULAR AND MOLECULAR MECHANISMS

The Adipocyte and Obesity: Cellular and Molecular Mechanisms

Editors

Aubie Angel, M.D., B.Sc. (Med.), M.Sc., F.R.C.P.(C).
Professor of Medicine and Attending Staff
Toronto General Hospital
University of Toronto
Toronto, Ontario, Canada

Charles H. Hollenberg, M.D., F.A.C.P., B.Sc., B.Sc. (Med)., F.R.C.P.(C).
Professor of Medicine
Director, Banting and Best Diabetes Center and Attending Staff
Toronto General Hospital
University of Toronto
Toronto, Ontario, Canada

Daniel A. K. Roncari, M.D., M.Sc., Ph.D., F.A.C.P., F.R.C.P.(C).
Professor of Medicine
Director, Institute of Medical Science and Attending Staff
Toronto Western Hospital
University of Toronto
Toronto, Ontario, Canada

Raven Press ■ New York

Raven Press, 1140 Avenue of the Americas, New York, New York 10036

Made in the United States of America

Library of Congress Cataloging in Publication Data
Main entry under title:

The Adipocyte and obesity.

  Proceedings of the International Conference on the Adipocyte and Obesity, held at the University of Toronto, June 1982, and sponsored by the Ontario Heart Foundation, et al.
  Includes bibliographical references and index.
  1. Obesity—Congresses.   2. Adipose tissues—Congresses.   I. Angel, Aubie.   II. Hollenberg, Charles H.
III. Roncari, Daniel A. K.   IV. International Conference on the Adipocyte and Obesity (1982 : University of Toronto)   V. Ontario Heart Foundation.   [DNLM:
1. Adipose tissue—Metabolism—Congresses.   2. Lipids—Metabolism—Congresses.   3. Obesity—Congresses.
QS 532.5.A3 A2347]
RC628.A33   1983   616.3′98   83-3372
ISBN 0-89004-946-7

Preface

This volume includes chapters originally presented at the International Conference on the Adipocyte and Obesity, held at the University of Toronto in June 1982. The contributors, scientists interested in adipose cell biology, were brought together to discuss major advances in this area. This meeting was the third in an ongoing series, focusing on cellular and molecular events, but differing somewhat from its predecessors in Nice, France (1979) and Göteborg, Sweden (1980) by its emphasis on research related to obesity. Major areas of adipose cell biology were considered under six topic headings (Fig. 1).

1. CELL GROWTH AND DEVELOPMENT
precursors
regional and sex variations
nutritional effects
massive obesity

6. ENERGY EXPENDITURE
metabolic efficiency
thermic effect of feeding
brown fat

2. INSULIN ACTION
mediators
receptor control
glucose transporter

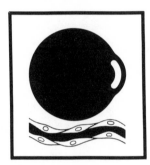

5. LIPOPROTEINS AND CHOLESTEROL
cholesterol storage
lipoprotein interactions
estrogen synthesis

3. LIPID ASSIMILATION
lipoprotein lipase
LPL activators
glyceride synthesis

4. LIPOLYSIS
adrenergic receptors
cyclic nucleotides
antilipolysis
obesity effects

FIG. 1. Major physiological functions of adipose tissue (Nos. 1–6 above) are mediated through coordinated structural and functional interactions between the fat cell and its capillary endothelial network. For this reason the adipocyte and an associated capillary may be viewed as the functional unit of adipose tissue and, in stylized form, serve as a logo for the conference and this proceeding.

Adipocyte growth and development is one of the important areas reviewed in this volume. This field of research began about 15 years ago with studies of control of fat cell number and of DNA synthesis in primordial fat cells and was stimulated considerably when adipocyte precursors were successfully cultured from human adipose tissue. The role of adipose tissue as a model system in the study of mechanisms of insulin action is highlighted by the presentation of evidence for the existence of new cellular mediators. Also discussed are newer insights in the regulation of triglyceride assimilation by lipoprotein lipase and fatty acid release through the lipolytic cascade which emphasizes the complex yet highly coordinated control of storage and release of nutrient by the fat cell. The role of adipose tissue in cholesterol turnover and storage as a newly recognized, important function of the adipocyte is presented. The relation of cholesterol metabolism to lipoprotein turnover and catabolism has attracted growing attention and is discussed in the following section. The final section describes the widespread interest in energy balance and thermoregulation in obesity. The possible role of brown adipose tissue in man prompted the inclusion of energy expenditure as a major topic area.

This volume presents a comprehensive update on the cellular and molecular mechanisms that control adipose cell function. It will be of interest to biochemists, particularly those interested in lipid metabolism, nutritionists, and all physicians and scientists interested in obesity and its management.

A. Angel
C .H. Hollenberg
D. A. K. Roncari

January 1983

Acknowledgments

The International Conference on the Adipocyte and Obesity and the publication of the proceedings were made possible by the generous support of major sponsors and supporters listed below. We wish to publicly thank these organizations for their assistance.

Sponsors:

Ontario Heart Foundation
Canadian Heart Foundation
Wintario Program Grant
Institute of Medical Sciences
Health and Welfare Canada
Banting and Best Diabetes Centre
Redpath Industries

Supporters:

Confederation Life
Ontario Wine Council
Ontario Ministry of Intergovernmental
  Affairs
Upjohn Company of Canada
Standard Brands Limited
Dairy Bureau of Canada
Metropolitan Toronto
City of Toronto

Contents

Perspectives 1

Adipose Cell Growth and Development

Insulin Action

Contributors

G. Ailhaud
Centre de Biochimie
Parc Valrose, Faculte des Sciences
Universite de Nice
06034 Nice, France

P. Alaupovic
Laboratory of Lipid and Lipoprotein Studies
Oklahoma Medical Research Foundation
Oklahoma City, Oklahoma 73104

A. Angel
Room 7368, Medical Sciences Building
University of Toronto
1 King's College Circle
Toronto, Ontario M5S 1A8, Canada

Alan D. Attie
Division of Metabolic Disease
Department of Medicine
University of California at San Diego
La Jolla, California 92093

P. Belfrage
Department of Physiological Chemistry 4
Box 750
S 220-7 Lund 7, Sweden

Gunilla Bengtsson
Department of Physiological Chemistry
University of Umea
S-901 87 Umea, Sweden

Per Björntorp
Department of Medicine
University of Goteborg
Sahlgren's Hospital
41345 Goteborg, Sweden

E. Joan Blanchette-Mackie
Laboratory of Cellular and Developmental
   Biology
NIADDK
National Institutes of Health
Bethesda, Maryland 20205

Conrad B. Blum
Arteriosclerosis Research Center
Departments of Medicine and Pediatrics
Columbia University College of Physicians
   and Surgeons
New York, New York 10032

J. Borensztajn
Northwestern Memorial Hospital
Wesley Pavilion, Room 407
Superior Street & Fairbanks Court
Chicago, Illinois 60611

George A. Bray
Department of Health Services
University of Southern California Medical
   Center
1200 North State Street
Los Angeles, California 90033

W. Carl Breckenridge
Department of Biochemistry
Dalhousie University
Halifax, Nova Scotia

David N. Brindley
Department of Biochemistry
University Hospital and Medical School
Clifton Boulevard
Nottingham NG7 2UH, England

Thomas W. Burns
Department of Pharmacology
University of Missouri-Columbia School of
   Medicine
M-523 Medical Sciences Building
Columbia, Missouri 65212

David B. Bylund
Department of Pharmacology
University of Missouri-Columbia School of
   Medicine
M-523 Medical Sciences Building
Columbia, Missouri 65212

George F. Cahill, Jr.
Director of Research
Howard Hughes Medical Institute
398 Brookline Avenue, Suite 8
Boston, Massachusetts 02215

Thomas E. Carew
Division of Metabolic Disease
Department of Medicine
University of California at San Diego
La Jolla, California 92093

T. P. Ciaraldi
Department of Medicine
University of Colorado Health Sciences Center
4200 East Ninth Avenue
Denver, Colorado 80262; and
Veterans Administration Hospital
Denver, Colorado 80222

William H. Cleland
Departments of Biochemistry and Obstetrics-
Gynecology and The Cecil H. and Ida
Green Center for Reproductive Biology
Sciences
The University of Texas Health Science Center
at Dallas
Dallas, Texas 75235

D. Cox
Research Institute
Hospital for Sick Children; and
Departments of Paediatrics and Medical
Genetics
University of Toronto
Toronto, Ontario, Canada

Samuel W. Cushman
Cellular Metabolism, Obesity Section
National Institute of Arthritis, Metabolism and
Digestive Diseases
National Institutes of Health
Danarc Building 4, Room 15
Bethesda, Maryland 20205

D. Czerucka
Centre de Biochimie
Universite de Nice
06034 Nice, France

Elliott Danforth, Jr.
University of Vermont
College of Medicine
Given Building
Burlington, Vermont 05405

Ralph B. Dell
Arteriosclerosis Research Center and the
Departments of Medicine and Pediatrics
Columbia University College of Physicians
and Surgeons
New York, New York 10032

P. Djian
Institute of Medical Science and Department
of Medicine
University of Toronto
Toronto, M5S 1A8 Canada

Irving M. Faust
Department of Medicine
The Rockefeller University
1230 York Avenue
New York, New York 10021

B. Fong
Department of Medicine
Toronto General Hospital and University of
Toronto
Toronto, Ontario, Canada M5S 1A8

C. Forest
Centre de Biochimie
(CNRS LP-7300)
Universite de Nice
06034 Nice, France

G. Fredrikson
Department of Physiological Chemistry
University of Lund
S-220 07 Lund, Sweden

J. S. Garrow
Department of Physiology
MRC Clinical Research Center
Harrow, England

DeWitt S. Goodman
Columbia University
College of Physicians and Surgeons
639 West 168th Street
New York, New York 10032

Howard Green
Department of Biology
Massachusetts Institute of Technology
77 Massachusetts Avenue
Cambridge, Massachusetts 02139

P. Grimaldi
Centre de Biochimie
Universite de Nice
06034 Nice, France

Jean Himms-Hagen
Department of Biochemistry
University of Ottawa
Alta Vista Health Science Centre
451 Smythe Road
Ottawa, Ontario K1H 8M5, Canada

Arthur D. Hartman
Department of Physiology
LSU Medical Center
1100 Florida Avenue
New Orleans, Louisiana 70119

Paul J. Hissin
Department of Chemistry
Mount Sinai Hospital
New York, New York 10029

C. H. Hollenberg
Toronto General Hospital
CW1-104
101 College Street
Toronto, Ontario M5G 1L7, Canada

L. Jarett
Department of Pathology, Laboratory of
*   Medicine*
University of Pennsylvania Hospital
3400 Spruce Street, Box 671
Philadelphia, Pennsylvania 19104

Lorna Joy
Division of Metabolic Disease
Department of Medicine
University of California at San Diego
La Jolla, California 92093

William B. Kannel
Department of Medicine
Boston University School of Medicine
80 East Concord Street
Boston, Massachusetts 02118

Eddy Karnieli
Metabolic Unit
Endocrine Institute
Rambam Medical Center
Haifa, Israel

K. Kawamura
Division of Metabolic Disease
Department of Medicine
University of California at San Diego
La Jolla, California 92093

J. C. Khoo
Division of Metabolic Disease
Department of Medicine M013
University of California at San Diego
School of Medicine
Basic Science Building
La Jolla, California 92093

F. L. Kiechle
University of Pennsylvania School of Medicine
Department of Pathology and Laboratory
*   Medicine*
Philadelphia, Pennsylvania 19104

S. Kindler
Institute of Medical Science
Department of Medicine
University of Toronto
Toronto, M5S 1A8 Canada

O. G. Kolterman
Department of Medicine
University of Colorado Health Sciences Center
Denver, Colorado 80262; and Veterans
*   Administration Hospital*
Denver, Colorado 80222

T. J. Kotlar
Department of Pathology
Northwestern University Medical School
Chicago, Illinois 60611

Brian R. Krause
Department of Pharmacology
Warner-Lambert/Parke-Davis
Pharmaceutical Research Division
Ann Arbor, Michigan 48105

A. Kuksis
Banting and Best Department of Medical
*   Research*
University of Toronto
Toronto, Canada

Lewis Landsberg
Beth Israel Hospital
330 Brookline Avenue
Boston, Massachusetts 02215

Paul E. Langley
Department of Medicine, Surgery, and
*   Pharmacology*
University of Missouri School of Medicine
Columbia, Missouri 65212

D. C. W. Lau
Institute of Medical Science and Department
*   of Medicine*
University of Toronto
Toronto, M5S 1A8 Canada

Nigel Lawson
Department of Biochemistry
University of Nottingham Medical School
Queen's Medical Centre
Nottingham, NG7 2UH England

F. T. Lindgren
Donner Laboratory
University of California
Berkeley, California 94720

J. A. Little
The Lipid Research Clinic Project
Department of Medicine
University of Toronto
St. Michael's Hospital
Toronto, Canada

John A. Little
Department of Biochemistry
University of Leeds
Leeds, LS2 9JT England

S. L. Macaulay
Department of Pathology and Laboratory
  Medicine
University of Pennsylvania
School of Medicine
Philadelphia, Pennsylvania 19104

Carole R. Mendelson
Department of Biochemistry
University of Texas Southwestern Medical
  School
5323 Harry Hines Boulevard
Dallas, Texas 75235

Wilson H. Miller, Jr.
The Rockefeller University
New York, New York 10021

Margaret L. Moule
Banting and Best Department of Medical
  Research
University of Toronto
Toronto, M5G 1L6 Canada

R. Négrel
Centre de Biochimie
Universite de Nice
06034 Nice, France

J. M. Olefsky
Department of Medicine
University of Colorado Medical Center
4200 East Ninth Avenue, Room 4629
Denver, Colorado 80262

Thomas Olivecrona
Department of Physiological Chemistry
University of Umea
S-90187 Umea, Sweden

H. Olsson
Department of Physiological Chemistry
University of Lund
S-220 07 Lund, Sweden

Robert H. Palmer
Arteriosclerosis Research Center
Departments of Medicine and Pediatrics
Columbia University College of Physicians
  and Surgeons
New York, New York 10032

J. C. Parker
Department of Pathology and Laboratory
  Medicine
University of Pennsylvania School of Medicine
Philadelphia, Pennsylvania 19104

Susan M. Parkin
Department of Biochemistry
University of Leeds
Leeds, LS2 9JT England

Ray C. Pittman
Division of Metabolic Disease
Department of Medicine
University of California at San Diego
La Jolla, California 92093

Rajasekhar Ramakrishnan
Arteriosclerosis Research Center
Columbia University College of Physicians
  and Surgeons
New York, New York 10032

Alli Reinila
Department of Pathology
University of Oulu
Oulu, Finland

Albert E. Renold
Institut de Biochimie Clinique
University of Geneva Medical School
Geneva, Switzerland

Donald S. Robinson
Department of Biochemistry
The University of Leeds
9 Hyde Terrace
Leeds, LS2 9LS, England

D. A. K. Roncari
University of Toronto
Room 7238, Medical Sciences Building
1 King's College Circle
Toronto, Ontario M5S 1A8, Canada

Lester B. Salans
Cellular Metabolism and Obesity Section
NIADDK
National Institutes of Health
Bethesda, Maryland 20205

J. A. Scarlett
Department of Medicine
University of Colorado Health Sciences Center
Denver, Colorado 80262

Robert O. Scow
National Institutes of Health
Building 10, 8D–14
Bethesda, Maryland 20205

David L. Severson
The University of Calgary
Health Sciences Center
3330 Hospital Drive, N.W.
Calgary, Alberta T2N 4N1, Canada

Evan R. Simpson
Departments of Biochemistry and Obstetrics-
    Gynecology
The Cecil H. and Ida Green Center for
    Reproductive Biology Sciences
The University of Texas Health Sciences
    Center at Dallas
Dallas, Texas 75235

Ian A. Simpson
Cellular Metabolism and Obesity Section
NIADDK
National Institutes of Health
Bethesda, Maryland 20205

Ethan A. H. Sims
University of Vermont
College of Medicine
Given Building
Burlington, Vermont 05405

Ulf Smith
Department of Medicine II
University of Goteborg
Sahlgren's Hospital
Goteborg, Sweden

Brian K. Speake
Department of Biochemistry
University of Leeds
Leeds, LS2 9JT England

Daniel Steinberg
University of California at San Diego
Basic Science Building, Room 4028
La Jolla, California 92093

P. Strålfors
Department of Physiological Chemistry
University of Lund
S-220 07 Lund, Sweden

Boyd E. Terry
Departments of Medicine, Surgery, and
    Pharmacology
University of Missouri School of Medicine
Columbia, Missouri 65212

C. Vannier
Centre de Biochimie
Universite de Nice
06034 Nice, France

Lawrence J. Wardzala
Cellular Metabolism and Obesity Section
NIADDK
National Institutes of Health
Bethesda, Maryland 20205

Mary G. Wetzel
Laboratory of Cellular and Developmental
    Biology
NIADDK
National Institutes of Health
Bethesda, Maryland 20205

M. Yamamoto
Division of Metabolic Disease
Department of Medicine
University of California at San Diego
La Jolla, California 92093

Cecil C. Yip
Banting & Best Department of Medical
    Research
University of Toronto
112 College Street
Toronto, Ontario M5S 1A8, Canada

D. K. Yip
Department of Medicine
Institute of Medical Science
University of Toronto
Toronto, Canada M5S 1A8

James B. Young
Charles A. Dana Research Institute and
    Thorndike Laboratory
Department of Medicine
Beth Israel Hospital
Harvard Medical School
Boston, Massachusetts 02215

The Adipocyte and Obesity: Cellular and Molecular Mechanisms, edited by A. Angel, C. H. Hollenberg, and D. A. K. Roncari. Raven Press, New York © 1983.

Adipose Tissue: A Brief History

George F. Cahill, Jr. and Albert E. Renold

Howard Hughes Medical Institute and the Harvard Medical School, Boston, Massachusetts 02115; and Institut de Biochimie Clinique, University of Geneva, Medical School, Geneva, Switzerland

Except for a few sporadic publications, adipose tissue was almost totally neglected by biomedical scientists until the past few decades. Virchow (43) in 1857 described the benign and malignant tumors of adipose tissue and initiated the concept that adipose cells were simply connective tissue cells containing fat. The same principle was supported by Flemming in 1879 (6); however, a publication by Toldt (38) in 1870 fostered the concept that adipose tissue might have its own origin in development and not simply be fat-laden connective tissue. It wasn't until an interesting case report was published in 1915 by Strandberg (37) that the individuality and embryonic destiny of adipose tissue began to be generally accepted. A twelve-year-old girl had sustained injury to her wrist and a transplant of skin was made from her abdomen. With her subsequent puberty and later obesity, the transplant also developed a marked increase in adipose tissue mass resulting in a 5 x 10 x 10 cm pad on the back of her hand. That adipose tissue is indeed a separate tissue was finally put on a firm anatomic and scientific basis by Wasserman in 1926 (45,46) who traced the embryonic development and subsequent maturation of primordial fat cells in man. At this same time Wertheimer (48,49), also in Germany, had initiated physiological and biochemical studies on the metabolism of adipose tissue. Accordingly we may date from 1926 the definition not only of a significant anatomic and embryogenic individuality of adipose tissue but also of its unique metabolic characteristics. The Strandberg observation that transplanted tissue retained primordial fat cells which would subsequently develop even though the anatomic location had been altered was confirmed by the other major pioneer in the field of adipose tissue metabolism, Dr. Franz Hausberger (16). He reported in 1938 that transplanted fetal tissues in experimental animals would maintain their adipose tissue for subsequent development parallel to that of the original location from where the tissue was removed.

That adipose tissue is more than a simple repository of fat was first suggested by von Gierke (44), of glycogen storage fame, who noted that glycogen accumulated in adipose tissue if an animal had been fasted and re-fed or else overfed from the start. He therefore inferred that the tissue has its own active internal metabolism. About the same time Rosenfeld (33) had noted that force-fed geese, which became obese, accumulated fat in their adipose tissue at a rate faster than could be explained by fat being formed in the liver and transported to adipose tissue by the blood. Although this was very inferential, he suggested that the fat might be synthesized in the adipose tissue itself.

In 1926 Wertheimer (48) demonstrated the extremely important role that innervation played in the storage of fat when he noted that cutting the nerve supply of adipose tissue resulted in extra fat accumulation. This had also been reported by Goering (11) who associated fat accumulation with clinical conditions in man where there was denervation. In 1934 Hausberger (15), who was working on his doctoral dissertation in Germany, described how denervation of one interscapular brown fat pad resulted in accumulation of fat in the denervated side but not in the other. Thus at this early stage in the biochemical and physiological characterization of adipose tissue, innervation was emphasized as a major control; however, Wertheimer's early studies (49) gave equal support to endocrine regulation, as will be discussed below.

The late 1930s saw the introduction of tracer methodology by Schoenheimer, Rittenberg (34,35) and their colleagues and during 1937-41 several papers were published demonstrating the incorporation of deuterium-labeled precursors into adipose tissue. This was subsequently reviewed in Schoenheimer's monograph published in 1942 (34). Wertheimer (39,50) and his colleagues then noted the lability of glycogen in adipose tissue, as earlier reported by von Gierke, and also observed that the respiratory quotient of adipose tissue was well above 1 after glycogen accumulation. This suggested that the adipose tissue might be synthesizing its own fat from precursors. Mirski (27) in Wertheimer's laboratory noted that insulin augmented this glycogen effect both in vitro and in vivo. These and other studies of Wertheimer and his associates were reviewed in a classic paper published in Physiological Reviews in 1948 by Wertheimer and Shapiro (51). A previous review had been assembled by Wells (47) in the Journal of the American Medical Association in 1940 entitled "Adipose Tissue, a Neglected Subject" but apparently little attention was paid to it, at least by investigators on the American continent and also in Europe with the two major exceptions discussed above: namely, by Wertheimer, who had emigrated in the mid-'30s from Germany to Jerusalem, and by Hausberger, who was still in Germany but who finally emigrated to Philadelphia in the 1940s, where he continues active today although in emeritus status at Jefferson Medical College.

Although the insulin effect on glycogen accumulation and, by inference, on fatty acid synthesis was demonstrated by Wertheimer and colleagues in Jerusalem, the importance of this effect as well as its exquisite sensitivity was not emphasized by the Jerusalem group. In 1950, stimulated by the clinical problems of fat atrophy and fat hypertrophy at the site of insulin injection in diabetic patients, the second author of this brief review (29) in collaboration with Drs. Alexander Marble and Don Fawcett noted that fat hypertrophied at the site of insulin injections in experimental animals. This subsequently prompted a more detailed study on the sensitivity of insulin on adipose tissue and lipogenesis and glycogenesis from radioactive substrates and, in 1958, Winegrad and Renold described the extremely important role played by insulin (52). Others, such as Favarger and Gerlach (4), had demonstrated in the whole animal that radioactive precursors, particularly glucose, were directly incorporated into adipose tissue triglyceride, and similar studies had been done in vitro by Feller (5) in Chaikoff's laboratory in San Francisco. At about this time a number of reviews on adipose tissue appeared on both sides of the ocean, in France by Vague et al. (40) and by Polonovski (28), in the USSR by Leites (25), and in America by Jeanrenand (19), Kinsell (21), and LeBoeuf (23). Finally, in 1965, the authors of this brief review edited the American Physiological Handbook Volume on Adipose Tissue (30). This last mentioned publication contained some 824 pages in 69 chapters with approximately 4,000 references.

In his classic study on fasting man published in 1915, Benedict (2) noted, using indirect calorimetry, that after the first day or two of starvation the respiratory quotient demonstrated that fat was the principal fuel. It is interesting that he never came to consider in detail how the adipose tissue relinquished its stored fat so that it could be metabolized by other parts of the body. Even more fascinating is the fact that this most important question was either not considered or else evaded by others active in intermediary metabolism until the mid-'50s, when the presence of free fatty acids in biological fluids was demonstrated. Independently, Dole (3) at the Rockefeller Institute and Gordon (12,9) at the National Institute of Health found that there was present in plasma, tightly bound to albumin, a very small component of fat which existed as a free fatty acid, and that this small component decreased on carbohydrate feeding and increased with fasting or with certain hormonal manipulations, such as epinephrine administration. Laurell (22) in Sweden had simultaneously described plasma free fatty acids and their increase in diabetic acidosis and starvation. It was soon demonstrated by a number of authors that free fatty acid release could be demonstrated in vitro from incubated adipose tissue and that a number of hormones stimulated this process, while insulin and glucose were inhibitory. LeBoeuf and colleagues (24) reported in 1959 that the glycerol of the triglyceride was also released. Vaughan (41,42) and her colleagues demonstrated how glycerol release could be used as an index of the rate of lipolysis and this simplified greatly the various assays designed to characterize lipolytic effects because of the relative ease of measuring glycerol as compared to free fatty acids. Also the fact that glycerol is poorly re-utilized, whereas the fatty acids may be re-esterified and are not therefore a true index of the rate of lipolysis, has given glycerol determinations added importance.

Thus, the technology of adipose tissue research had moved very rapidly in the Fifties, both with the use of radioactive substrates and the capacity to analyze free fatty acids and glycerol, as well as the physiological characterization of the incubated epididymal or parmetrial fat pad systems. A major methodological advance was subsequently made by Rodbell (31,32) when he found that the use of collagenase permitted the disruption of fat tissue and that the isolated fat cells could then be incubated and studied in vitro. This isolated fat cell preparation is now the standard system for the study of the physiology and biochemistry of adipose tissue in vitro.

The extreme sensitivity of adipose tissue in vitro to insulin, as evidenced by glucose incorporation into fat or glucose oxidation to CO_2, was used by Renold and his colleagues as a bioassay for insulin activity in biological fluids. This assay, however, was soon replaced by the immunoassay of insulin by Berson and Yalow. However, Froesch et al. (10) capitalized on the interesting fact that there were at least two components of insulin activity in plasma or serum, and one of these was inhibitable by antibody specific to insulin whereas the other was not. This led to the isolation and chemical characterization of insulin-like growth factors by Froesch and Humbel. The large number of recent studies on the insulin-like growth factors, the somatomedins, epidermal growth factors, nerve growth factors, etc., has sprung from these initial observations of the original adipose tissue studies in the late '50s and early '60s (10,1).

Two more technological advances deserve comment. One was the methodology to study the size and number of fat cells originally developed by

Hirsch and Gallian (17) and modified by Björntorp, Salans and others.
This technology permitted the calculation of the number of lipid-laden fat
cells in an organism, such as an experimental animal or man, and led to
the concept that obesity in the formative years in man is associated with
both hypertrophy and hyperplasia, whereas obesity after completion of the
growth phase is mainly hypertrophic. This topic continues to be an extremely interesting, active and controversial one, as discussed by a number
of contributors to this volume.

Another major technological advance was made by Green and colleagues
(13,14) who noted that a tissue cell line, namely the 3T3 cell, could be
changed from being a connective tissue-like cell into one which takes on
all the enzymatic and morphologic characteristics of adipose tissue cells.
Since the mid-1970s, the 3T3 cell continues as a model both for tissue
differentiation as well as an outstanding topic for research into the
characterization of the control of enzyme levels responsible for fat metabolism in adipose cells.

This brief review of the history of adipose tissue would not be complete without one or two words concerning brown fat. The anatomists of 100
years ago noted that with starvation adipose tissue lost its single, large
central vesicle (which gave it a signet-ring appearance) and instead developed a mulberry-type appearance with numerous small fat droplets in
each cell. As the fat was reaccumulated on refeeding, again the signet-
cell appearance returned. With starvation, fat tissue became brown in
color and this was partly due to the loss of triglyceride as well as to
the relative increase in vascularity and connective tissue content. However, it was noted that in certain areas of the rodent, particularly in
the interscapular area, the brown appearance and mulberry-type distribution of fat would persist even on refeeding. Hypotheses were put forth
that this might be an endocrine organ rather than specialized adipose
tissue, but again it was noted at the turn of the century that this tissue
is more prominent in certain rodents which undergo hibernation. As discussed in this volume and in a number of recent reviews (20,36), brown fat
is now considered as a "radiator" or the "central heating system" used by
hibernating animals to rapidly rewarm when the occasion warrants arousal
or for small rodents which live in a cold environment and require extra
(non-shivering) heating (18,8,7). Its presence has also been identified
in non-hibernating animals and Dr. Himms-Hagen discusses this further in
her chapter. Whether brown adipose tissue is embryogenetically distinct
from white adipose tissue and achieves its unique physiological role
thanks to its excessive innervation still awaits definitive study, but an
interesting observation was made 25 years ago when a pathologist, Melicow
(26), noted that in man the perirenal white adipose tissue developed all
the anatomic characteristics of brown adipose tissues in those subjects
who developed tumors of the adrenal medulla, producing excessive epinephrine or norepinephrine. In a similar fashion, it had been noted that
denervation of brown adipose tissue would induce it to turn into cells
containing central vacuoles, in other words, to the signet-ring type indistinguishable from otherwise normal white adipose tissue.

This volume summarizes a large number of very active areas still facing
adipose tissue research. One of the most important is the recruitment of
new mesenchymal cells into becoming adipose cells after the growth phase
has ceased in both animals and man, and whether or not these cells can
revert with weight loss back to their mesenchymal state. Still unanswered,
however, is the most challenging question of all: How does an animal control its entire triglyceride mass? Although brown adipose tissue was and

still is on occasion considered to have an endocrine function, the system whereby white adipose tissue, the major depot of triglyceride in the mammal, communicates its mass to the feeding centers in the brain to maintain total caloric homeostasis remains to be described. This last and as yet unanswered question remains a major challenge to adipose tissue physiology, one that is certain to entail tremendous agricultural and clinical implications in addition to its purely scientific nature.

REFERENCES

1. Antoniades, H.N., and Gundersen, K. (1962): Studies on the state of insulin in blood: materials and methods for the estimation of "free" and "bound" insulin-like activity in serum. Endocrinology 70:95-98.
2. Benedict, F.G. (1915): A study of prolonged fasting. Carnegie Institute of Washington, publication 203.
3. Dole, V.P. (1956): A relation between non-esterified fatty acids in plasma and the metabolism of glucose. J. Clin. Invest. 35:150-154.
4. Favarger, P., and Gerlach, J. (1955): Studies on the synthesis of fats from acetate or glucose. II. The relative roles of adipose tissue and other tissues in lipogenesis in mice. Helv. Physiol. Pharmacol. Acta 13:96-105.
5. Feller, D.D. (1952): Synthesis of lipids from radioactive acetate by surviving adipose tissue slices. Federation Proc. 11:45-46.
6. Flemming, W. (1879): On the development of the fat cell and of fatty tissue. Arch. Anat. Physiol. Anat. Abt.:pp.401-454.
7. Foster, D.O., and Frydman, M.L. (1978): Nonshivering thermogenesis in the rat. II. Measurements of blood flow with microspheres point to brown adipose tissue as the dominant site of the calorigenesis induced by noradrenaline. Can. J. Physiol. Pharmacol. 56:110-122.
8. Foster, D.O., and Frydman, M.L. (1979): Tissue distribution of cold-induced thermogenesis in conscious warm or cold-acclimated rats regulated from changes in tissue blood flow: The dominant role of brown adipose tissue in the replacement of shivering by nonshivering thermogenesis. Can. J. Physiol. Pharmacol. 57:257-270.
9. Fredrickson, D.S., and Gordon, R.S. (1958): Transport of fatty acids. Physiol. Rev. 38:585-630.
10. Froesch, E.R., Burgi, H., Ramseier, E.G., Bally, P., and Labhart, A. (1963): Antibody-suppressible and non-suppressible insulin-like activities in human serum and their physiologic significance. An insulin assay with adipose tissue of increased precision and specificity. J. Clin. Invest. 42:1816-1834.
11. Goering, D. (1922): On the influence of the nervous system on adipose tissue. Zschr. Ges. Anat. Konstit. Lehre. 8:312-335.
12. Gordon, R.S., Jr., and Cherkes, A. (1956): Unesterified fatty acid in human blood plasma. I. J. Clin. Invest. 35:206-212.
13. Green, H., and Kehinde, O. (1974): Sublines of mouse 3T3 cells that accumulate lipid. Cell 1:113-116.
14. Green, H., and Kehinde, O. (1976): Spontaneous heritable changes leading to increased adipose conversion in 3T3 cells. Cell 7:105-113.
15. Hausberger, F.X. (1934): On the innervation of adipose tissue. Z. Mikranat. Forsch. 36:231-266.
16. Hausberger, F.X. (1938): On the ability of transplanted fetal adipose tissue from rats to grow and develop. Virchows Arch. Pathol. Anat. Physiol. Klin. Med. 302:640-656.

17. Hirsch, J., and Gallian, E. (1968): Methods for the determination of adipose cell size in man and animals. J. Lipid Res. 9:110-119.
18. Jansky, L. (1973): Non-shivering thermogenesis and its thermoregulatory significance. Biol. Rev. 48:85-132.
19. Jeanrenand, B. (1961): Dynamic aspects of adipose tissue metabolism: A review. Metab. Clin. Exp. 10:535-581.
20. Joel, C.D. (1965): The physiological role of brown adipose tissue. In: Handbook of Physiology, edited by A.E. Renold, and G.F. Cahill, Jr., ch. 9, pp.59-85.
21. Kinsell, L.W., editor (1962): Adipose Tissue as an Organ. Charles C. Thomas, Springfield, Illinois.
22. Laurell, S. (1956): Plasma free fatty acids in diabetic acidosis and starvation. Scand. J. Clin. Lab. Invest. 8:81-82.
23. LeBoeuf, B. (1963): Controle Hormonal du Métabolisme du tissue adipeux. Union Med. Can. 92:241.
24. LeBoeuf, B., Flinn, R.B., and Cahill, G.F., Jr. (1959): Effect of epinephrine on glucose uptake and glycerol release by adipose tissue in vitro. Proc. Soc. Exp. Biol. Med. 102:527-529.
25. Leites, S.M. (1954): Physiology and Pathology of Adipose Tissue. Medgiz, Moscow.
26. Melicow, M.M. (1957): Hibernating fat and pheochromocytoma. Arch. Pathol. 63:367-372.
27. Mirski, A. (1942): Metabolism of adipose tissue in vitro. Biochem. J. 36:232-241.
28. Polonovski, J. (1957): Biochemistry of adipose tissue. Path. Biol. (Paris) 5:1595-1605.
29. Renold, A.E., Marble, A., and Fawcett, D.W. (1950): Action of insulin on deposition of glycogen and storage of fat in adipose tissue. Endocrinology 46:55-66.
30. Renold, A.E., and Cahill, G.F., Jr., editors (1965): Handbook of Physiology, Section 5: Adipose Tissue. American Physiological Society, Washington, D.C.
31. Rodbell, M. (1964): Metabolism of isolated fat cells. I. Effects of hormones on glucose metabolism and lipolysis. J. Biol. Chem. 239: 375-380.
32. Rodbell, M. (1965): The metabolism of isolated fat cells. In: Handbook of Physiology, edited by A.E. Renold, and G.F. Cahill, Jr., ch. 47, pp.471-482. American Physiological Society, Washington, D.C.
33. Rosenfeld, G. (1902-3): The formation of fat. Parts I and II. Ergeb. Physiol. 1:651-678, 1902 and 2:50-94, 1903.
34. Schoenheimer, R. (1942): The Dynamic State of Body Constituents. Harvard University Press, Cambridge.
35. Schoenheimer, R., and Rittenberg, D. (1937): Deuterium as an indicator in the study of intermediary metabolism. IX. The conversion of stearic acid into palmitic acid in the organism. J. Biol. Chem. 120: 155-165.
36. Smith, R.E., and Horwitz, B.A. (1969): Brown fat and thermogenesis. Physiol. Rev. 49:330-425.
37. Strandberg, J. (1915): Hudtransplantation med sagreget resultat. Hygiea 77:372-374.
38. Toldt, C. (1870): Contribution to the histology and physiology of adipose tissue. Sitzber. Akad. Wiss. Wien. Math. Naturwiss. Kl.Abt 2 62:445-467.

39. Tuerkischer, E., and E. Wertheimer. (1942): Glycogen and adipose tissue. J. Physiol. 100:385-409.
40. Vague, J., Garrigues, J., Teitelbaum, M., Miller, G., and Favier, G. (1956): Notions on the physiology of adipose tissue. Marseille Med. 93:497-540.
41. Vaughan, M. (1962): The production and release of glycerol by adipose tissue incubated in vitro. J. Biol. Chem. 237: 3354-3358.
42. Vaughan, M., and Steinberg, D. (1965): Glyceride biosynthesis, glyceride breakdown and glycogen breakdown in adipose tissue: mechanisms and regulation. In: Handbook of Physiology, Chap. 24 (Renold, A.E. and Cahill, G.F., Jr., eds.) American Physiological Society, Washington, D.C. p. 239-251.
43. Virchow, R. (1857): On malignant tumors of adipose tissue. Virchow Arch. Path. Anat. 11:281-288.
44. von Gierke, E. (1906): About the metabolism of adipose tissue. Verh. Deutsch. Ges. Path. 10:182-185.
45. Wassermann, F. (1926): The fat organs of man: development, structure and systematic place of the so-called adipose tissue. Z. Zellforsch. Mikroskop. Anat. Abt. Histochem. 3:235-328.
46. Wasserman, F. (1965): The development of adipose tissue. In: Handbook of Physiology, Chap. 10 (Renold, A.E. and Cahill, G.F., Jr., eds.) American Physiological Society, Washington, DC, p. 87-100.
47. Wells, H.G. (1940): Adipose tissue, a neglected subject I. J.A.M.A. 114:2177-2183 and 2284-2289.
48. Wertheimer, H.E. (1926): Regulation of metabolism. I. Regulation of fat metabolism: the central regulation of fat mobilization. Pfluegers Arch. Ges. Physiol. 213:262-279.
49. Wertheimer, H.E. (1926): Regulation of metabolism. II. The endocrine regulation of fat mobilization. Pfluegers Arch. Ges. Physiol. 213: 280-286.
50. Wertheimer, H.E. (1943): Glycogen in adipose tissue after insulin injections. Nature 152:565-566.
51. Wertheimer, E. and Shapiro, B. (1948): The physiology of adipose tissue. Physiol. Rev. 28:451-464.
52. Winegrad, A.I. and Renold, A.E. (1958): Studies on rat adipose tissue in vitro. I. Effects of insulin on the metabolism of glucose, pyruvate and acetate. J. Biol. Chem. 233:267-272.

The Adipocyte and Obesity: Cellular and Molecular Mechanisms, edited by A. Angel, C. H. Hollenberg, and D. A. K. Roncari. Raven Press, New York © 1983.

Obesity in Man: A Risk Factor in Metabolic and Cardiovascular Disease

William B. Kannel

Section of Preventive Medicine and Epidemiology, Boston University School of Medicine, Boston, Massachusetts 02118

ABSTRACT SUMMARY

Obesity is a health hazard with major metabolic and cardiovascular consequences. Despite uncertainty about its determinants and hazards, the pathogenetic mechanism involved and the efficacy of correcting it, obesity control constitutes the chief hygienic means for the control of a number of major chronic disabling and lethal diseases. No other single measure can simultaneously improve all of the major atherogenic precursors of cardiovascular disease including: hypertension, impaired glucose tolerance, the LDL/HDL cholesterol ratio and hyperuricemia. No better recommendation is currently available for avoidance of gallbladder disease, diabetes, gout or degenerative arthritis.

Overall mortality tends to increase with relative weight and the excess mortality reported for too lean persons is confined to cigarette smokers. There is a distinct excess of cardiovascular morbidity and mortality in the obese, which is proportional to the degree of overweight, occurs in either sex and wanes with advancing age. Not all of the effect is attributable to associated increases in blood pressure, blood sugar, and lipid abnormalities. The obese ($>$ 20% overweight) have a doubled risk of brain infarction and cardiac failure, and are impressively predisposed to sudden death and angina pectoris.

Because of its high prevalence, metabolic concomitants and cardiovascular consequences, obesity constitutes a powerful force of morbidity and mortality. Framingham data suggest that if everyone could be maintained at optimal weight, there would be 25% less coronary heart disease and 35% less cardiac failure or strokes.

Overweight is a well-documented but poorly understood hazard to health. Because of its epidemic proportions, the problem of obesity constitues a major public health concern. Although many epidemiologic investigations have been undertaken to gain insights into its determinants, health consequences, risks and disadvantages, many unresolved issues remain. Despite extensive actuarial and epidemiologic evidence, some investigators remain skeptical about the medical hazards (13,16).

PREVALENCE

Issues of prevalence, biological concomitants, and hazards of obesity are clouded by controversy about how to measure adiposity. Precise determination of body fat composition, while technically feasible, requires procedures not applicable in clinical practice or epidemiologic investigation. For general clinical use in the United States, measurement of body weight in relation to height is still the method of choice. However, obesity may be generalized or central, hyperplastic or hypertrophic, early or late in onset, and endomorphic or mesomorphic. Little information is available on the biological features or disease potential of each of these varieties of obesity. Also, the optimal or ideal weight for delineating the morbidly obese from the non-obese remains elusive.

However, it is clear that by any definition, obesity is highly prevalent in the United States and weights tend to increase with age in both sexes until late in life (1,8). Despite psychosocial influences, youth cultism and health concerns, obesity in men is more prevalent than formerly (5). The epidemic of obesity continues in most subgroups of the population, in women more than men, and in black women more than white women. Depending on definitions, obesity or excess body fat afflicts from one-tenth to one-third of the adult population on the United States (19). It appears to be more prevalent in low rather than high income subgroups of the population. While genetics are a factor, obvious environmental variables include food intake and physical activity. Hence, while genetic, metabolic, endocrine and nutritional influences are all probably involved, the evolution of obesity is strongly influenced by social, economic, racial and ethnic factors. Marked secular trends in weight and geographic variation in obesity attest to the environmental influences.

MORTALITY

Insurance statistics have since the turn of the century consistently indicated excessive mortality in the obese (2,15,23). Except for the massively obese, this excess mortality has in general been greater for men than women. The relationship of relative weight to mortality is, however, complex. Some epidemiologic data have indicated an inverse relationship to weight and a quadratic relationship with excess mortality at both extremes of weight (24). Considering the rather striking relationship of obesity to potentially lethal conditions such as coronary heart disease, cardiac failure, strokes, gallbladder disease and diabetes, the mortality risk gradients associated with obesity are in general suprisingly modest. However, overall mortality tends to increase with relative weight and the excess mortality reported for too lean persons is seen only in cigarette smokers. There appears to be insufficient data to allow inferences about mortality at less than ideal weights in men who have not been exposed to tobacco. As long as the confounding between cigarette smoking and leanness exists, interpretation of mortality data in relation to relative weight will be difficult.

CARDIOVASCULAR HAZARDS

Although the relationship between obesity and the severity of atherosclerosis seen at post-mortem is not clearly demonstrated, there is substantial evidence linking obesity with an increased risk of cardiovascular disease. Post-mortem data may suffer from assessments of weights obtained during the chronic terminal illnesses. This may explain why long range predictions involving relative weight are more distinct than those based on biennial reassessments.

In the Framingham Study there was a distinct excess incidence of cardiovascular morbidity in the obese, demonstrable in either sex (Table 1).

Table 1. RISK OF CARDIOVASCULAR EVENTS ACCORDING TO RELATIVE WEIGHT. 20-YEAR FOLLOW-UP. FRAMINGHAM STUDY. SUBJECTS 45-74.

	CARDIAC FAILURE		BRAIN INFARCTION		CORONARY DISEASE		CARDIOVASCULAR MORBIDITY*	
	MEN	WOMEN	MEN	WOMEN	MEN	WOMEN	MEN	WOMEN
65-109	28	16	17	12	119	58	165	86
110-124	34	21	19	16	144	67	193	99
125-272	57	28	22	20	180	80	226	117

T-VALUES

AGE-ADJUSTED	2.60	4.81	1.05	3.72	4.47	4.09	3.72	4.69
MULTI-VARIATE	1.51	2.80	-0.13	1.20	3.41	1.06	1.95	1.22

* CARDIAC FAILURE, STROKE, CORONARY DISEASE, OCCLUSIVE PERIPHERAL ARTERIAL DISEASE

The risk increased in proportion to the degree of overweight (12,11,22). This association which is as strong in women as in men, tended to diminish with advancing age in both sexes and beyond age 65 no association can be demonstrated. To a considerable extent the excess of cardiovascular morbidity is attributable to the fact that as people gain weight, their blood pressure, blood lipids and glucose tend to rise. However, recent observations of cardiovascular disease occurrence over a 26-year follow-up in the Framingham Study indicate that obesity at initial exam is a significant independent precursor of cardiovascular disease, particularly in women. Multiple logistic regression analysis has indicated that relative weight predicts cardiovascular disease, including coronary disease, coronary deaths and cardiac failure in men independently of age, cholesterol, systolic blood pressure, cigarette smoking habit, left ventricular hypertrophy and glucose intolerance. Relative weight in women was also positively and independently associated with coronary disease, stroke, cardiac failure, and coronary and cardiovascular mortality (Table 2). These results serve to emphasize the importance of obesity as a long-term predictor of cardiovascular disease operating not only as a precursor to the established major known risk factors, but through some unique mechanism yet to be identified as well. The obese (i.e. > 20% overweight) have almost a doubled risk of brain

infarction and cardiac failure, and a more modest excess risk of coronary heart disease (Table 1). Sudden death and angina pectoris are most
impressively related to obesity. Also, the proportion of coronary
deaths that are sudden increases with degree of overweight, suggesting a
rather specific relationship to sudden death in particular.

Table 2. RISK GRADIENTS FOR RELATIVE WEIGHT. 26-YEAR FOLLOW-UP.
          FRAMINGHAM STUDY. SUBJECTS 50-62.

CARDIOVASCULAR HAZARDS	MULTIVARIATE LOGISTIC REGRESSION COEFFICIENTS	
	MEN	WOMEN
CORONARY DISEASE	.012***	.008**
CARDIAC FAILURE	.014**	.015***
BRAIN INFARCTION	.004	.012**
CHD MORTALITY	.009*	.010**
C-V MORTALITY	.006	.008**

REGRESSIONS ADJUSTED FOR: AGE, SYSTOLIC BLOOD PRESSURE, SERUM CHOLES-
TEROL, CIGARETTES/DAY, GLUCOSE INTOLERANCE, AND ECG-LVH AT INITIAL EXAM.

From: Hubert et al. Presented at 22nd Conference on Cardiovascular
                      Epidemiology

METABOLIC CONCOMITANTS

In addition to overt abnormalities severe enough to be labelled diseases, obesity produces changes in blood pressure, blood lipids, glucose tolerance, and uric acid values. Changes in blood volume and
cardiac output and pulmonary function have also been noted with morbid
obesity. A relationship between overweight and blood pressure elevation
is well established (4,25,26). Intervention trials indicate that weight
reduction is usually accompanied by a corresponding reduction in blood
pressure and that this is independent of salt intake (20). Positive
correlations exist between blood pressure and various indices of adiposity including percent body fat, fat cell number, and total body fatness
(26,6). Changes in relative weight were the most potent factors associated with longitudinal trends in blood pressure discerned in the
Framingham Study. Spontaneous weight fluctuations were associated with
corresponding changes in blood pressure (Figure 1). One standard deviation change in weight was associated with a 6.5 mm Hg change in blood
pressure in ten years. This is not a fat arm artifact, since it can be
demonstrated in blood pressures taken in the forearm and documented
using intra-arterial blood pressure measurements. This well-established
relationship of blood pressure to weight change is of uncertain pathogenesis, and may be related to enhanced sympathetic nervous activity,
and expanded intra-vascular volume or an altered handling of a salt load
(13,17,16,9,19). Fat distributed prominently to the trunk has been
alleged to be more closely correlated with blood pressure than
limb fat (3).

FIGURE 1

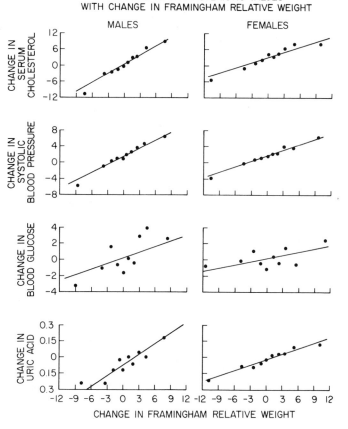

CHANGES IN CHARACTERISTIC VALUES
WITH CHANGE IN FRAMINGHAM RELATIVE WEIGHT

CHANGE IN FRAMINGHAM RELATIVE WEIGHT

Development of obesity affects various blood lipids including the LDL and VLDL which are positively correlated and HDL which is inversely related. The association in the Framingham data was strongest for HDL, with the relationship varying little by age and sex. Triglyceride was a close second, and this association with obesity was more prominent in men than women and in the young than in the old. In particular, the total cholesterol/HDL ratio was realted to degree of adiposity. This is important since this ratio is the best lipid profile for predicting coronary heart disease (9) (Fig. 2). Health surveys consistently link obesity to the development of diabetes. The severity and duration of obesity is the factor most strongly related to adult onset diabetes in the United States (19). In the Framingham Study multivariate analysis of the precursors of diabetes indicated that in either sex future glucose tolerance was highly related to not only the casual blood glucose values within the normal range, but to relative weight and VLDL (Table 3) In women obesity influenced the risk of developing glucose intolerance over a 14 year period of observation were in the top 20% of the weight distribution in the Framingham cohort. Weight alone was able to predict 45% of the future glucose intolerance in women and those in the upper quintile of weight distribution developed four times as much glucose intolerance as those in the lower quintile. Since weight loss was also mirrored by a reduction in the blood glucose (Fig. 2) and since weight loss corrects the glucose intolerance and hyperinsulinemia of the obese, a causal association seems likely. It is not clear whether the pathogenesis involves a cell membrane receptor problem or intracellular metabolic dysfunction. However, whatever the mechanism, obesity clearly impairs glucose metabolism and affects insulin secretion.

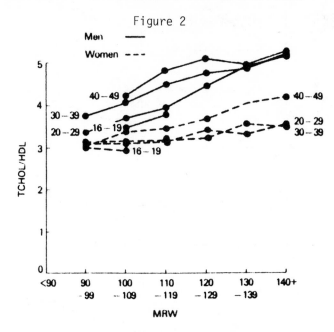

Figure 2

Mean TCHOL/HDL by MRW class and age group for men and woman.

Table 3   STANDARDIZED MULTIVARIATE LOGISTIC REGRESSION COEFFICIENTS PREDICTING GLUCOSE INTOLERANCE OVER 14 YEARS: THE FRAMINGHAM STUDY

CHARACTERISTIC	MEN COEFFICIENT	WOMEN COEFFICIENT
AGE	0.16	-0.11
METROPOLITAN RELATIVE WEIGHT	0.38***	0.48***
CLAUDICATION	0.17**	0.08
URIC ACID	-0.06	0.18
LDL	-0.18	-0.03
VLDL	0.22	0.27**
HEMOBLOBIN	0.07	0.34**
SYSTOLIC BLOOD PRESSURE	-0.03	0.16
GLUCOSE	0.50***	0.33***

** $P < 0.01$; *** $P < 0.0001$ using two tailed Student's t tests.

Although the connection between purine metabolism and adiposity is poorly understood, gout has long been linked to overweight. In the Framingham Study, both uric acid values and clinical gout have been snown to be related to relative weight (Fig. 3). Again, since change in weight is associated with a corresponding change in uric acid values (Fig. 1), a causal relationship seems likely.

Figure 3

--Prevalence of gout at exam 2 by relative weight. Framingham Study: men (age-adjusted rates: 45-64).

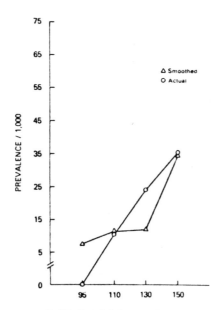

RELATIVE WEIGHT (Percent of Desirable Weight)

Obese persons tend to hypersecrete lithogenic biliary cholesterol because of a disproportionate saturation with cholesterol relative to bile salt and phospholipid. As a consequence, gallbladder disease has been found to be strongly related to obesity in autopsy studies, case reports and prospective population studies (21). The relationship of obesity to gallbladder disease in women is found at all ages and even after adjusting for parity.

There is also a substantial body of evidence linking obesity to various menstrual disturbances in women (21). Teenage obesity has also been connected with increased risk of endometrial carcinoma. Excessive estrogen stiumlation leading to cystic glandular hyperplagia has been implicated. Prolonged estrogen stimulation associated with obesity is also believed to promote anovulatory cycles and polycystic ovaries (7).

Thus, many medical conditions have been found to be associated with obesity including cardiovascular disease, gallbladder disease, menstrual irregularities, gout, and arthritis, among others.

PREVENTIVE IMPLICATIONS

Many unresolved questions exist concerning the determinants and hazards of obesity, the pathogenesis of its adverse metabolic effects, and
the efficacy of correcting the condition. Nevertheless, obesity control
constitutes a promising means of intervention for prevention-minded physicians and health officials. No other measure can correct so many of
the underlying metabolic disorders which predispose to accelerated
atherogenesis. For diseases such as gallbladder disease, adult-onset
diabetes, gout or degenerative arthritis, no other measure holds as much
promise for hygienic control.

Avoidance of obesity would seem a useful means for reducing the
annual toll of cardiovascular mortality. Medical science would be well
served by greater attention to overweight, its atherogenic metabolic
effects, and its hemodynamic effects on the cardiovascular system.
Weight control is the logical first approach for the correction of mild
to moderate hypertension, hyperlipidemia and impaired glucose tolerance,
particularly in persons susceptible to cardiovascular disease. Correction of overweight should improve the exercise tolerance of patients
with with established coroanry heart disease or cardiac failure. Control of obesity should be a prominent feature of a comprehensive
approach to the prevention of cardiovascular disease.

Only a trial demonstrating the efficacy of correcting long-standing
obesity in prolonging life will suffice to convince the skeptic. Because of difficulty in achieving and sustaining long-term control of
obesity such evidence is not likely to become available in the forsee-
able future. Because of the soundness of the rationale, and the great
potential benefit. avoidance of obesity would appear to merit a high
priority in the lexicon of preventive recommendations.

It is estimated from Framingham Study data that if everyone could be
maintained at optimal weight there would be 25% less coronary heart
disease and 35% less cardiac failure or strokes in the general population. The benefits in terms of avoidance of diabetes and gallbladder
disease should also be considerable.

Because of this potential benefit a continuing effort to seek better
ways to control or avoid obesity is warranted. The unsatisfactory state
of the treatment of obesity is attested to by the perennial fad diets
and continued high prevalence of the condition in the general population.
Formidable barriers to control of obesity are our ignorance of the
pathogenesis of the condition, some indifference, ingrained cultural
patterns and commercial vested interests. A greater sense of urgency
about beginning obesity is warranted since long-standing massive obesity
is a virtually incurable condition. The causes, prevention and patho-
logic physiology of obesity are probably the least well understood of
the major contributors to cardiovascular disease. A more intense research effort would appear to be amply justified.

REFERENCES

1. Abraham S, Johnson CL (1980): Prevalence of Severe Obesity in Adults in the United States. Am J Clin Nutr 33:364-369.

2. Stamler J, Rhomberg P, Schoenberger JA, Shekelle RB et al (1975): Multivariate Analysis of the Relationship of 7 variables to Blood Pressure. J Chron Dis 28:527-548.

3. Blitzer PH, Blitzer EC, Rimm AA (1976): Association Between Teen-age Obesity and Cancer in 56,111 Women. Prev Med 5:20-31.

4. Boe J, Humerfelt S, Wedervang F (1957): The Blood Pressure in a Readings and Height and Weight Determinations in the Adult Population of the City of Bergen. Acta Med Scand 157 (Suppl 321):1-336.

5. Bray GA, ed (1976): Obesity in Perspective, Parts 1 and 2. Fogarty Internationsl Center Series on Preventive Medicine, Vol 2. DHEW Publication No. 76-852. Washington, DC. US Government Printing Office.

6. Chiang BN, Perluran LV, Epstein FH (1969): Overweight and Hypertension: A Review. Circ 39:403-421.

7. Fisher ER, Gregorio R, Stephan T, Nolan S, Danowski TS (1974): Ovarian Changes in Women with Morbid Obesity. Obstet Gynecol 44:839-844.

8. Gordon T, Kannel WB (1973): The Effects of Overweight on Cardiovascular Diseases. Geriatrics 28:80-88.

9. Kannel WB, Castelli WP (1980): Prognostic Implications of Blood Lipid Measurements. In, Prognosis (Eds., JF Freis, GE Ehrlich) Pp 263-268, Charles Press Publications.

10. Kannel WB, Gordon T (1979): Obesity and Some Physiological and Medical Concomitants. In, Obesity in America (Ed., GA Bray) NIH 79-359.

11. Kannel WB, Gordon T, Castelli WP (1979): Obesity, lipids and Glucose Intolerance: The Framingham Study. Am J Clin Nutr 32:1238-1245.

12. Keys A, Aravanis C, Blackburn H, VanBuckem FSP, Busina R, Bjordevic BS, Findanza FF, Karvonen MJ, Menotti A, Puddu V, Taylor HL (1972): Coronary Heart Disease: Overweight and Obesity as Risk Factors. Ann Int Med 77:15-27, 1972.

13. Landsberg L, Young JB (1981): Diet-Induced Changes in Sympathoadrenal activity: Implications for Thermogenesis and Obesity. Obesity and Metab 1:5-33.

14. Lew EA (1961): New Data on Underweight and Overweight Persons. J Am Diet Assoc 38:323-327.

15. Mann GV (1974): The Influence of Obesity on Health. N Engl J Med 291:226-232.

16. Marx JL (1981): Natriuretic Hormone Linked to Hypertension. Science 212:1255-1257.

17. Messerti FH, Christie B, DeCarvellio JG et al (1981): Obeisty in Essential Hypertension. Hemodynamice, Intravascular Volume, Sodium Excretion, and Plasma Renin Activity. Arch Int Med 141:81-85.

18. National Center for Health Statistics (1977). Weight by Height and Age of Adults 18-74 Years: United States, 1971-1974. Vital and Health Statistics Advance Data No. 14.

19. National Commission on Diabetes Report, Vol 3, Part 1 (1975). DHEW Publication No. (NIH) 76-1021. Washington DC, U.S. Government Printing Office.

20. Reisen E, Abel R, Modan M et al (1978): Effect of Weight Loss Without Salt Restriction in the Reduction of Blood Pressure in Overweight Hypertensive Patients. N Engl J Med 298:106.

21. Rim AA, White PL (1979): Obesity: Its Risks and Hazards. In, Obesity in America. Ed., GA Bray. NIH Public No. 79-359. Pp 103-124.

22. Shurtleff D: Some Characteristics Related to the Incidence of Cardiovascular Disease adn Death: The Framingham Study, 18-Year Follow-up. In, The Framingham Study, WB Kannel and T Gordon, eds., Section 30. DHEW Publication No. (NIH) 74-599. Washington, DC US Gov't Printing Office, 1974.

23. Society of Actuaries (1960): Build and Blood Pressure Study, 1959. Chicago.

24. Sorlie P, Gordon T, Kannel WB (1980): Body Build and Mortality. JAMA 243:1828-1831.

25. Stamler J, Rhomberg P, Schoenberger JA, Shekelle RB et al (1975): Multivariate Analysis of the Relationship of 7 Variables to Blood Pressure. J Chronic Dis 28:527-548.

26. Tobian L (1978): Hypertension and Obesity. New Eng J Med 298:46.

The Adipocyte and Obesity: Cellular and Molecular Mechanisms, edited by A. Angel, C. H. Hollenberg, and D. A. K. Roncari. Raven Press, New York © 1983.

Obesity: What Comes First

George A. Bray

Division of Diabetes and Clinical Nutrition, Department of Medicine, University of Southern California School of Medicine, Los Angeles, California 90033

Obesity, that is excess stores of body fat, results from cumulative ingestion of more calories than the body uses to meet its energy needs (25). The consequences of this process of energy storage have been examined in both experimental animals; as well as clinical studies with human beings. The usual animal models are the rat with injury to the ventromedial hypothalamus (16), rats or mice with genetically transmitted obesity (16) animals fed a high fat diet (60) or rats which are force-fed (18, 45). The introduction of the supermarket or cafeteria diet (56) has expanded the number of animal models available for study of obesity.

While Sims and his collaborators pioneered the studies on the effects of conscious overeating in otherwise lean healthy men (63), these studies have been expanded in other laboratories (70,50). This paper will examine some of the metabolic consequences of excess calorie intake with special attention to human beings.

One response to eating extra calories is an expansion of the total body fat stores (7). Since adipose tissue is the major expandable depot for energy storage, excess calories, whether derived from carbohydrate, fat or protein, are converted into fatty acids and then stored as triglycerides in fat cells.

A number of important insights into the sequence of events resulting from weight gain have come from carefully controlled studies in normal individuals. In one study, four healthy young men consumed a basal diet containing 1800 kCal/M^2 prior to the period of weight gain. Throughout the period of overeating they were hospitalized on a metabolic unit. After 7 to 14 days on the basal diet, a daily supplement of 4000 kcal was provided, making a total daily intake of just over 7000 kcal. The weight gain during this period of time ranges fro 4 to 10 kg (7). If all of this added weight were triglyceride, this would represent storage of 40,000 to 91,000 kcal, assuming a caloric value for fat of 9.1 kcal/g. Since 112,000 extra kcal were ingested a maximum of 81 per cent of the ingested energy could be accounted for by stored energy. Since fluid and other tissue components were retained as part of this weight gain, the calories added to the body would be correspondingly reduced and there would be a larger discrepancy between ingested and stored calories.

The composition of the tissue formed during weight gain has been analysed by Brozek et al (17) and again by Salans, Horton, and Sims (58). These latter authors found that fat accounted for about 70 per cent of the total weight gain in the normal individuals who overate. The remainder was distributed between intra-and extracellular fluid and other cellular components. If one assumes that 75 per cent of the weight added by the normal subjects was triglyceride, then only 30,000 to 70,000 kcal or less than 65 per cent of the ingested calories would be stored as triglyceride during the 28 days of overeating. The difference between the amount stored and the 112,000 calories ingested are partially accounted for, by the caloric requirements to add new body tissue. These data on caloric retention during weight gain are in reasonable agreement with the observations of Blaxter (6) who found that in growing animals between two-thirds and three-quarters of the ingested calories are added to body stores as fat and lean tissue. This discrepancy between ingested and stored calories is best referred to as dietary thermogenesis, although it has also been called 'luxusconsumption'. This concept was proposed over 50 years ago, and was revived by Miller et al, (40, 41). They proposed that the extra ingested calories might be dissipated by heat loss during exercise (40). Detailed studies of caloric expenditure during exercise either before or after a meal have shown this effect to be small and not increased by overeating (14, 28, 27). More recently Rothwell and Stock have suggested that luxusconsumption or dietary thermogenesis can be demonstrated in experimental animals and that it might be due to enhanced metabolism by brown adipose tissue (55, 8).

Evidence for dietary thermogenesis has been reported in several studies in which subjects ate the extra calories as carbohydrate and protein and when the period of overeating lasted more than 10-14 days (25). Studies of shorter duration or when the dietary supplement was only fat did not show this effect (27). In an analysis of studies during overeating, Garrow concluded that at least 7 days of overfeeding were needed to detect any increase in metabolism (25). Norgan and Durnin (47) have re-explored the energy balance during overeating and have concluded that there is no evidence for luxusconsumption and no dissipation of calories above what can be accounted for by energy storage and carrying extra weight.

Thyroid hormones play an important role in regulating body metabolism. Approximately 75 per cent of the 3,5,3'-triiodothyronine (T3) and essentially all of the reverse T3 (3,3',5'-triiodothyronine) are made from thyroxine by deiodi-nation in peripheral tissues. The concentration of T3 and rT3 is altered both by under and over feeding (22). During starvation or with diets containing less than 800 kcal/d diets T3 falls, and rT3 rises. Thyroxine which is secreted by the thyroid gland usually remains unchanged (69, 66, 68, 26). During overfeeding there are effects opposite to those of starvation. That is, T3 rises and rT3 stays the same or falls (12, 22). Both obese and normal weight volunteers who overeat show a rise in T3 which results primarily from increased production of this hormone (22). It is conceivable that the rise in T3 plays a role in the increased heat production observed during overfeeding, but this has not yet been conclusively shown.

Another factor accounting for the discrepancy between ingested and stored calories is the extra calories used to move the heavier body. In careful studies before and after weight gain in normal men neither Goldman (28) Whipp et al (70, 14) nor Norgan and Durnin (47) could find any alteration in the efficiency for performing physical work on a cycle ergometer.

From adipose tissue biopsies obtained before and after weight gain and the simultaneous measurements of body fat, Salans, Horton, and Sims (58) calcula-ted the total number of adipocytes, and found that during short-term acute weight gain, the storage of fat was accomplished almost entirely by an increase in the size of the preexisting fat cells which were present already. There was no apparent increase in the number of fat cells.

The formation of triglyceride in adipose tissue requires the availability of fatty acids and a source of sn-glycerol-3-phosphate (αGP) (7). Although both liver and adipose tissue can synthesize fatty acids, the importance of each site varies with species and age (5, 61, 30, 52, 10, 29, 15, 1). The rate of incorporation of radioactivity from ^{14}C-pyruvate into fatty acids by adipose tissue obtained after weight gain was diminished (15). This finding would suggest that synthesis of fatty acids by adipocytes was reduced after the acute gain in weight. This implies that the liver may be the primary site for the synthesis of the new fatty acids. Fatty acids of hepatic origin would then be incorporated into lipoproteins for transport to the adipose tissue where they could be incorporated into triglycerides after hydrolysis by lipoprotein lipase. Incorporation of fatty acids into adipose tissue triglyceride from lipoprotein-triglyceride is more rapid than the de novo synthesis of fatty acids from glucose. However, recent data comparing human liver slices and slices of human adipose tissue indicate that adipose tissue may indeed be a significant site for de novo synthesis of fatty acids in both normal weight and obese subjects (1).

The hallmark of obesity is increased body fat which is stored in large adipocytes (7, 33). One metabolic consequence of obesity is an impaired response to the action of insulin. In 1968, Salans, Knittle and Hirsch hypothesised that this resistance to the action of insulin might be due to the unresponsiveness of the large fat cells. They found that large fat cells have a smaller response to insulin than small fat cells (59). This concept has been reexamined recently by comparing adipocytes obtained before and after weight gain (57). From these studies, it is now clear that the sensitivity of fat cells to insulin in vitro is determined by at least two variables: (1) the size of the adipose cell and (2) the nutritional intake of the subject from whom the adipocytes were obtained for study. As fat cells enlarge, their sensitivity to insulin is diminished (63, 19). When the diet is constant, the stimulation of glucose metabolism by insulin is less in small fat cells than in large fat cells obtained after weight gain. However, the stimulation of glucose metabolism by insulin in large or small fat cells can be increased by feeding a high carbohydrate diet in the period prior to the study (57). Indeed, the effects of a high carbohydrate intake may by greater than the effects of enlargement of the fat cells.

The mechanism of the insensitivity to insulin could reside in many sites (19). The possibility that the circulating insulin was inactive has been eliminated (31, 38). However, the interaction of insulin with its receptors has been one area of considerable interest sparked by the observation that insulin binding was reduced in fat cells and liver membranes from obese (ob/ob) mice (65). Studies with cell membranes from obese humans (36, 21, 2) or animals have shown a modest or marked reduction in the number of receptors for insulin on the cell surface. These changes in receptor number have been correlated with the changes in physiological effects of insulin (35). Although the number of receptors may be reduced on cell membranes from obese humans the effect of insulin on glucose entry or metabolism may be even further impaired. This suggests that the block in insulin metabolism may be intracellular as well as at the cell membrane (35).

The release of free fatty acids and glycerol from adipose tissue is also influenced by the size of the fat cell (13, 64). The rate of basal lipolysis, that is, the rate at which glycerol is released from adipocytes, is increased with increasing size of the fat cell. This has been noted in both experimental animals (71) and man (13, 64). When adipocytes are reduced in size, their rate of basal lipolysis decreases along with the decrease in size. Conversely, large adipocytes show a greater basal release of glycerol.

One consequence of the increased rate of lipolysis is an increase in the concentration of free fatty acids (4). The turnover of free fatty acids in obese subjects has been examined in several studies (42). The rate of metabolism of free fatty acids is higher in obese subjects than in lean individuals, whether expressed in absolute terms or in relation to body size or fat (42). There is also an increase in the metabolism of cholesterol (43, 39). Cholesterol production and excretion are significantly correlated with body fat. Each extra kilogram of triglyceride is associated with production of an extra 20 mg of cholesterol (39). When this cholesterol is excreted in the bile it tends to become more lithogenic accounting for the higher risk of gallstones in obesity (7, 53).

Suppression of growth hormone which is usually observed in obesity (37) might result from the increase in the concentration of free fatty acids. An increased supply of fatty acids to the liver might also provide a stimulus to gluconeogenesis in this organ.

The correlation of plasma triglycerides with obesity has been documented in clinical studies (51). Increases in triglyceride have been obeserved by in experiments with acute overfeeding of normal human beings (62). Triglycerides usually fall with weight loss (54). These effects of obesity on triglyceride are explained at least in part by the increased supply of free fatty acids to the liver. The increase in this substrate results from the increased rate of lipolysis associated with the large adipocytes which reflects the increased storage of calories. A second factor may be the high levels of insulin.

Hyperinsulinemia is characteristic of obesity (3). An increase in insulin occurs in all forms of obesity, although that produced by feeding a high fat diet may be small (16, 63). The concentration of insulin can be increased with an increase in body fat. This has been shown in human and animal experiments. When fat was the supplement used to increase caloric intake in human volunteers during weight gain the fasting plasma insulin increased from nine to sixteen μU/ml (63). There also was a small but significant increase in plasma glucose; however, proportionately, the rise in insulin was greater. One investigative group failed to find a rise in insulin levels of rats fed a high fat diet, but when the experiments were replicated using a pair-fed control group, insulin was significantly increased (48). For these studies three groups of animals were used. One group ate a high carbohydrate diet and the second ate a high fat diet. The third group was limited in its intake of the high fat diet to the number of calories eaten by the animals on the high carbohydrate diet. Under these circumstances the rats fed a high fat diet gained more weight and had a higher insulin level than the restricted animals on the high fat diet.

Sims et al (63) have examined the effects of feeding two different levels of carbohydrate before and after weight gain in normal volunteers. The level of carbohydrate intake influenced both the concentration of fatty acids in the plasma and the concentration of insulin. Plasma insulin was higher on the high carbohydrate diet. When the carbohydrate intake increased from 100 g/M^2 to 300 g/M^2 the insulin levels rose from 8.3 % 1.0 and rose to 13.1 ± 2.3 μU/ml. Similar differences have been observed in obese subjects (32).

To obtain further insight into the influence of calories and carbohydrate on plasma insulin and triglyceride, we fed four obese patients on a diet which contained either 1800 or 1400 kCal/M^2. For two weeks at each caloric intake the diet contained 300 g/M^2 of carbohydrate and for the other two weeks the diet had 100 g/M^2. Basal concentrations of insulin were significantly higher on the high carbohydrate diet at each level of caloric intake. However, the insulin levels were reduced significantly for corresponding carbohydrate intakes when the total calories were reduced. Thus, both the level of caloric intake and the carbohydrate content of the diet are important in determining the basal levels of insulin.

The circulating levels of free fatty acids also were affected by the changes in carbohydrate content of the diet. When lean or obese subjects were fed high carbohydrate diets, free fatty acids were lower than when they ate a high fat diet (63). Triglyceride levels also changed in relation to the intake of carbohydrate. Caloric intake per se had very little effect. At both of the caloric levels, the circulating triglycerides were lower when the subjects were fed the high fat diet than when they received the high carbohydrate diet. These data indicate that the effects of calories and carbohydrate on insulin and triglycerides have a complex interrelationship.

Hyperinsulinemia in obesity may be explained in at least two ways, one involving humoral and the other neural mechanisms. Among the humoral controls is the hyperglycemia which is associated with both experimental and clinical obesity. Sims et al. (63) observed a significant increase in blood glucose in the studies of volunteers who overate and gained weight. The explanation for this rise in glucose cannot be simply because extra or carbohydrates were eaten because a rise in glucose was also observed in individuals whose caloric supplement was made up entirely of fat. The most likely source for the increased glucose is thus from enhanced gluconeogenesis stimulated by the increased concentration of free fatty acids entering the liver and augmented by the increased supply of glycerol released from the enlarged adipocytes. These effects might be sufficient to raise the concentration of glucose and increase basal levels of insulin.

A second humoral explanation for the hyperinsulinemia might be the increased levels of five amino acids in both spontaneous and experimentally induced obesity (24). These five amino acids are leucine, isoleucine, valine, phenylalanine, and tyrosine. Leucine is a potent stimulator of insulin secretion and acts synergistically with glucose in stimulating insulin release. In order to document this further, we infused two normal subjects with a mixture of these five amino acids during one experiment, glucose during a second experiment and the combination of glucose and amino acids during a third experiment. A marked increase in insulin levels occurred when the amino acids and glucose were infused together.

Enhanced secretion of gastric inhibiting polypeptide (GIP) provides a final hormonal mechanism which might increase insulin secretion. This peptide is released in higher quantities in obese people than in normal ones (GIP).

Alterations in the autonomic nervous system also may play a role in controlling insulin secretion in obesity. The suppression of insulin by epinephrine is well known in lean subjects but is even more pronounced in obese individuals (9). In five lean and five massively obese individuals who were infused sequentially with saline, epinephrine (6 µg/min) or epinephrine with propranolol (80 µg/min), the percentage rise in glucose was higher in the lean than in the obese during infusion of epinephrine. Propranolol did not lower glucose levels. Epinephrine infusion lowered insulin significantly in the obese, but the effect could not be detected in the lean individuals. Adding propranolol was without effect. When the infusion was terminated there was a sharp rebound in insulin in the obese individuals but not in the lean ones. This may imply that the normal suppressive effects of the sympathetic nervous system are less evident in obese individuals. Whether there is any effect of obesity on the parasympathetic nervous system is not known. In rats with ventromedial hypothalamic lesions, both vagal hyperactivity (34) and reduced sympathetic activity (46) have both been observed. In man, however, there is no direct evidence for alterations in the vagal system.

To complete the story of the metabolic responses to increased caloric intake we need to add some recent data on the effects of overfeeding on the autonomic nervous system. Young and Landsberg (72) have shown that increased food intake can enhance the turnover of catecholamines in peripheral tissues. This suggests that under some circumstances the sympathetic nervous system an increase in firing rate following bouts of overeating. With starvation the sympathetic nervous system appears to become less active. (72).

In summary, we have sketched some of the effects of excessive caloric intake on the metabolism of carbohydrate, lipids and amino acids. From the changes which are produced it is possible to gain some insight into pathogenetic mechanisms for the increased incidence of diabetes mellitus and gall stones in obese patients. The high level of fatty acid turnover results in increased cholesterol production, increased cholesterol excretion and a change in the composition of bile towards greater lithogenicity. The hyperinsulinemia may be related to increased glucose and amino acids or the changes in the autonomic nervous system. If the pancreatic capacity for insulin secretion is reduced when the load imposed by obesity occurs then diabetes mellitus may develop. Finally, hypertension and cardiovascular disease may result directly from the increased load on the heart and circulatory system, or indirectly from increased salt intake accompanying the higher intake of calories.

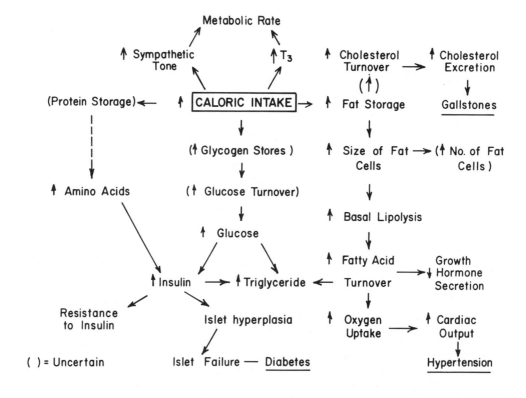

FIG. 1. Diagram of metabolic response to overeating. This diagram shows some of the effects of excess caloric intake on the metabolism of lipids, carbohydrates and proteins on the control of the thyroid hormones and the autonomic nervous system.

REFERENCES:
1. Angel, A. and Bray, G.A.(1979): Europ J Clin Invest 9:355-62.
2. Archer, J.A., Gorden, P. and Roth, J. (1975): J Clin Invest 55:166.
3. Bagdade, J.D., Bierman, E.L. and Porte, D. (1967): J Clin Invest 46: 1549-57.
4. Bjorntorp, P., Bergman, H. and Varnauskas, E. (1969): Acta Med Scand 185:351-6.
5. Bjorntorp, P. and Sjostrom, L. (1978): Metabolism 27:1853.
6. Blaxter, K.L. (1975):. "Obesity in Perspective." In Fogarty International Center Series on Preventive Medicine, Vol. II, Part I and Part II, edited by G.A. Bray, pp. Washington D.C.:U.S. Government Printing Office.
7. Bray, G.A. (1982): "Current Concepts." Kalamazoo, MI: The Upjohn Co.
8. Bray, G.A. (1981): Triangle 20:145-9.
9. Bray G.A. (1979): Disease-a-Month 26:1-85.
10. Bray G.A. (1972): J Clin Invest 51:537-48.
11. Bray, G.A. (1969): J Clin Invest 48:1413-22.
12. Bray, G.A., Chopra,I.J. and Fisher, D.A. (1976): Lancet 1:1206-8.
13. Bray,G.A., Glennon,J.A. Salans,L.B. Horton,E.S. Danforth,E. Jr. and Sims, E.A.H. (1977): Metabolism 26:739-47.
14. Bray, G.A., Whipp,B.J. and Koyal, S.N. (1974): Am J Clin Nutr 27:254-59.
15. Bray, G.A., Whipp,B.J., Koyal, S.N. and Wasserman, K. (1977): Metabolism 26:403.
16. Bray, G.A., and York, D.A. (1979): Physiol Rev 59:719-809.
17. Brozek, J., Grande,F. Taylor,H.L. Anderson,J.T. Buskirk, E.R. and Keys, A. (1957): J Appl Physiol 10:412-20.
18. Cohn, C. and Joseph, D. (1962): Yale J Biol Med 34:598.
19. Crofford, O.B. (1976): "Insulin resistance: A commentary of definitions and on current methods of assessment." In Obesity in Perspective, edited by G.A. Bray DHEW Publication No. (NIH) 75-708, 297.
20. Czech, M.P. (1976): J Clin Invest 57:1523.
21. Czech, M.P., Richardson, D.K. and Smith, C.J. (1977): Metabolism 26: 1057.
22. Danforth, E., Horton,E.S. O'Connell,M. Sims, E.A.H. (1979): J Clin Invest 64:1336-47.
23. Danforth, E., Burger,A.G. Goldman,R.F. Sims, E.A.H. (1978): In Recent Advances in Obesity Research II, Proceedings of the 2nd International Congress on Obesity, edited by G. A. Bray pp. 229-36. London:Newman Publishing Ltd.
24. Felig, P., Marliss, E. and Cahill,G.F. Jr. (1969): N Engl J Med 281:811-16.
25. Garrow, J. S. (1978): "The Regulation of Energy Expenditure in Man." In Recent Advances in Obesity Research II, Proceedings of the 2nd International Congress on Obesity, edited by G. A. Bray pp. . London:Newman Publishing Ltd.
26. Glass, A.R., Burman,K.D. Dahms, W.T. and Boehm, T.M. (1981): Metabolism 30:89-104.
27. Glick, Z., Shvartz,E. Magazanik, A. and Modan, J. (1977): Am J Clin Nutr 30:1026.
28. Goldman, R.F. (1975): "Obesity in Perspective." In Fogarty International Center Series on Preventive Medicine, Vol. II, Part I and Part II, edited by G.A. Bray, pp. Washington D.C.:U.S. Government Printing Office.
29. Goldrick, R.B., Ashley, B.C.E. and Lloyd, M.L. (1969): J Lipid Res 10: 253.
30. Goldrick, R.B. and Galton, D.J. (1974): Clin Sci Mol Med 46:469.
31. Gordon, P. and Roth, J. (1969): J Clin Invest 48:2225.
32. Grey, N. and Kipnis, D.M. (1971): N Engl J Med 285:827-31.

33. Hirsch, J. and Knittle, J.L. (1970): Fed Proc 29:1516.
34. Inoue, S., Mullen, Y. and Bray, G.A. (1979): The Endocrine Society 104: A-187.
35. Kolterman, O.B., Insel,J. Sacknow, M. and Olefsky, J.M. (1980): J Clin Invest 65:1272-84.
36. Livingston, J.N., Purvis, B.J. and Lockwood, D.H. (1978): Metabolism 27: 2009-14.
37. Londono, J., Gallagher,T.F. Jr., and Bray, G.A. (1969): Metabolism 18: 996.
38. Melani, F., Rubenstein,A.H. and Steiner, D.F. (1970): J Clin Invest 49: 497.
39. Miettinen, T.A. (1971): Circulation. 44:842-850.
40. Miller, D.S. and Mumford, P. (1967): Am J Clin Nutr 20:1212.
41. Miller, D.S., Mumford,P. and Stock,M.J. (1967): Am J Clin Nutr 20:1223.
42. Nestel, P., Ishikawa, J.T. and Goldrick, R.B. (1978): Metabolism 27:589-97.
43. Nestel, P.J. and Whyte, H.N. (1968): Metabolism 17:1122.
44. Neumann, R.O. (1902): Archiv fur Hygiene 45:1.
45. Nishizawa, Y. and Bray, G.A. (1980): Am J Physiol 239:R344-51
46. Nishizawa, Y. and Bray, G.A. (1978): J Clin Invest 61:714.
47. Norgan N.G. and Durnin, I.G.A. (1980): Am J Clin Nutr 33:978-88.
48. Ogundipe, O.O., and Bray, G.A. (1974): Horm Metab Res 6:351.
49. Olefsky, J.M. (1976): J Clin Invest 57:842.
50. Olefsky, J., Crapo,P.A. Ginsberg, H. and Reaven, G.M. (1975): Metabolism 24:495.
51. Olefsky, J., Reaven, G.M. and Farquhar, J.W. (1974): J Clin Invest 53:64-76.
52. Patel, M.S., Owen,O.E. Goldman, L.I. and Hanson, R.W. (1975): Metabolism 24:161.
53. Rimm, A.A., Werner,L.H. Van Yserlos, B. and Bernstein, R.A. (1975): Public Health Report 90:44-51.
54. Robertson, R.P., Favareski,D.J. Henderson,J.D. Porte,D.R. and Bierman, E.L. (1973): J Clin Invest 52:1620
55. Rothwell, N.J. and Stock, M.J. (1979a): Nature (Lond.) 281:31-5.
56. Rothwell, N.J. and Stock, M.J. (1979b): J Comp Physiol Psychol 93:1024-34.
57. Salans, L.B., Bray,G.A. Cushman,S.W. Danforth,E. Glennon,J.A. Horton, E.S. and Sims, E.A.H. (1974): J Clin Invest 53:848.
58. Salans, L.B., Horton, E.S. and Sims, E.A.H. (1971): J Clin Invest 50: 1005-11.
59. Salans, L.B., Knittle, J.L. and Hirsch,J. (1968): J Clin Invest 47:153-65.
60. Sclafani, A (1978): In Recent Advances in Obesity Research II, Proceedings of the 2nd International Congress on Obesity, edited by G. A. Bray pp. . London, England:Newman Publishing Ltd.
61. Shrago, E. and Spennetta, T. (1976): Am J Clin Nutr 29:40.
62. Sims, E.A.H., Goldman,R.F. Gluck, C.M. (1968): Assoc Am Phys 81:153-70.
63. Sims, E.A.H., Danforth,E. Horton,E.S. Bray,G.A. Glennon, J.A. and Salans, L.B. (1973): Rec Prog Horm Res 29:457.
64. Smith U. (1972): Anat Res 112:597-602.
65. Soll, A.H., Kahn, C.R. and Neville,D.M. Jr (1975): J Biol Chem 250: 4702-07.
66. Spaulding, S.W., Chopra,I.J. Sherwin, R.S. and Lyall, S.S. (1976): J Clin Endocrinol Metab 42:197.
67. Sturdevant, R.A.L., Pearce, M.L. and Dayton, S. (1973): New Engl J Med 288:24-7.

68. Suda, A.K., Pittman,C.S. Shimizu, T. and Chambers, J.B. (1978): J Clin Endocrinol Metab 47:1311.
69. Vagenakis, A.G., Burger,A. Portnay,G.I. Rudolph,M. O'Brien,J.T. Azizi,F. Arky,R.A. Nicod,P. Ingbar, S.H. and Braverman, L.E. (1975): J Clin Endocrinol Metab 41:191.
70. Whipp, B.J. (1975): "Obesity in Perspective." In Fogarty International Center Series on Preventive Medicine, Vol. II, Part I and Part II, edited by G.A. Bray, pp. Washington D.C.:U.S. Government Printing Office.
71. York, D.A. and Bray, G.A. (1973): Metabolism 22:443.
72. Young, J.B. and Landsberg, L. (1980): J Clin Invest 65:1086-94.

The Adipocyte and Obesity: Cellular and Molecular Mechanisms, edited by A. Angel, C. H. Hollenberg, and D. A. K. Roncari. Raven Press, New York © 1983.

Adipogenic Factors and the Formation of Adipocytes

Howard Green

Department of Physiology and Biophysics, Harvard Medical School, Boston, Massachusetts 02115

The total number of adipose cells in an animal is regulated within fairly narrow limits. Adipose cells begin to form in late fetal life and additional cells are added during subsequent growth. New adipocytes cannot be formed by multiplication of existing mature adipocytes, since these cells seem to be incapable of multiplying. In culture, immature adipocytes are capable of limited multiplication, but it is not clear whether the extent of this multiplication can be regulated. Probably differentiation of preadipose cells is an important means by which new adipocytes are generated both before and after birth. This differentiation is obviously regulated by chemicals reaching preadipose cells from remote sites. Two possible kinds of regulatory system can be imagined:

1. The preadipose cell might respond directly to the external metabolite concentration. Adipocyte formation in early life, or following over-feeding, would be a direct response of preadipocytes to an elevated concentration of lipids or glucose in the fluid bathing the cells.

2. The preadipose cell might not respond to metabolites directly but rather through an intermediate agent designated as an adipogenic factor. Such a factor could be made in any organ and reach preadipocytes through the blood. The concentration of the factor could be regulated according to the stage of development of the animal and the metabolite concentration at the remote site at which the adipogenic factor is produced.

The existence of a substance possessing adipogenic activity became clear several years ago, when it was found that sera of different animals have different capacity to support adipose conversion of 3T3 cells. This activity was associated with a macromolecule, since it was retained during dialysis of the serum. The action of the adipogenic factor seemed to be positive in nature: when cultured cells were exposed to a mixture of serum low in adipogenic activity (cat serum) together with one high in adipogenic activity (fetal calf serum) the effect of the mixture was nearly as adipogenic as the highly adipogenic serum alone.

When purification of the adipogenic factor of serum proved difficult, extracts of different organs were surveyed in the hope of identifying the origin of the serum adipogenic factor. Of all the organs tested, only the pituitary possessed such an activity. The macromolecule responsible for this activity was eventually identified as growth hormone. Although this result seemed surprising at first, there had actually been earlier studies, on both animals and humans, implicating the pituitary and even growth hormone itself as a determinant of fat cell number.

These earlier studies focussed on a possible role for growth hormone in supporting multiplication of preadipose cells. Such a role could not explain the effect of the hormone on the adipose conversion of cultured 3T3 cells. In this process, growth hormone promotes the different-iation of the target preadipose cells. Since these preadipose cells are a cloned population, growth hormone obviously acts directly on those cells, and not through somatomedin production by an intermediate cell type.

It would seem that it is time to reexamine the traditional view of how growth hormone acts. Is the action of the hormone on the adipose conversion similar to its action on other cells and tissues? Can the growth induced by the hormone in those tissues be the result of the creation of new differentiated cells from their precursors, as seems to be the case in the adipose conversion?

Returning to the problem of regulation of adipose cell number, it seems essential to determine whether the entire adipogenic activity of serum is due to its growth hormone content. If so, the serum of hypophysectomized animals should be devoid of adipogenic activity. From experiments recently carried out by Dr. Tracy Nixon, it seems unlikely that this is the case; and there may therefore exist adipogenic factors in addition to growth hormone.

As mentioned, multiplication of immature adipose cells may also make an important contribution to the total number of adipose cells. It seems possible that this proliferation might either not be regulated at all i.e. consist of a fixed number of cell divisions, or be regulated separately from the process by which new adipose cells are formed by differentiation of preadipose cells.

References

Bjorntorp, P. (1982). Adipocyte Development in Adipose Tissue in Childhood. ed. F. P. Bonnet, CRC Press, Boca Raton, Florida, pp 9-28.

Bonnet, F., Vanderschueren-Lodeweyckx, M., Eckels R. and Malvaux, P.. (1974). Subcutaneous adipose tissue and lipids in blood in growth hormone deficiency before and after treatment with human growth hormone. Pediatr. Res. 8:800-805.

Green, H.. (1979). Adipose Conversion: A program of differentiation. Les Colloques de l'Inserm. Obesity - Cellular and Molecular Aspects 87:15-24.

Hayasni, I., Nixon, T., Morikawa, M., and Green, H. (1981). Adipogenic and anti-adipogenic factors in the pituitary and other organs. Proc. Natl. Acad. Sci. USA 78:3969-3972.

Hollenberg, C. H., and Vost, A. (1968). Regulation of DNA synthesis in fat cells and stromal elements from rat adipose tissue. J. Clin. Invest. 47:2485-2498.

Kuri-Harcucn, W. and Green, H. (1978). Adipose conversion of 3T3 cells depends on a serum factor. Proc. Natl. Acad. Sci. USA 75:6107-6109.

Klyde, B. J. and Hirsch, J. (1979). Increased cellular proliferation in adipose tissue of adult rats fed a high-fat diet. J. Lipid Res. 20:705-715.

Morikawa, M., Nixon, T., and Green, H. (1982). Growth hormone and the adipose conversion of 3T3 Cells. Cell 29:783-789.

Pairault, J., and Green, H. (1979). A study of the adipose conversion of suspended 3T3 cells by using glycerophospnate dehydrogenase as differentiation marker. Proc. Natl. Acad. Sci. USA 76:5138-5142.

The Adipocyte and Obesity: Cellular and Molecular Mechanisms, edited by A. Angel, C. H. Hollenberg, and D. A. K. Roncari. Raven Press, New York © 1983.

Development of Adipose Tissue *In Vivo* and *In Vitro*

Per Björntorp

Department of Medicine I, Sahlgren's Hospital, University of Göteborg, S-413 45 Göteborg, Sweden

Previous methodological and physiological work with adipose precursor cells reported at two previous similar meetings (1,4) has shown that new adipocytes are found from such precursor cells under certain conditions. A partly hypothetical regulation of adipose tissue growth has been suggested. This will first be briefly summarized in order to provide a background for further work both in the rat and in the human.

Upon start of overfeeding with fat available fat cells begin to enlarge, and there is an increase in the formation of new cells in adipose tissue. Some of these cells are probably non-determined adipose precursor cells (adipoblasts), and some are probably cells or precursor cells for supply and support of adipocytes. This is a generalized phenomenon all over adipose tissue. When adipose tissue is "full", that is, available adipocytes have reached a certain "critical size", then non-determined adipose precursor cells from the pool of newly formed cells are determined to adipocytes which fill up, and are rapidly incorporated into the pool of monovacuolar adipocytes. This determination seems to be locally regulated because it occurs at different times in different fat depots, depending on the adipocyte size of the depot in question.

Two regulating signal systems can then be visualized, one distributed generally to all adipose depots, producing an increase in new cell formation, and another probably produced locally to recruit adipoblasts by determination to adipocytes.

The first, generally distributed signal is not of neural origin, because gangliectomy in the rat does not prevent new fat cell formation with overfeeding (Faust and Koopmans, personal communication). It is therefore likely that this is a signal distributed in the circulation. Consequently we started to examine the stimulatory activity of serum and plasma in rats under experimental conditions known previously to stimulate or inhibit new fat cell formation. (Björntorp, Faust and Mitler, to be published).

33

First a method was worked out which allowed quantitative assays of such activity. The tissue culture technique was utilized with adipose precursor cells in primary cultures, and with addition of the serum or plasma to be assayed. The assay was performed either as measurements of triglyceride per unit protein or per cell, or as a count of the number of lipid-containing cells formed. The both first-mentioned assays seemed to give best precision.

Preliminary experiments showed that essentially platelet-free heparin plasma gave higher activity than other plasmas or serum. Furthermore, there was a marked species variation with little or no activity in cat serum, as previously described for the 3T3 cells undergoing adipose conversion (7). With this background each heparin plasma was assayed in a dose-response curve with cat serum constituting a background for support of cellular multiplication and growth.

Adult, male Osborne-Mendel rats were utilized. Groups fasted for 4 days, fed ordinary carbohydrate-rich laboratory chow, or overfed with a fat cafeteria-type diet for 5, 10 and 21 days were examined. Blood was drawn by aortic cannulation, with all plastic material to prevent platelet destruction, into plastic tubes with heparin to a final concentration of 5 IU/ml. Essentially platelet-free plasma was then prepared by centrifugations at 1085 xg for 15 minutes, and 22000 xg for 30 minutes respectively.

Fig. 1 shows that fasting rats were devoid of activity stimulating triglyceride accumulation in adipose precursor cells. The activity increased with 10 and 21 days of fat feeding. Citrate inhibited activity.

The nature of the activity in question is not known. The end-point for measurements is rather unspecific and might mean either an increased rate of multiplication of the adipoblasts specifically, or a determination effect on these cells, or simply that the availability of substrate was higher in the fat-fed rat plasmas. The last alternative is highly unlikely, however, fat-feeding resulted in no or very slight increase in plasma triglycerides. The remaining alternatives are now being studied.

The postulated local regulatory factor for adipose tissue growth by new adipocyte formation can be studied with the developed methodology, where non-determined and determined adipose precursor cells as well as adipocytes of various sizes can be obtained. In addition, capillaries and capillary endothelial cells at different stages of development can also be obtained (4,5). The main cellular components of adipose tissue are thus available for reconstitution experiments where potential interactions can be studied.

A first idea was to study if endothelial cell growth influenced on the growth and development of the adipocyte series of cells. The background to this idea was the old observations that the first visible identifyable structure in a developing fat lobulus seems to be a capillary (6).

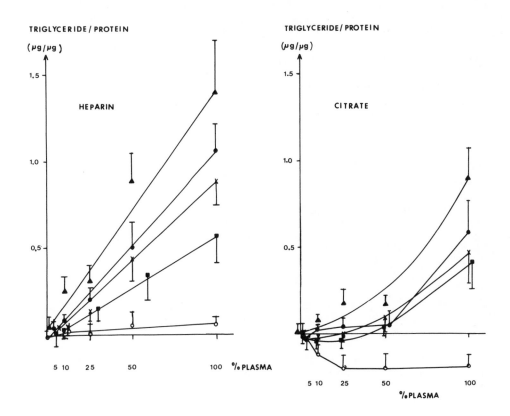

Fig. 1. Effects of different volumes of platelet-poor rat heparin or citrate plasmas on lipid accumulation in adipose tissue precursor cells. Open circles: Fasted 4 days. Crosses: Fed laboratory chow. Filled squares: Fat fed 5 days. Filled circles: Fat fed 10 days. Filled triangles: Fat fed 21 days. Significant (p <0.05) differences between regression coefficients in heparin plasma experiments: Fasted lower than all other groups. 21 day fat-fed higher than controls and 5 day fat-fed. Means ± SEM.

Isolated fragments of capillaries had no effect on the growth and development of adipocyte precursor cells. Next endothelial cells were allowed to start to grow and develop from the capillary fragments, and then adipocyte precursor

cells were added. Again, no effect was observable on the
preadipose cells. There was, however, a strong stimulatory
effect on the growth of the endothelial cells when the preadipose cells were added. The stimulatory activity was not
transferrable in growth medium from the adipose precursor
cells. The specificity of this phenomenon is now examined.
In addition, a number of other combinations of cells of
different sorts and degree of development with addition of
plasma with high or low stimulating activity on adipocyte
formation are now tested.

Studies in humans

The ultimate goal in this research project has been to
study adipose tissue development in severely obese humans
with a hyperplastic adipose tissue. The policy has been,
however, to develop methodology and examine regulatory factors first in the rat, where technical problems of various
sorts are smaller. In the following some initial attempts
will be described.
A specific method has been developed to attempt to quantitate cells which have already been determined to adipocytes in vivo, but not been filled with lipid. These cells
have been called preadipocytes. They are allowed to fill up
with lipid in a suspension culture system to be identifyable,
and at the same time to prevent multiplication. In adipose
tissue of growing, small rats many such cells are found (2).
They can also be found temporarily when adipose tissue is
expanding by the formation of new fat cells in adult rats
(4).
Examining adipose tissue from non-obese subjects has not
resulted in the finding of any such cells. In preparations
from severely obese subjects, however, they can be found
although in a very limited number. This is the case also in
fat from non-obese children (Table 1).
The conclusion from this work is that preadipocytes normally do not seem to be present in neither non-obese nor
obese human adipose tissue. Therefore, the attempts to estimate fat cell number is probably not hampered by such a potential error.
In the same type of adipose tissue cell preparation the
cells multiplying in an ordinary monolayer culture have been
examined after a long period of time in primary culture.
These experiments were performed in a system with a feeding
layer to allow full expression ("pastry culture", 3). There
are no doubt adipocytes formed here, presumably by division
of adipoblasts. We have the impression that more of these
cells are found in material from severely obese subjects.
Roncari (8) has already reported that adipose precursor
cells from obese subjects divide much more rapidly than such
cells from normals.
Finally,"adipogenic activity"from human plasma has been
examined in the same way as with rat plasma described above.
The patients examined have been followed up with adipocyte

Table 1. <u>Number of cells filling up with lipid in suspension</u>
        <u>culture (in vivo determined preadipocytes)</u> in humans.

	Number per 10^6 adipocytes
Adult, nonobese (n:10)	0
Adult, obese (n:10)	$< 0.02 \times 10^4$
Children, nonobese (n:10)	$0.18 \pm 0.02 \times 10^4$
Sprague-Dawley rats (15 wks)(n:18)	$30 \pm 10 \times 10^4$
Sprague-Dawley rats (3 wks)(n:14)	$210 \pm 20 \times 10^4$

Adipose tissue was obtained from abdominal subcutaneous in
obese and non-obese adults, and/or omental tissue in non-
obese adults. In children (age 1 month - 15 years) adipose
tissue was obtained from various subcutaneous regions. In
rats the epididymal fat pad was used. (Means $\pm$ SEM).

number determinations in their adipose tissue (9) and the
activity in plasma could then be set in relation to what has
actually seemed to happen in their adipose tissue during a
long observation time. In addition, non-obese sex- and age
matched controls were examined. Fig. 2 shows these results.
The activity was assayed here on the fat cell precursors
from about 300 g male Sprague-Dawley rats. The activity in
the obese subjects was higher than in controls. The activity
showed little dispersion from the average in the controls.
Three of the obese subjects showed similar activity (1,5,7),
but in the rest there was an elevated activity. The elevation in activity was not associated with degree of obesity,
fat cell proliferation over 3-7 years or blood glucose.
There was, however, a striking relationship with the weight
history for the preceding few months, subjects increasing
in weight having high values and vice versa. Fasting plasma
insulin followed this pattern also.
    These early results with human material show so far that
the methodology developed in the rat is applicable for human studies which are now continuing.

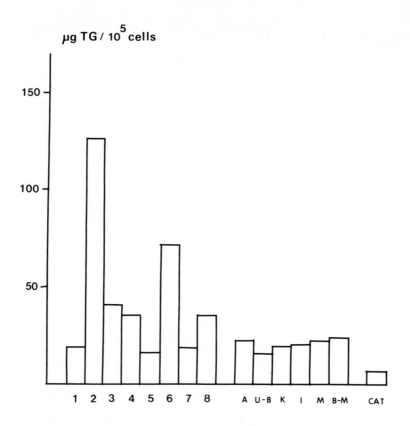

Fig. 2. Heparin plasma activity to promote triglyceride accumulation in adipose precursor cells in 8 (left) obese and 6 non-obese (right) subjects. Cat serum activity for comparison. All controls and obese subjects 1 and 7 were weight stabile. Obese subject 5 was decreasing in weight and the remaining obese (2,3,4,6,8) were in a period of weight gaining.

Acknowledgements:
   Supported by grants from the Swedish Medical Research Council (B82-19X-251-20C) and the National Institutes of Health (5 R01 AM25173-03-MET). Part of this work was performed during a sabbatical year at the Rockefeller University, New York, N.Y.

References

1. Björntorp, P. (1979a): Development of adipocytes from pre-
   cursor cells obtained from epididymal fat pads of rats.
   In: Obesity, cellular and molecular aspects, edited by
   G. Ailhaud, pp 89-102. INSERM, Paris.
2. Björntorp, P., Karlsson, M., Gustafsson, L., Smith, U.,
   Sjöström, L., Cigolini, M., Storck, G., and Pettersson,
   P. (1979b): Quantitation of different cells in the epi-
   didymal fat pad of the rat. J. Lipid Res. 20:97-106.
3. Björntorp, P., Karlsson, M., Pettersson, P., and
   Cypniewska, G. (1980): Differentiation and function of
   rat adipocyte precursor cells in primary culture. J.
   Lipid Res. 21:714-723.
4. Björntorp, P. (1981a): Adipose precursor cells. In:
   Recent Advances in Obesity Research III, edited by P.
   Björntorp, M. Cairella, and A. Howard, pp 58-69. Libby,
   London.
5. Björntorp, P., Hansson, G.K., Pettersson, P., and
   Sypniewska, G. (1981b): Isolation and characterization
   of endothelial cells from the epididymal fat pad of the
   rat. Submitted for publication.
6. Toldt, C. (1870): Contribution to the histology and physiology of adipose tissue. Sitzber. Akad. Wiss. Wien.
   Math. Naturwiss. Kl. 62:445.
7. Kuri-Harcuch, W., and Green, H. (1978): Adipose conversion of 3T3 cells depends on a serum factor. Cell Biol.
   75:6107-6109.
8. Roncari, D.A.K. (1981): Characterization of cultured human precursors. In: Recent Advances in Obesity Research
   III, edited by P. Björntorp, M. Cairella, and A. Howard,
   pp 70-74. Libby, London.
9. William-Olsson, T., and Sjöström, L. (1980): Development
   of adipose tissue cellularity in adult obese women over
   a 6 to 9 years period. Third Intern. Congress of Obesity
   (Abstract). Alim. Nutr. Metab. 1:382.

The Adipocyte and Obesity: Cellular and Molecular Mechanisms, edited by A. Angel, C. H. Hollenberg, and D. A. K. Roncari. Raven Press, New York © 1983.

Hyperplastic Growth of Adipose Tissue in Obesity

Irving M. Faust and Wilson H. Miller, Jr.

The Rockefeller University, New York, New York, 10021

Obesity is the manifestation of at least one of two morphological abnormalities of the adipose tissue: hypertrophy of the fat cells and an excessive number of fat cells. If an individual has fat cells that are larger than normal, but there is no abnormality of fat cell number, the total fat mass may be two to three times greater than normal. For the average 120 pound woman, with about 20% body fat and an average fat cell lipid content of about .55 µg, an extremely large increase to 1.50 µg would correspond to a weight gain of about 50 pounds (consisting primarily of lipid and a small amount of water and protein). To return to normal body weight, the woman would need only to reattain the normal average fat cell size. Both fat cell size and number would then be the same as if there had been no obesity. Metabolic abnormalities (such as hyperinsulinemia) that were probably present during the time the woman was obese would most likely also be rectified as a result of the reattainment of normal body weight.

Obesity that is the result not only of hypertrophied fat cells, but of excessive numbers of fat cells as well, can be much more severe in its magnitude and involves a morphological alteration in adipose tissue that is not erased with weight reduction (21). Fat cell number can easily be several times greater than normal in severely obese people, and weight loss involves only a reduction of fat cell lipid content (see below). Thus, if a person with four times the normal number of fat cells were to lose all his excess weight, his adipose tissue would still have its full complement of excess cells, but the cells would be one fourth the normal size. Such a small fat cell size, in turn, appears to lead to metabolic and psychological alterations. For example, metabolic rate (R.L. Leibel et al., unpublished) and levels of T3 (B.S. Schneider et al., unpublished) decrease as a function of degree of weight loss, and are greatly decreased in reduced obese patients in which body weight is stable but fat cell size is very small. Such patients have aberations in self-perception (18), and are often severely depressed (16). Since similar alterations occur in fasted non-obese people (26,43), they may well reflect the normal action of physiologic mechanisms that serve to resist depletion of the fat cell lipid stores and become increasingly active as fat cell size declines. The available clinical evidence suggests that diet has a better chance of long-term success in moderating the weight of severely obese people if the degree of weight reduction is moderate, i.e., is discontinued at about the time normal fat cell size is achieved (4,32).

ATTEMPTS TO ERADICATE FAT CELLS

Surgical removal of adipose tissue is not very practical and can only reduce excess adipose tissue mass by a small percentage in cases of severe obesity, but it may be an effective procedure for people who desire reduction only of a disproportionately large mass of adipose tissue in some particular part of the body (38). However, compensatory regrowth or regeneration of the extirpated tissue may occur, with variation across individuals and across lipectomy sites. The degree of restoration of adipose tissue in lipectomized rats and mice has been seen to vary widely as a function of many factors such as the site of surgery, hormonal status and the age and strain of the animal at the time of surgery (7,8,30,34 and Faust, et al., unpublished). A more desirable way to eradicate fat cells, especially in the severely obese, would be through alterations of the diet. Therefore, it is of interest to know whether a sufficient degree of food restriction can cause the loss of fat cells. The earliest studies to address this issue found no evidence of such an effect (20,23), but the results of more recent studies at least suggest that it is possible (25,47).

To help resolve this issue, we subjected rats to the most severe long-term food deprivation we could devise and then analyzed adipose tissue cellularity to determine whether a detectable reduction in the number of fat cells had occured. We fasted male rats for seven days and then fed them only a calorically inadequate glucose-electrolyte solution for another 40 days, causing them to lose nearly 50% of their initial body weight. Their fat depots could barely be seen; depots that normally weigh 10-20 grams weighed only a few milligrams. Nevertheless, there was no detectable loss or turnover of fat cells. The wisp of tissue that was an epididymal fat pad in these rats contained as many adipocytes as epididymal fat pads of non-fasted controls. It also contained as many cells as contralateral pads in the same rats after ad libitum refeeding had resulted in restoration of much of the lost body weight (36). Analysis of the pads by autoradiography showed that many non-parenchymal cells were formed in the adipose tissue during the course of refeeding, presumably to replace cells lost during the fast, but no newly formed fat cells were found. Those fat cells present after refeeding were the same cells that were present prior to the fast (see figure 1). If eradication of fat cells by food restriction were feasible, the degree and duration of food restriction employed in this experiment surely should have achieved some reduction in the number of fat cells. That it did not suggests that alterations of diet cannot be used to eliminate existing fat cells.

REDUCTION OF FAT CELL SIZE

If we cannot eliminate existing fat cells by dietary means, perhaps diet can be used to reset the lipid storage mechanism so that each cell is inclined to store a subnormal amount of lipid. Restriction of food intake in adults can surely achieve a small fat cell size, but the small size is maintained only as long as the restriction continues. "Set points" for fat cell size are not affected by food restriction. Upon refeeding, a previously restricted or fasted adult rat quickly gains weight until its normal average fat cell size is restored (20). People also show such restoration following a fast (26).

The results of several early experiments suggested that it might be possible to reset the level of lipid storage per fat cell by malnourishing very young rats (28). However, it now appears that the effects on cell size seen in these experiments were transitory. In a more recent experiment it was found that average fat cell size is perfectly normal in one year old rats severely malnourished during the suckling period (12). It appears that the physiological mechanisms governing the degree of fat cell lipid storage cannot be altered at any time of life by food intake restriction. The only way to achieve and maintain a reduced fat cell size is by some form of continuous action. Dieting is one such action. Protocols of sustained alteration of activity or diet composition and/or long-term use of appropriate pharmacologic agents can also be at least moderately effective at keeping fat cells smaller than they otherwise would be. Unfortunately, these actions require a life-long commitment and are generally successful only when the degree of overweight is moderate.

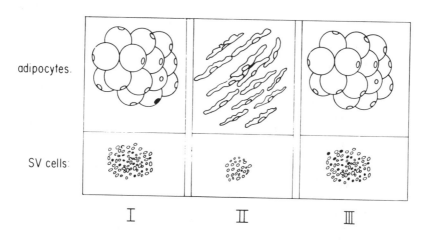

Figure 1. Schematic representation of effects of severe long-term food deprivation and refeeding on cells in adipose tissue of adult rats. Cells with darkened nuclei have incorporated injected ³H-thymidine in their DNA and thus have been recently produced. I- Ad Libitum feeding: very slow production of adipocytes and slow production or turnover of stromal-vascular (SV) cells. II- At the end of the deprivation period, adipocytes have virtually no lipid, but all are present. SV cell number is diminished. No new cells are seen. III- During refeeding, adipocytes refill with lipid and many new SV cells are formed. However, no new adipocytes are formed.

PREVENTING THE PRODUCTION OF EXCESS FAT CELLS

If we accept the notion that fat cells are permanent fixtures of the body, and that fat cell size can, realistically, only be reduced a certain amount by some form of continuous action, a primary goal of therapeutic intervention should be the prevention of the formation of excess fat cells. To have a basis for such intervention it is essential that we understand normal fat cell production as well as when, how, and under what circumstances excess fat cells are formed.

In the ordinary laboratory rat, the most rapid and extensive proliferation of fat cells occurs during the first few weeks of life (17,20). When overall growth continues into adulthood, as it does in the male rat, fat cell production continues as well (2,14). Fat cell production also continues during growth of cattle (39) and during the adolescent growth spurt in man (29,33). There is no evidence that fat cell production normally continues in any animal or in man when growth of lean body mass has ceased.

It has been known for some time that malnourishment of rats during the suckling period restrains production of fat cells (28). Under normal circumstances most fat cells are produced during this period, so this effect is not surprising. However, many other cells are also normally produced in the rat during the suckling period, so malnourishment during this stage of life impairs overall body growth as well. Effects of early malnourishment of the genetically obese Zucker rat are even more discouraging. There is relatively less restriction of fat cell production and greater restriction of growth of lean tissue (6). If food restriction is ever to be used for the purpose of limiting production of fat cells in man, care will surely have to be taken with regard to timing and degree of severity of restriction to insure that growth of other organs is not impeded as well.

In rats, the normal increases in fat cell number that occur during adulthood can also be limited by weight control. When adult male rats are fed 60% of normal ad libitum food intake, the usual age-related increases in fat cell number are substantially restricted (3). More severe food restriction might prevent such increases entirely. Age-related increases in the number of fat cells are also impeded in rats that lose weight as a result of being housed in the cold. When they are raised in a 4^0C environment, their body weight declines and remains lower than that of controls for several months even though food intake is sharply increased. During this period of lowered body weight, normal, age-related increases in fat cell number do not occur in most adipose tissue depots (35).

EFFECTS OF HORMONES ON PROMOTION AND INHIBITION OF FAT CELL PRODUCTION

The results of the above study of adipose cellularity in rats reared in the cold illustrate another feature of fat cell production in adults: variation across depots. While increases in fat cell number were found to be essentially arrested in retroperitoneal and inguinal depots, they were found to be greatly enhanced in epididymal pads. The factor (or factors) responsible for the heterogeneous response are not known, but this issue is currently being addressed. Studies in several laboratories have shown that different hormones produce different patterns of adipose tissue hypertrophy across depots. Progesterone stimulates enlargement of parametrial pads almost exclusively (48), while insulin primarily stimulates enlargement of the subcutaneous fat (31,41). While the effects produced in these experiments were primarily on the size of fat cells, the periods of hormone treatment were of relatively short duration. Changes in the number of fat cells might very well have occurred if the studies had been of longer duration.

In the adolescent human female, high levels of sex hormones are surely responsible, at least in part, for extensive growth of adipose tissue in certain areas of the body, such as breasts, thighs and buttocks. It is thus not surprising to find that when estrogen is added to cultures of human preadipocytes, proliferation and differentiation of the cells become accelerated (40). The sex hormones also appear to affect regrowth of adipose tissue in male rats from which subcutaneous-inguinal fat depots have been removed. The degree of such regrowth is substantially greater in rats that have been castrated (Faust, I.M., et al., unpublished).

An extremely interesting experiment suggesting powerful hormonal restraint of adipocyte production in the woodchuck has recently been reported by Young et al (49). Woodchucks, like all animal hibernators, experience a period of pre-hibernation hyperphagia during which body fat stores are greatly increased. Since hibernation usually occurs at least once a year, production of new fat cells during each episode of pre-hibernatory weight gain would cause regular increases in baseline body fat mass (i.e., fat mass maintained at times other than during pre-hibernation and hibernation). Such permanent increases in body fat could well be disadvantageous to animals that must often move quickly to avoid predators. Excessive amounts of fat may also interfere with reproduction (19). Thus, some device may have evolved in these animals specifically to interfere with the usual stimulatory impact of adipocyte hypertrophy on fat cell production (discussed below). Observations of the lack of long-term body weight change over the course of several hibernatory cycles support this possibility (37). The study by Young et al supports it more directly. Pre-hibernatory weight gain in the woodchuck was found to involve increases only in fat cell size, while relatively moderate weight gain at other times, resulting from captivity and the feeding of a laboratory diet, involved increases in fat cell number as well. The adult woodchuck can produce new fat cells, but such production appears to be prevented by some factor (or factors) present during pre-hibernation.

EFFECTS OF DIET COMPOSITION AND FAT CELL SIZE ON PROMOTION AND INHIBITION OF FAT CELL PRODUCTION

In certain strains of rats the feeding of a high-fat diet results in the development of obesity (42). Diets high in sucrose and diets containing a variety of snack foods also cause rats to become obese (9,45). Typically, when such diets are first introduced, overeating occurs and average fat cell size increases in all depots. Several weeks later, significant increases in fat cell number appear in some depots. During ensuing weeks, increases appear in other depots as well (9). Body weight rises during the initial, relatively short, period of fat cell enlargement as well as during the more prolonged subsequent period of fat cell number increase. But only the weight gain due to fat cell enlargement is reversible. If Osborne-Mendel rats are fed a fattening diet, fat cell size approximately doubles in a few weeks and fat cell number doubles in about six months. Refeeding of ordinary chow causes weight loss only until normal fat cell size is achieved. Fat cell number remains twice normal, so total body fat mass also remains twice normal (11).

In juvenile onset obesity in man, there is usually fat cell hypertrophy and excessive numbers of fat cells, while in moderate adult onset obesity there is primarily fat cell hypertrophy (22). However, when adult onset obesity is severe, there may be a substantial increase in the number of fat cells (1,22). Unfortunately, there is no clear boundary of body weight or adiposity separating moderate and severe adult onset obesity, and studies of adipose cellularity are much more difficult to conduct in man than in animals. So we can only guess, at this time, the degree of weight gain an individual may experience as an adult before there is a likelihood that increases in the number of fat cells will occur. However, we do know that very large increases in the number of fat cells can occur in rats when the average fat cell becomes particularly large, at least when the rats are fed certain diets (9). Since fat cell number begins to increase at about the time that fat cell size peaks, it has been suggested that at some level of enlargement the cells begin to produce locally acting signals which stimulate production of new fat cells (5,9). By so doing, the fat cells would help to relieve themselves of the burden of having to store increasingly greater amounts of lipid. It is thus reasonable to speculate that production of new fat cells will occur in man when fat cells get very large, and that the critical degree of enlargement will vary among individuals as well as across fat depots. If the specific parameters of such a link were to be established for an individual, important clinical advice could be offered as to the maximum body weight that could be attained before a risk of stimulating fat cell production would be incurred.

Two points must be emphasized with regard to the possible promotion of adipocyte production by signals from large fat cells. First, large fat cells are not the only source of stimuli which cause increases in the number of fat cells: most fat cells are produced in young, growing animals in which average fat cell size is usually very small; adipose tissue regrowth (which includes formation of many new fat cells) occurs in adult rats in which fat cell size is normal (10); and, as mentioned above, fat cell number in epididymal pads of rats reared at 4^0C for six months increases about 50%, even though average fat cell size is substantially smaller than normal during all, or most, of that time (35). Second, large fat cells, by themselves, do not provide the most effective stimulus for rapid and extensive production of fat cells. Chow-fed rats made obese by means of lesions of the ventromedial hypothalamus (VMH) achieve an extremely large fat cell size, but fail to show any increases in fat cell number three months following lesioning, even in the retroperitoneal depots (which typically show the greatest such increases in rats fed high-fat diets) (13,20). On the other hand, we have found that an occasional group of rats in our laboratory (either Sprague Dawley or Osborne Mendel) fails to show the usual increase in body weight in response to a high-fat, high-sucrose diet. When this happens, the rats also fail to show increases in fat cell number (unpublished). Diet content alone may therefore also be ineffective as a stimulus of major increases in fat cell number. It is most likely that signals from large fat cells work in conjunction with substrates provided by certain diets to stimulate maximal fat cell production.

We have found that when we feed VMH-lesioned rats a high-fat diet, fat cell number increases rapidly and dramatically. Furthermore, when we feed VMH-lesioned rats sweetened-condensed milk, but pair-gain them to lesioned rats fed chow, they show significantly greater numbers of fat cells than the chow-fed rats (Faust et al., unpublished). A recently reported study by Sclafani et al. (46) illustrates how synergism between signals from large fat cells and substrate provided by diet may act to affect changes in body weight. VMH-lesioned rats were alternately fed chow and snack foods. Body weight increased rapidly during the initial period of chow feeding, but then plateaued (presumably when signals from the extremely enlarged fat cells became strong enough to cause food intake to subside.) As soon as snack food feeding began, body weight resumed its rapid ascent (presumably reflecting the rapid production of new fat cells). Return to chow feeding caused only a small decline in body weight, to a level well above the previous plateau. The combination of substrate provided by the snack food diet and signals from greatly enlarged fat cells appears to have provided a powerful and immediate stimulus for the rapid production of new fat cells.

THE SOURCE OF NEW FAT CELLS IN ADIPOSE DEPOTS OF ADULTS

Early studies of fat cell production in rats showed that rapid proliferation of cells destined to become adipocytes occured in the stromal-vascular fraction of epididymal pads of rats from the time of birth until about 60 days of age (17,23). More recently, it has been shown that extensive production of cells occurs in the adipose tissue of older rats during the first week that they are fed a high-fat diet (27). However, the rate of production of fat cell progenitors is probably much lower than the rate for supporting stromal-vascular cells. This makes production rates of the progenitors difficult to determine, especially since available cell separation techniques cannot fully separate adipocytes from non-adipocytes.

Thus, we recently decided to obtain a qualitative assessment of rates of progenitor production by measuring changes in DNA synthetic rates in two fat depots that show markedly different levels of fat cell number increase in response to high-fat feeding: the retroperitoneal and the epididymal (Miller, W.H., Jr., et al., unpublished). We confirmed the earlier finding that during the first week of high-fat feeding, DNA synthetic rates are greatly increased in both depots. The degree of increase was indistinguishable between them. However, we also found that the level of DNA synthesis in epididymal pads decreased toward control levels during ensuing weeks, while in retroperitoneal depots it remained significantly elevated. This is fully consistent with the changes in fat cell number that are seen in these two depots during the initial months of high-fat feeding. These different patterns of cell production were found in studies conducted in vivo as well as in studies of pieces of the fat depots incubated in vitro with ^{3}H-thymidine. Figure 2 presents a scheme of what may be happening at the cellular level.

We can draw several conclusions about production of cells in adipose tissue from these observations. First, the initial response to high-fat feeding is very likely a rapid burst of proliferation of supporting stromal-vascular cells. Such support is apparently provided regardless of whether the major impending change in the depot is increased fat cell size (as in the epididymal pad) or increased fat cell size and number (as in the retroperitoneal depot). This conclusion was also reached by Bjorntorp (5) as a result of his studies of collagenase-separated adipose tissue cells maintained in suspension culture. Second, new adipocytes in a depot arise from the maturation of precursor cells that have recently proliferated in that depot, rather than from the maturation of cells produced earlier in life or from cells produced elsewhere and transported to the fat depots. Third, while quantitative studies of this sort are extremely difficult, it is nevertheless possible to assess relative rates of adipocyte precursor production, at least at those times when the production rate of stromal-vascular cells is low. Since such assessment can be made with small pieces of tissue in vitro, it can also be used in studies of adipose tissue growth in man. With the in vitro technique, it may now be possible to determine whether there is indeed a relationship between fat cell size and the production of new fat cells in man. Effects of manipulations of diet, exercise or drugs on fat cell production in individuals at risk for hyperplastic growth of adipocytes could also be assessed.

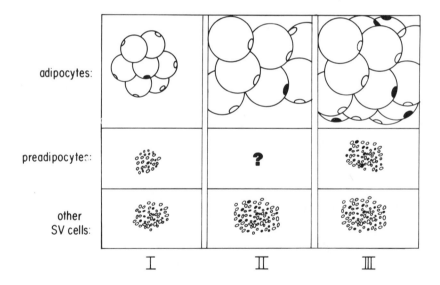

Figure 2. Schematic representation of growth of cells in adipose tissue of adult rats fed a high-fat, high-sugar diet. Cells with darkened nuclei are newly synthesized. I-Ad Libitum chow-feeding: very slow production of adipocytes and slow production or turnover of stromal-vascular (SV) cells. II-During the initial few days of high-fat, high-sugar feeding, production of SV cells increases dramatically. Level of production of pre-adipocytes and adipocytes is not discerned. III-After five weeks on the diet, production of SV cells is back to control levels. Rate of production of pre-adipocytes is increased (substantially in retroperitoneal depots and moderately, if at all, in epididymal pads) and new adipocytes are formed.

ADIPOCYTE HYPERPLASIA AS A COMPENSATORY RESPONSE TO
ADIPOCYTE HYPERTROPHY

Excessively hypertrophied fat cells appear to be responsible for hyperinsulinemia which, in turn, may cause pancreatic beta-cell "exhaustion" (44). Adipocyte hyperplasia may compensate for the hypertrophy, and thereby ameliorate the hyperinsulinemia, by allowing the excess lipid stores to be more widely distributed. Studies of rat models of obesity indicate that adipocyte hyperplasia may or may not be an effective compensatory response depending upon the underlying cause of the obesity.

As mentioned above, VMH-lesioned rats fed only chow achieve an extremely large average fat cell size, but show no increase in fat cell number for at least three months following lesioning. Feeding such rats a high-fat diet for six months causes the most dramatic adipocyte hyperplasia we have ever seen. However, fat cell size is as enlarged in VMH-rats fed high-fat as it is in VMH-rats fed chow (Faust et al., unpublished). In this model, increases in fat cell number help little, if at all, to reduce the size of the fat cells.

On the other hand, increases in fat cell number may be the basis for dramatic reduction of fat cell size in genetically obese Zucker rats. In these rats, adipocyte hypertrophy and hyperplasia are seen almost from the time of birth. Fat cell size increases greatly until a peak is reached at about 14 weeks of age, and then declines and plateaus at a level about 25% below the peak. Plasma insulin levels (and thus presumably peripheral insulin resistance) correspondingly increase, peak, decline and plateau (24). We do not know whether the 25% drop in fat cell size after 14 weeks of age in the Zucker rat is contingent upon the increases in fat cell number. However, we do know that further increases in fat cell number, promoted by high-fat or snack-food feeding, cause fat cell size to drop another 30% (15).

We do not know whether the relationship between hyperplastic growth of adipose tissue and reduction of adipocyte hypertrophy in obese people is usually more like that of VMH or Zucker obesity. Perhaps hyperplastic adult onset obesity will be found to be usually of one sort and juvenile onset usually the other. In any case, the possibility that adipocyte hyperplasia may be an important compensatory response to adipocyte hypertrophy suggests that therapies directed solely at the prevention of adipocyte hyperplasia may have unexpected metabolic repercussions.

References

1. Ashwell, M., Durrant, M., and Garrow, J.S.(1977): <u>Proc. Nutr. Soc.</u>, 36:111A.
2. Bertrand, H.A., Masoro, E.J., and Yu, B.P.(1978): <u>Science</u>, 201: 1234-1235.
3. Bertrand, H.A., Lynd, F.T., Masoro, E.J., and Yu, B.P.(1980): <u>J. Gerontol.</u>, 35:827-835.
4. Bjorntorp, P., Carlgren, G., Isaksson, B., Krotkiewski, M., Larsson, B., and Sjostrom, L.(1975): <u>Am. J. Clin. Nutr.</u>, 28: 445-452.
5. Bjorntorp, P.(1981): In: <u>Recent Advances in Obesity Research III</u>, edited by P. Bjorntorp, M. Cairella, and A.N. Howard, pp.58-69. John Libbey, London.

6.   Cleary, M.P., Vasselli, J.R., and Greenwood, M.R.C.(1980): <u>Am. J.</u>
     <u>Physiol.</u>, 238:E284-E292.
7.   Faust, I.M., Johnson, P.R., and Hirsch, J.(1976): <u>Am. J.</u>
     <u>Physiol.</u>, 231:538-544.
8.   Faust, I.M., Johnson, P.R., and Hirsch, J.(1977): <u>Science</u>, 197:
     391-393.
9.   Faust, I.M., Johnson, P.R., Stern, J.S., and Hirsch, J.(1978):
     <u>Am. J. Physiol.</u>, 235:E279-E286.
10. Faust, I.M., Johnson, P.R., and Hirsch, J.(1979): <u>Proc. Soc.</u>
     <u>Exp. Biol. Med.</u>, 161:111-114.
11. Faust, I.M.(1980): <u>Int. J. Obesity</u>, 4:314-321.
12. Faust, I.M., Johnson, P.R., and Hirsch, J.(1980): <u>J. Nutr.</u>, 110:
     2027-2034.
13. Faust, I.M., Triscari, J., Sclafani, A., Miller, W.H., Jr., and
     Sullivan, A.C.(1980): <u>Fed.Proc.</u>, 39:887 (abstract).
14. Faust,I.M., and Miller, W.H., Jr.(1981): <u>Int. J. Obesity</u>,
     5:593-596.
15. Gale, S.K., Van Itallie, T.B., and Faust, I.M.(1981): <u>Metabolism</u>,
     30:105-110.
16. Glucksman, M.L., Hirsch, J., McCully, R.S., Barron, B.A., and
     Knittle, J.L. (1968): <u>Psychosom. Med.</u>, 30:359-373.
17. Greenwood, M.R.C., and Hirsch, J.(1974): <u>J. Lipid Res.</u>,
     15:474-483.
18. Grinker, J., and Hirsch, J.(1972): In: <u>Physiology Emotion and</u>
     <u>Psychosomatic Illness</u>, CIBA Foundation Symposium 8,
     pp. 349-373. ASP, Amsterdam.
19. Hemmes, R., Faust, I.M., and Hirsch, J.(1979): <u>Eastern Psychol.</u>
     <u>Assoc.</u>, 50:125 (abstract).
20. Hirsch, J., and Han, P.W.(1969): <u>J. Lipid Res.</u>, 10:77-82.
21. Hirsch, J., and Knittle, J.L.(1970): <u>Fed.Proc.</u>, 29:1516-1521.
22. Hirsch, J., and Batchelor, B.(1976): <u>Clin. Endocrinol. Metab.</u>,
     5:299-311.
23. Hollenberg, C.H., and Vost, A.(1968): <u>J. Clin. Invest.</u>,
     47:2485-2495.
24. Johnson, P.R., Stern, J.S., Greenwood, M.R.C., and Hirsch, J.
     (1978): <u>Metabolism</u>, 27:1941-1954.
25. Kasubuchi, Y., Mino, M., Yoshioka, H., and Kusunoki, T.(1979):
     <u>J. Nutr. Sci. Vitaminol.</u>, 25:419-426.
26. Keys, A., Brozek, J., Herschel, A., Mickelsen, O., and Taylor,
     H.L.(1950): <u>The Biology of Human Starvation</u>. University of
     Minnesota Press, Minneapolis, Minn.
27. Klyde, B.J., and Hirsch, J.(1979): <u>J. Lipid Res.</u>, 20:691-704.
28. Knittle, J.L. and Hirsch, J.(1968): <u>J. Clin. Invest.</u>,
     47:2091-2098.
29. Knittle, J.L., Timmers, K., Ginsberg-Fellner, F., Brown, R.E.,
     and Katz, D.P.(1979): <u>J. Clin. Invest.</u>, 63:239-246.
30. Kral, J.G.(1976): <u>Am. J. Physiol.</u>, 231:1090-1096.
31. Krotkiewski, M., and Bjorntorp, P.(1976): <u>Acta Physiol. Scand.</u>,
     96:122-127.
32. Krotkiewski, M., Sjostrom, L., Bjorntorp, P., Carlgren, G.,
     Garellick, G., and Smith, U.(1977): <u>Int. J. Obesity</u>, 1:395-416.
33. Leibel, R.L., Berry, E.M., and Hirsch, J.(1982): In: <u>Health and</u>
     <u>Obesity</u>, edited by H.L. Conn, Jr., E.A. DeFelice, and P. Kuo,
     pp.21-48. Raven Press, New York.

34. Lemmonier, D., and Alexiu, A.(1974): In: The Regulation of Adipose Tissue Mass, edited by J. Vague, and J. Boyer, pp.158-173. Excerpta Medica, Amsterdam.
35. Miller, W.H., Jr., and Faust, I.M.(1982): Am. J. Physiol., 242: E93-E96.
36. Miller, W.H., Jr., Goldberger, A.C., and Faust, I.M.(1982): Fed. Proc., 41:714 (abstract).
37. Mrosovsky, N.(1971): Hibernation and the Hypothalamus. Appleton-Century-Crofts, New York.
38. Pitanguy, I.(1977): In: Reconstructive Plastic Surgery, edited by J.M. Converse, pp. 3800-3823. Saunders, Philadelphia.
39. Robelin, J.(1981): J. Lipid Res., 22:452-457.
40. Roncari, D.A.K., and Van, R.L.R.(1978): J. Clin. Invest., 62: 503-508.
41. Salans, L.B., Zarnowski, J.M., and Segal, R.(1972): J. Lipid Res., 13:616-623.
42. Schemmel, R., Mickelson, O., and Gill, J.L.(1970): J. Nutr., 100:1041-1048.
43. Schiele, B.C., and Brozek, J.(1948): Psychosom. Med., 10:31-50.
44. Schneider, B.S., Faust, I.M., Hemmes, R., and Hirsch, J. (1981): Am. J. Physiol., 240:E358-E362.
45. Sclafani, A., and Springer, D.(1976): Physiol. Behav., 17:461-471.
46. Sclafani, A., Aravich, P.F., and Landman, M.(1981): J. Comp. Physiol. Psychol., 95:720-734.
47. Sjostrom, L.(1981): In: Recent Advances in Obesity Research III, edited by P. Bjorntorp, M. Cairella, and A.N. Howard, pp. 85-93. John Libbey, London.
48. Steingrimsdottir, L. Brasel, J., and Greenwood, M.R.C.(1980): Am. J. Physiol., 239:E162-E167.
49. Young, R.A., Salans, L.B., and Sims, E.A.H.(1982): J. Lipid Res., 23: (in press).

The Adipocyte and Obesity: Cellular and Molecular Mechanisms, edited by A. Angel, C. H. Hollenberg, and D. A. K. Roncari. Raven Press, New York © 1983.

Metabolic Characteristics of Murine Adipocyte Precursor Clones

C. Forest, D. Czerucka, P. Grimaldi, C. Vannier, R. Négrel, and G. Ailhaud

Centre de Biochimie, Université de Nice, 06034 Nice, France

The factors which are involved in vivo in the dysregulation of adipose tissue development are largely unknown. In spite of multiple causes leading to obesity (4), it could be hypothesized that some biological signals common to these different situations might be active at the cellular level and might control the proliferation of preadipose cells and their differentiation into adipocytes. In that respect, the isolation of preadipocyte cell strains from adipose tissue (3,16), and the establishment of preadipocyte cell lines from embryonic and adult mouse, have been useful tools with which to study in vitro the process of adipose cell differentiation (1).

Proliferation and differentiation of preadipocyte clonal lines are regulated by extracellular signals (present in the culture medium) and by intracellular signals (1). The characterization and the isolation of external signals rely upon the biological properties of the cell system used. In order to investigate the role of known hormones in adipose conversion, it is equally important that the cell responses occur within the physiological range of hormone concentrations. During the last few years preadipocyte clonal lines from the epididymal fat pad of the genetically-obese adult C 57 BL/6J ob/ob mouse (clone Ob17) and of its lean +/? counterpart (clone HGFu) (9,16) were established in this laboratory.

Among our objectives were i) to establish preadipocyte cell lines from a known tissular origin ii) to control the cell environment in vitro which, in vivo, varies dramatically between genetically-obese and non-obese animals iii) to analyze, on a long-term basis, the effects of known hormones on adipose conversion.

The establishment of Ob17 and HGFu cell lines has allowed us to delineate their metabolic characteristics in response to the long-term action of insulin and triiodothyronine(T3). It has also allowed us to perform a comparative study under identical environmental conditions and to examine the existence of "intrinsic" differences, if any, between cell lines established from genetically-obese and non-obese mice.

MATERIALS AND METHODS

Methods of cell growth, cell numbering and determination of cell protein content were as previously described (16). Briefly, cells were grown in Dulbecco's Modified Eagle's Medium (DMEM) supplemented with 10% Fetal Calf Serum (FCS). At confluence, cells were maintained under standard conditions in DMEM + 10% FCS (standard medium) containing 17 nM insulin, 1.5 nM triiodothyronine, 8 μg.ml^{-1} biotin and 4 μg. ml^{-1} pantothenate. [^{125}I]insulin binding assays were performed as previously described (12). "Crude" membranes of differentiated HGFu and Ob17 cells were used for the [^{3}H] ouabain binding assays whereas intact cells were used for the determinations of [^{86}Rb]uptake (10). The binding of [^{125}I] triiodothyronine was measured after isolation of nuclei from Ob17 and HGFu cells (2) according to a described procedure (11). Biochemical determinations and enzyme assays were identical to those previously reported (11). All determinations were performed on at least duplicate aliquots of the same preparation obtained from two to four pooled dishes. Interassay variability did not differ by more than 10% whereas variability among mean values from three separate dishes never exceeded 20%. The sources of materials have been already given (11).

RESULTS

Main Features of Adipose Conversion of Ob17 Cells

Differentiated Ob17 cells are present in fat cell clusters which are separated by insusceptible cells. Similar observations can be made for HGFu cells. The adipose conversion in both cell lines involves a limited number of cells (< 90%). In Ob17 cells, recent experiments led to the conclusion that the commitment of insusceptible cells to cells susceptible to adipose conversion can occur during the exponential phase of growth in the absence of added insulin. After confluence and a resting period of 1-3 days, only susceptible cells divide for a limited period of time (7-10 days) whether or not insulin is present. These post-confluent mitoses, which are dependent upon an adipose conversion factor(s) (ACF) present in fetal calf serum and in bovine pituitary extract (13), amplify the proportion of adipose cells relative to non-adipose cells, but are not essential for adipose conversion (7). In contrast to ACF, triiodothyronine is essential for adipose conversion of Ob17 cells (13). Insulin at *physiological* concentrations accelerates the rate of adipose conversion (number of lipid-filling cells within a given period of time) but has no effect upon the extent of adipose conversion (maximal number of adipose cells attained within 3-4 weeks after confluence).

Binding Properties of Ob17 and HGFu Cells

Exponentially-growing, as well as resting, Ob17 and HGFu cells possess insulin binding sites. Curvilinear Scatchard plots of insulin binding at equilibrium were obtained and resolved into high affinity-low capacity and low affinity-high capacity binding sites (12 and unpublished). Since both cell lines show a down-regulation of their receptor levels after chronic exposure to insulin, comparisons were made on confluent cells never exposed to the hormone. The number of high-affinity binding sites is 2.7 fold higher in HGFu cells than in Ob17 cells, but the K_d values are very similar (Table 1).

T3 binding sites were compared in Ob17 and HGFu cells since i) an extensive study of Ob17 cells has previously shown the existence in growing and differentiated cells of a single class of high-affinity binding sites (11). The binding studies on isolated nuclei are strongly in favor of nuclear binding sites (2) ii) adipose conversion does *not* occur in the absence of T3 in the culture medium of confluent Ob17 cells.

Comparative data for the binding of T3 on nuclei from confluent Ob17 and HGFu cells are given in Table 1. A low but statistically significant difference is found in the number of $[^{125}I]T3$ binding sites between the two cell lines (4,825+250 sites and 6,038+466 sites per cell of Ob17 and HGFu lines, respectively) whereas the K_d values are very similar in both cases ($< 10^{-10}M$).

The number of $[^3H]$ouabain binding sites on "crude" membrane proteins and the $[^{86}Rb]$uptake on intact cells were also examined under carefully controled conditions. It is known that the (Na^+,K^+)ATPase is inhibited by the cardiac glycoside, ouabain, and that the amount bound correlates directly with the enzyme activity. The potassium uptake was followed by employing $[^{86}Rb]$ as a substitute for K^+.

The maximal values for $[^3H]$ouabain binding sites per cell were found to be 140,000 and 110,000 for Ob17 and HGFu lines respectively, with identical K_d values. In agreement with these data, the ouabain-suppressible component of $[^{86}Rb]$ uptake was slightly lower in HGFu cells than in Ob17 cells (Table 1).

Comparative Time Course of Adipose Conversion of Ob17 and HGFu Cells

As shown in Table 2, considerable changes in activity occur as a function of adipose conversion in both cell lines for lipoprotein lipase, acid:CoA ligase and glycerophosphate dehydrogenase. A large increase in the cellular triglyceride content is also observed. Prior to confluence, with the limited amounts of cell homogenate or cell supernatant available, the activities were below the limits of detection of the different assays. The activity ratios of late confluent cells over early confluent cells vary dramatically. It should be pointed out that significant levels of lipoprotein lipase activity are already present in early confluent HGFu cells as well as in early confluent Ob17 cells (Table 2). In contrast to lipoprotein lipase, the most significant enhancement in the other enzyme activities occurs later during

Table 1 : Binding properties of Ob17 and HGFu cells

PREADIPOCYTE CLONAL LINE	INSULIN BINDING SITES[b]		TRIIODOTHYRONINE BINDING SITES[a,b]		(Na^+,K^+)ATPase[b]		
					[^{3}H]ouabain binding sites		Ouabain-suppressible [^{86}Rb]uptake
	K_d(nM)	Sites/cell	K_d($\times 10^{-10}$M)	Sites/cell	K_d(nM)	Sites/cell	(nmol/min/10^6 cells)
Ob17 (ob/ob mouse)	1.0	7,000	0.8 ±0.12	4,825±250	50	140,000	0.34±0.03
HGFu (+/? mouse)	1.1	19,000	0.69±0.12	6,038±466	50	110,000	0.3 ±0.03

[a]Data from A. Anselmet, J. Gharbi-Chihi, and J. Torresani (2).

[b]Binding of insulin and triiodothyronine, and the uptake of [^{86}Rb], were performed on confluent cells as described in "Materials and Methods". [^{3}H]ouabain binding to crude membrane proteins was determined on 13 day post-confluent cells (50-60% adipose converted cells).

TABLE 2 : Enzyme markers during adipose conversion of Ob17 and HGFu cells

DIFFERENTIATION MARKER	CHANGES IN SPECIFIC ACTIVITY (mU.mg^{-1} of protein) AND IN TRIGLYCERIDE CONTENT (nmol/10^6 CELLS)								ACTIVITY RATIOS OF Late confluent cells / Early confluent cells			
	Ob17				HGFu				Ob17		HGFu	
	Early confluent		Late confluent		Early confluent		Late confluent					
	INS.	INS.+T3	INS.	INS.+T3	INS.	INS.+T3	INS.	INS.+T3	INS.	INS.+T3	INS.	INS.+T3
LIPOPROTEIN LIPASE	1.9	2.4	8.0[a]	11.1[a]	1.8	1.5	9.2	11.3	4.2	4.6	5.1	7.5
ACID:CoA LIGASE	0.2	0.2	23.9[b]	25.7[b]	0.24	0.31	17.6	28.3	120	129	73	91
GLYCEROL-3-P DEHYDROGENASE	und.	und.	1162[b]	1100[b]	und.	und.	1099	1770	–	–	–	–
ACYL CoA: DIGLYCERIDE ACYLTRANSFERASE	0.12	0.18	2.4[b]	3.4[b]	n.d.	n.d.	n.d.	n.d.	20	18.9	n.d.	n.d.
TRIGLYCERIDE CONTENT	50	50	880[b]	1065[b]	22	26	550	886	17.6	21.3	25	34

Ob17 and HGFu cells were grown in standard medium and were shifted at confluence in the same medium containing 17 nM insulin without or with 1.5 nM triiodothyronine. The different parameters in Ob17 cells were determined after confluence at day 1 (early confluent cells) or at day 11 (a) and day 23 (b) (late confluent cells). The determinations for HGFu cells were performed after confluence at day 1 (early confluent cells) and at day 24 (late confluent cells). und., undetectable ; n.d., not determined.

adipose conversion. In addition to insulin, inclusion of triiodothyronine on a long-term basis leads to an increase in the specific activities
of the different enzymes and also to an increase in the cellular
triglyceride content.
     Since differentiation of Ob17 and HGFu cells occurs with the
formation of fat cell clusters separated by undifferentiated cells,
one should keep in mind that the maximal values obtained are dependent
upon the proportion of adipose versus non-adipose cells and upon enzyme
activities (or the triglyceride content) per adipose cell. Since
separate experiments have shown that T3 is not required for post-
confluent mitoses (13), it is most likely that T3 in the above experiments is only active on adipose cells. Moreover, since the proportion
of late confluent differentiated Ob17 and HGFu cells is similar, data
of Table 2 indicate no significant difference in their responsiveness
to optimal concentrations of insulin and T3.

Long-term Effects of Insulin on Adipose Conversion of Ob17 and HGFu Cells

     Chronic exposure of confluent Ob17 and HGFu cells to insu-
lin, in the presence of a maximally effective concentration
of triiodothyronine (1.5 nM), leads to increased activity levels of enzyme markers of adipose conversion and to increased
cellular triglyceride contents (Fig.1 to Fig.3).
Prolonged exposure to concentrations of insulin above 1.7nM
significantly increases the number of Ob17 and HGFu cells
while the mitogenic effect of the hormone is rather weak
within a physiological range of concentrations. In contrast,
supraphysiological concentrations of insulin are highly mitogenic for Ob17 and HGFu cells. In order to assess this
point, DNA synthesis reinitiation experiments were performed
on Ob17 cells which had been previously maintained in serum-
free medium for 24 hours. The results have shown that the
EC50 values for pork insulin and for pork proinsulin are
0.5 μM in each case whereas the EC50 value for IGF-1 is 1nM
(data not shown). Thus, it is likely that the mitogenic effect of insulin is mediated in Ob17 cells by the receptors
of insulin-like growth factors (14).

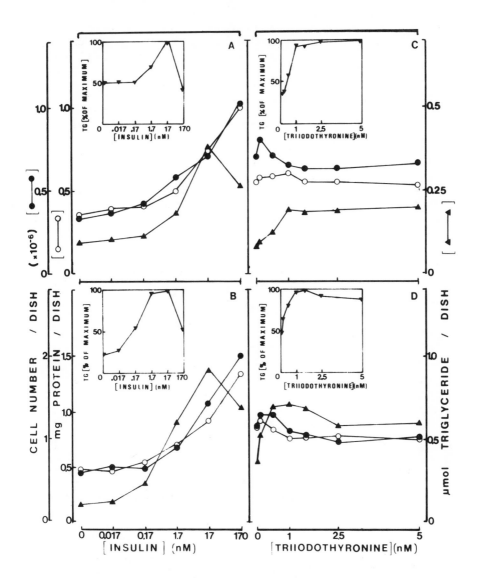

FIG.1 : <u>Changes in cell number and in protein and triglyceride contents during adipose conversion of Ob17 and HGFu cells as a function of insulin and triiodothyronine concentrations</u>

Ob17 (A and C) and HGFu cells (B and D) were grown in standard medium and shifted at confluence to standard medium containing either 1.5nM triiodothyronine and varying concentrations of insulin (A and B) or 17nM insulin and varying concentrations of triiodothyronine (C and D). The different parameters were determined 11 days (C), 15 days (A), 17 days (D), 21 days (B) after confluence (see "Materials and Methods"). Two series of Ob17 cells (A and C) and two series of HGFu cells (B and D) were used. <u>Insets</u> : 100% correspond to 513 (A), 660 (B), 306 (C) and 712 (D) nmol of triglyceride (TG) per 10^6 cells.

The role of insulin as a lipogenic hormone is clearly visible within a physiological range of concentrations. In both cell lines, insulin is already effective at 17 pM and is maximally effective at 17nM. The concentrations of hormone required for half-maximal effects, determined on i) the cellular triglyceride content (Fig.1) ii) the increase in lipoprotein lipase activity (Fig.2) iii) the increase in acid: CoA ligase and glycerophosphate dehydrogenase activities (Fig.3), are between 1 and 2nM. These concentrations are within the K_d values determined for the high-affinity binding sites of insulin on these cells (Table 1). The above experiments strongly suggest that the insulin receptors <u>per se</u> mediate the lipogenic effects of insulin, and that no significant differences in the sensitivity to this hormone on a long-term basis seem to exist between Ob17 and HGFu cells.

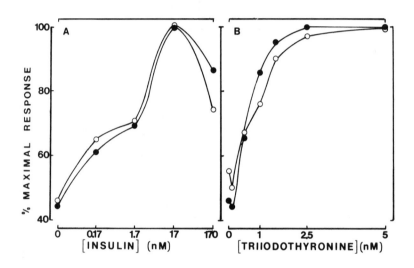

FIG.2 : <u>Long-term effects of insulin (A) and triiodothyronine (B) on lipoprotein lipase activity of Ob17 (●) and HGFu (O) cells</u>
Lipoprotein lipase was determined 11 days (B) and 15 days (A) after confluence, on the same series of cells as described in Fig.1. Values taken as 100% correspond to 6.7 (A) and 7 mU.mg^{-1} (B) for Ob17 cells and to 5.1 (A) and 6.2 mU.mg^{-1} (B) for HGFu cells.

Long-term Effects of Triiodothyronine on Adipose Conversion

In contrast to insulin, triiodothyronine below and above the physiological concentration of 1.5nM (bound plus unbound) is not mitogenic for Ob17 and HGFu cells (Fig.1). The maximally effective concentration of T3 for triglyceride accumulation is found to be 1.5nM (Fig.1).

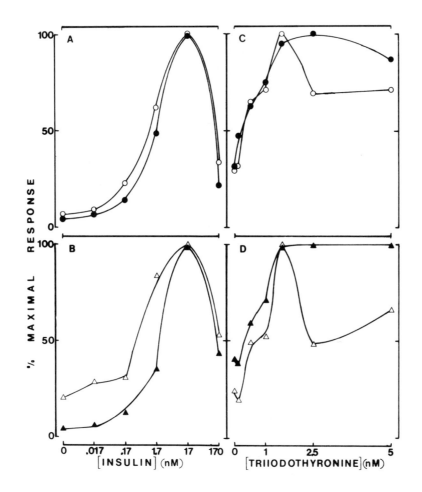

FIG.3 : Long-term effects of insulin (A and B) and triiodothyronine (C and D) on the glycerophosphate dehydrogenase and acid:CoA ligase activities of Ob17 and HGFu cells
Glycerophosphate dehydrogenase ($\bullet$,$\circ$) and acid:CoA ligase ($\blacktriangle$,$\triangle$) activities were determined at day 11 (C and D) and at day 15 (A and B) in Ob17 cells ($\bullet$,$\blacktriangle$) and HGFu cells ($\circ$,$\triangle$). The four series of cells were identical to those of Fig.1. Values taken as 100% correspond for acid:CoA ligase at day 11 to 14.4 (Ob17) and 8.8 mU.mg^{-1} (HGFu) and at day 15 to 10.5 (Ob17) and 3.6 mU.mg^{-1} (HGFu). The corresponding figures for glycerophosphate dehydrogenase were 605, 649, 1040 and 380 mU.mg^{-1} respectively.

After prolonged exposure to varying concentrations of T3 in
the presence of 17nM insulin, dose-dependent curves are obtained for the activities of the different enzyme markers
(Figs. 2 and 3). The maximal effects are again observed at
1.5nM T3 for both Ob17 and HGFu cells. Half-maximal effects
of T3 are observed at a concentration around 0.5nM for both
cell lines, which is in agreement with the expected concentration of unbound (active T3) and with K_d values for the
nuclear receptors of triiodothyronine characterized on Ob17
and HGFu cells (Table 1).

DISCUSSION

The clonal Ob17 and HGFu cell lines exhibit after differentiation both morphological and biochemical properties characteristic of mature adipocytes. Differentiated Ob17 cells
accumulate triglycerides and contain high activity levels of
enzymes required for the triglyceride assimilation, i.e. lipoprotein and monoglyceride lipases (15), as well as the full
enzyme equipment necessary for the mobilization of intracellular triglycerides, which includes the hormone-sensitive lipase (J. Khoo, personal communication). Similarly differentiated HGFu cells contain lipoprotein and monoglyceride lipases and are capable to respond to lipolytic hormones with release of unesterified fatty acids. The sensitivity to a pure
β-agonist (isoproterenol) was found to be similar in Ob17 and
HGFu cell lines (8,9).
   Regarding the expression of the differentiation program,
it is of interest that lipoprotein lipase emerges rather early as compared to acid:CoA ligase and glycerophosphate dehydrogenase, and is found to be present in cells *before* any
triglyceride accumulation. These observations would suggest
that better estimates of the adipose tissue cellularity during development in rodents should be obtained by determining
the lipoprotein lipase-containing cells rather than the tri-
glyceride-filled cells. In support of this proposal is the
fact that lipoprotein lipase-containing cells can be directly
detected by indirect immunofluorescence and that changes in
lipoprotein lipase activity are directly correlated with
changes in enzyme content (17).
   It must be stressed that both Ob17 and HGFu cells respond
on a long-term basis to *physiological* concentrations of insulin and triiodothyronine. The EC50 values found for each
hormone regarding the enhancement of the activity levels of
enzyme markers and of the triglyceride content per cell are
in agreement with the affinities for their respective receptors. Therefore both cell lines i) fail to show any significant difference regarding post-receptor events ii) represent
useful tools to study at the molecular level the mechanisms
of action of insulin and triiodothyronine on adipose conversion.
   The availability of established cell lines from genetically-obese and non-obese mice has allowed us to carry out a
comparative study. The differences observed between Ob17
and HGFu cells in the number of insulin and triiodothyronine
receptors are not "translated" into differences in their li-

pogenic responses.

The levels of (Na^+,K^+)ATPase were examined in both cell lines in spite of the controversy regarding the contribution of the sodium pump in energy expenditure (5). The reduction of the number of Na^+,K^+-pump units in the genetically-obese mouse has been proposed as a primary defect in the development of obesity (4). Our data show that no significant differences (in favor of the HGFu cell line) are found in the number of [^{3}H]ouabain binding sites and in the rate of the ouabain-suppressible [^{86}Rb] uptake. These results are in agreement with recent data obtained in vivo on genetically-obese and lean C57 BL/6J mice (6).

In conclusion our data would indicate that, despite some "intrinsic" differences regarding the levels of insulin and triiodothyronine receptors, the metabolic characteristics of Ob17 and HGFu cells are not in favor of an "innate" increased sensitivity or responsiveness of Ob17 cells to both hormones. Thus, it is tempting to postulate that the numerous differences in the metabolic properties of adipose tissue, or of isolated adipocytes, observed between the ob/ob mouse and its lean counterpart, should be mainly a reflection of environmental conditions occurring in vivo.

ACKNOWLEDGEMENTS

This work was supported by the "Centre National de la Recherche Scientifique", by the "Délégation Générale à la Recherche Scientifique et Technique" (Grant n° 4162) and by the "Fondation pour la Recherche Médicale". Thanks are due to A. Anselmet et al. (2) for sending us their manuscript prior to publication. IGF-1 was a kind gift from Dr. R. Humbel (Zürick - Switzerland).

REFERENCES

1. Ailhaud,G. (1982): Mol.Cell.Biochem., in press.
2. Anselmet, A., Gharbi-Chihi, J., and Torresani, J. (1982), submitted.
3. Björntorp, P., Sjöström, L., and Smith, U. (1978): J. Lipid Res. 19:316-324.
4. Bray, G.A., York, D.A.(1979): Physiol.Reviews 59:719-809.
5. Clark, D.G., Brinkman, M., Filsell, O.H., Lewis, S.J., and Berry, M.N. (1982): Biochem.J. 202:661-665.
6. Clausen, T., and Hansen, O. (1982): Biochem.Biophys.Res. Commun. 104:357-362.
7. Djian, P., Grimaldi, P., Négrel, R., and Ailhaud, G. (1982), Exp.Cell Res., in press.
8. Forest, C., Négrel, R., and Ailhaud, G. (1981): Biochem. Biophys.Res.Commun. 102:577-587.
9. Forest, C., Grimaldi, P., Czerucka, D., Négrel, R., and Ailhaud, G. (1982), submitted.
10. Forest, C., Ponzio, G., Rossi, B., Lazdunski, M., and Ailhaud, G. (1982), Biochem.Biophys.Res.Commun., in press.

11. Gharbi-Chihi, J., Grimaldi, P., Torresani, J., and Ailhaud, G. (1981): J.Receptor Res. 2:153-173.
12. Grimaldi, P., Négrel, R., Vincent, J.P., and Ailhaud, G. (1979): J.Biol.Chem. 254:6849-6852.
13. Grimaldi, P., Djian, P., Négrel, R., and Ailhaud, G. (1982), EMBO Journal, in press.
14. King, G.L., Kahn, C.R., Rechler, M.M., and Nissley, S.P. (1980): J.Clin.Invest. 66:130-140.
15. Murphy, M., Négrel, R., and Ailhaud, G. (1981): Biochim. Biophys. Acta 664:240-248.
16. Négrel, R., Grimaldi, P., and Ailhaud, G. (1978): Proc. Natl.Acad.Sci.USA 75:6054-6058.
17. Vannier, C., Jansen, H., Négrel, R., and Ailhaud, G. (1982), submitted.

The Adipocyte and Obesity: Cellular and Molecular Mechanisms, edited by A. Angel, C. H. Hollenberg, and D. A. K. Roncari. Raven Press, New York © 1983.

Culture and Cloning of Adipocyte Precursors from Lean and Obese Subjects: Effects of Growth Factors

D. A. K. Roncari, D. C. W. Lau, Ph. Djian, S. Kindler, and D. K. Yip

Institute of Medical Science and Department of Medicine, University of Toronto, Toronto, M5S 1A8 Canada

The cell biology of adipocyte lineages and the factors controlling the development and turnover of fat cells have been recent foci of intense interest and investigation. Impetus for this research sprang from the development of methods for in vivo labelling of adipocytes and their precursors by injecting animals with radioactive thymidine (1), and by the elaboration of cell culture systems for adipocyte precursors, first reported for those of human origin (3,4, 10,11).

In this paper, we will describe methods enabling colony formation from single adipocyte progenitors; these approaches, which are based on principles of clonality, are enabling the elucidation of distinct stages of adipocyte lineages, encompassing the spectrum from stem cells to differentiated adipocytes. These methods are also enabling the isolation and characterization of determination and commitment factors in the differentiative program. We will also present further studies on the mitogenic effect of pituitary fibroblast growth factor (FGF), and on the more elaborate purification of pituitary "adipocyte growth factors". In the last section, we will describe an extension of our investigations indicating that adipocyte precursors from massively obese persons proliferate excessively in culture; we will also contrast differing clones of these cells.

METHODS

Source and Culture of Adipocyte Precursors

All subjects, whose adipose tissue was obtained at elective surgery, were older than 20 years. The 110 massively obese subjects exceeded by more than 70% the desirable values for body weight, as specified by the Metropolitan Life Insurance Company Tables. The range of excess weight was 72-269%, with a mean of 127% (could also be expressed as a mean 227% of desirable body weight). The age range of the 110 massively obese subjects was 21-62, with a

mean of 38 years; 72% were women. The age and gender dis-
tributions were similar for the 36 lean subjects, who were
within 15% of desirable body weight.
  Isolation as well as primary and secondary culture of
adipocyte precursors were conducted by reported methods (5,
10,11). Cell counting and sizing by Coulter systems, and
quantification of radioactive thymidine incorporation into
DNA were also carried out at reported (5,7,10,11). In most
cases, omental adipose tissue was the source of precursors.
In some instances, which will be indicated, abdominal subcutaneous fat tissue was used.

Colony formation and cloning

  In the case of primary culture, fresh adipose tissue was
completely disaggregated into single cells with a collagenase preparation, the stromal-vascular cells were harvested
by gentle centrifugation, and plated on flasks containing
alpha medium supplemented with 10% fetal calf serum. Twelve
hours later, the adherent cells were detached with trypsin-
Na$_2$EDTA. They were then plated, at an inoculum size of 50-
100 cells per 100-mm culture dish (or 15-60 cells per 35-mm
dish), and grown in alpha medium supplemented with 10% fetal
calf serum and "conditioned medium" or "feeder layers". To
prepare "conditioned medium", fresh pieces (about 100 mg) of
omental adipose tissue were incubated in alpha medium for 4
days. Cell-free "conditioned medium" was then obtained by
centrifugation and passage through 0.25 µm Millipore
filters. "Feeder layers" were prepared by irradiating fresh
pieces of adipose tissue with 2000 rads. For cloning of
adipocyte precursors from massively obese persons, irra-
diated precursors from the same subject, were used as
"feeder cells".
  After 12-15 days of culture in alpha medium supplemented
with 10% fetal calf serum and "conditioned medium" or
"feeder layers" (or growth factor added at 4 days in primary
culture), the cells, which constituted colonies of varying
size, were either fixed and stained, or colonies were isolated with "cloning cylinders", and subculture was carried
out to obtain relatively large quantities of cloned cells.
  Similar procedures were used for colony formation and
cloning, starting with adipocyte precursors in secondary
culture.

Purification and initial characterization of pituitary "adipocyte growth factors"

  The initial purification steps of bovine anterior pituitary "adipocyte growth factors" were similar to those
already described for bovine pituitary fibroblast growth
factor (9). Briefly, the homogenizing solution included
0.25 mM phenylmethylsulfonylfluoride and 0.4 mg/l each of
leupeptin and pepstatin A. After ammonium sulfate fractionation, serial carboxymethyl-Sephadex and Sephacryl S-200
steps were implemented. Further procedures for the

purification of "adipocyte growth factors" will be reported elsewhere; they include chromatofocusing as well as analytical and preparative polyacrylamide gel electrophoresis in sodium dodecyl sulfate.

The growth factors were assayed for their influence on the number of human (and rat) adipocyte precursors and on the incorporation of radioactive thymidine into DNA. For the latter assay, the precursors were grown in alpha medium supplemented with 20% fetal calf serum for 18 hours. Medium H199 was then substituted and the serum concentration decreased to 0.5%. Under these conditions, the cells are quiescent but viable. Eighteen hours later, putative mitogenic fractions were added and incubation was carried out for 16 more hours. Finally, [^{3}H]thymidine (sp. radioact. 70 Ci/mmole, 7.5 μCi/5 ml flask) was added and cell culture was continued for an additional 24 hours. The incorporation of radioactive thymidine into DNA and cell counts were then quantified as reported (7).

RESULTS AND DISCUSSION

Colony Formation and Cloning

When the growth medium is supplemented not only with fetal calf serum, but also with "conditioned medium" or "feeder layers", colonies form readily from cells in either primary or secondary culture (Fig. 1). When alpha medium is supplemented with serum only, the cloning efficiency is 0.5%. Upon addition of either "conditioned medium" or "feeder layers", the cloning efficiency increases to about 40%, and the colonies are larger, but still vary from about 200 to 8000 cells, most around 5000 cells (Fig. 1).

Under the conditions of medium enrichment that have been reported (4,11), and which include a higher concentration of fetal calf serum and the presence of methylcellulose, most cells in almost all colonies mature into adipocytes. Rather uniform differentiation occurs not only in secondary culture, but also in primary culture, under conditions in which each colony should be derived from a single cell present in the stromal fraction of adipose tissue both in vivo and ex vivo. These findings suggest that most of the "fibroblastoid cells" present in fat tissue are adipocyte precursors. This occurrence would represent an example of organ and regional specialization of a mesenchymal cell type. Thus, adipose depots would contain stromal cells that are similar to skin fibroblasts, but, in contrast to fibroblasts, would all share the unique potential property of differentiation into adipocytes. With regard to nomenclature, it is of course most probably that different stages of differentiation exist in a spectrum encompassing pluripotent stem cells and mature adipocytes. However, pending proper identification and characterization of each stage, the collective term "adipocyte precursors" is still most accurate in describing all the cells that are capable of differentiation into mature fat cells.

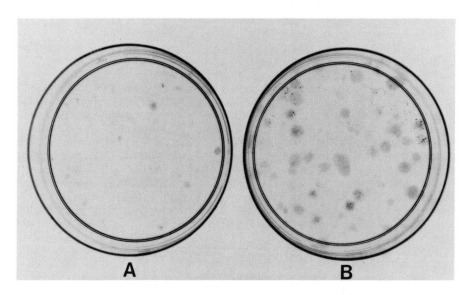

FIG. 1. Formation of colonies consisting of human omental
adipocyte precursors in the absence (A) or presence of
"conditioned medium" (B). The colonies were at two weeks
in primary culture. The "conditioned medium" was obtained
by incubation with pieces of human adipose tissue.

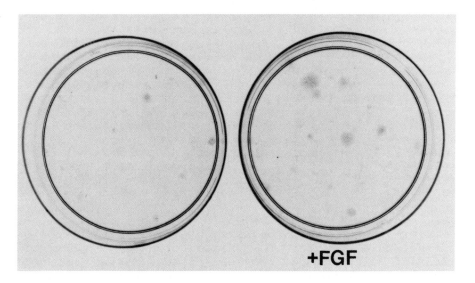

FIG. 2. Formation of human omental adipocyte precursor
colonies in the absence and presence of bovine pituitary
fibroblast growth factor (50 ng/ml growth medium). The
colonies were at two weeks in primary culture. "Conditioned
medium" was not present.

Purification and initial characterization of pituitary adipocyte growth factors

As we reported previously, pituitary fibroblast growth factor promotes the replication of adipocyte precursors (8). In addition to its mitogenic influence on cells grown in secondary culture, FGF stimulates the multiplication of precursors present in the stromal fraction of adipose tissue. When these cells were isolated and grown in primary culture as described, the resulting colonies were much larger when the growth medium was supplemented with FGF (Fig. 2). These findings indicate and confirm the mitogenic effect of this pituitary polypeptide on human adipocyte precursors. The increase in cell number is not significantly different from that observed with skin fibroblasts.

Pituitary polypeptides distinct from fibroblast growth factor promote the replication of adipocyte precursors (6,8). These anterior pituitary principles, which we have termed "adipocyte growth factors" have now been purified to a high degree. They are relatively stable to sodium or lithium dodecyl sulfate, and to mild acidic or alkaline conditions, properties facilitating their purification. At least some of these factors are selectively more potent on adipocyte precursors than on skin fibroblasts, i.e., the mitogenic effect per mg of protein is significantly higher. In view of the similarities between skin fibroblasts and adipocyte precursors during early differentiation, the relative selectivity of these pituitary factors is notable. The adipocyte growth factors are a series of both acidic and basic polypeptides ranging in isoelectric point between 4 and 10, and in molecular weight between 8,200 and 55,000 daltons. The complete purification of some of these polypeptides will be described elsewhere.

The putative physiologic role of "adipocyte growth factors" requires proof in vivo. In the meantime, we propose that this family of anterior pituitary polypeptides, possibly in concert with fibroblast growth factors, regulates in complementary fashion the growth of adipose tissue.

Adipocyte precursors from lean and massively obese persons

Adipocyte precursors from most massively obese persons replicate in culture to an excessive degree. The current

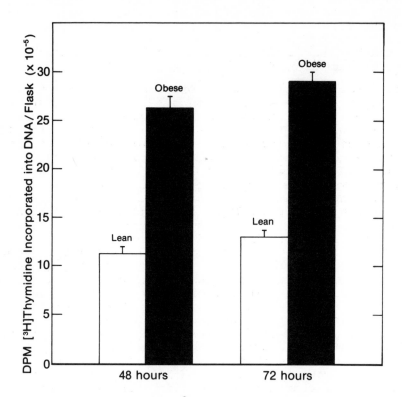

FIG. 3. Incorporation of [³H]thymidine into trichloroacetic acid-insoluble macromolecules, by adipocyte precursors (in second subculture) from lean and massively obese subjects. Mean±SEM.

studies of 110 massively obese subjects extends and confirms our previous report on 34 patients (7). As shown in Fig. 3, cultured omental adipocyte precursors from the massively obese incorporated radioactive thymidine into DNA to a significantly greater (p<0.001) extent than cells from lean persons. Direct cell counting confirmed the fact that these findings indicate excessive proliferation. Abdominal subcutaneous adipocyte precursors also multiply to a greater extent when compared to corresponding cells from the lean; however, the difference was less pronounced than that observed for omental precursors. As reported, precursors from most moderately obese subjects have similar replicative indices as those from the lean (7). Within the polyclonal mixture of precursors within adipose tissue of the massively obese, an in vivo and in culture selection of a rapidly dividing population of cells might be occurring.

Exaggerated replication of adipocyte precursors from the massively obese persists in successive subcultures, cells during the first five passages having been studied to date. Similar degrees of excessive proliferation, moreover, are still observed in precursors from persons whose massive obesity has been corrected. Of possibly major prospective significance, a few young adults who were moderately obese, but had a family history of massive corpulence, had adipocyte precursors that replicate excessively in successive subcultures; it may be relevant that massive obesity developed after age 18 in about one-third. In secondary culture, cells are of course removed from such in vivo influences as circulating growth factors, which might be present at elevated levels in some obese persons. These lines of evidence suggest that the exaggerated proliferation in vitro of adipocyte precursors from massively corpulent persons, reveals the presence of a primary, genetic abnormality in this subset of the obese population. We are currently investigating whether factors produced within adipose tissue mediate the inordinate proliferation of precursors in massive obesity by paracrine or autocrine mechanisms.

The exaggerated replication of adipocyte precursors probably accounts, at least partly, for the excessive total number of mature fat cells characteristic of massive obesity. One must consider that the adipocyte hyperplasia is probably not causally related to massive obesity, but might be associated with such a fundamental, but as yet unproven abnormality as excessive conservation of energy.

Clones of adipocyte precursors from massively obese subjects

After developing colonies in primary culture under clonal conditions, clones of human adipocyte precursors were propagated in secondary culture, as described. Like their parent cells, clones of precursors from the massively obese replicate excessively in vitro (2). As shown in Fig. 4, some of these clones revealed "spontaneous" differentiation in culture, i.e., without the need to enrich the growth medium with the supplements generally required for complete maturation (2). It is of potentially profound significance that clones derived from the same person, differed in their potential to undergo "spontaneous" differentiation in culture (Fig. 4). "Spontaneous" differentiation was indicated by the marked triglyceride accretion that was evident upon microscopic inspection of living cells (Fig. 4) and upon staining with Oil-Red-O. Biochemical characterization of adipocyte precursor clones from massively obese as compared to those from lean subjects, is in progress. Preliminary findings, at equivalent stages in subculture,

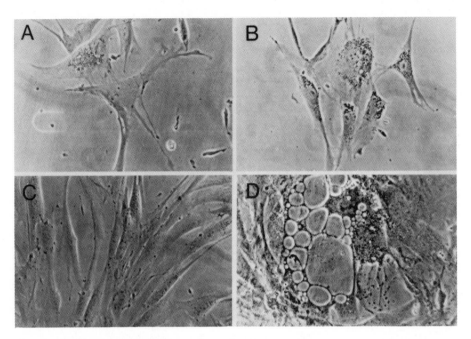

FIG. 4. Clones of omental adipocyte precursors from one
massively obese person. The panel on the reader's left
shows a clone on day 4 (Panel A) and day 14 (Panel C) of
culture. The panel on the reader's right shows another
clone, grown under identical conditions, on day 4 (Panel B)
and day 14 (Panel D) of culture. Original magnification
x 400.

suggest higher rates per mg protein of enzymes catalyzing
fatty acid and triglyceride synthesis in some clones of
precursors from the massively obese.

The pathophysiologic significance of "spontaneous" differentiation in culture of some clones of adipocyte precursors from massively corpulent subjects, is unknown. One
hypothesis to be tested is that it reflects the selection of
mutant clones that in vivo not only proliferate excessively,
but also have a special proclivity to differentiate into
mature adipocytes.

One of our major interests is the elucidation of abnormalities, at the level of the gene, that might, when coupled
to appropriate environmental conditions, lead to excessive
adipocyte precursor proliferation, and possibly to their
inordinate degree of differentiation.

ACKNOWLEDGMENTS

This work is supported by the Medical Research Council of Canada (MT-5827) and the Ontario Heart Foundation (T1-46). D.C.W.L. is a Centennial Fellow of the Medical Research Council of Canada. Ph.D. was a Fellow of the Banting and Best Diabetes Centre, University of Toronto.

REFERENCES

1. Hollenberg, C.H., and Vost, A. (1968): J. Clin. Invest., 47:2485-2498.

2. Lau, D.C.W., and Roncari, D.A.K. (1981): Clin. Invest. Med., 4:32B (Abstract).

3. Poznanski, W.J., Waheed, I., and Van, R. (1973): Lab. Invest., 29:570-576.

4. Roncari, D.A.K., and Van, R.L.R. (1978): Clin. Invest. Med., 1:71-79.

5. Roncari, D.A.K., and Van, R.L.R. (1978): J. Clin. Invest. 62:503-508.

6. Roncari, D.A.K. (1979): In: Systematic Endocrinology, edited by C. Ezrin, J.O. Godden, and R. Volpé, pp. 458-490. Harper and Row, Publishers, Hagerstown, MD.

7. Roncari, D.A.K., Lau, D.C.W., and Kindler S. (1981): Metabolism, 30:425-427.

8. Roncari, D.A.K. (1981): Int. J. Obesity, 5:547-552.

9. Thomas, K.A., Riley, M.C., Lemmon, S.K., Baglan, N.C., and Bradshaw, R.A. (1980): J. Biol. Chem., 255:5517-5520.

10. Van, R.L.R., Bayliss, C.E., and Roncari D.A.K. (1976): J. Clin. Invest., 58:699-704.

11. Van, R.L.R., and Roncari, D.A.K. (1978): Cell Tiss. Res., 195:317-329.

The Adipocyte and Obesity: Cellular and Molecular Mechanisms, edited by A. Angel, C. H. Hollenberg, and D. A. K. Roncari. Raven Press, New York © 1983.

Insulin Action Mediated by Plasma Membrane Components

L. Jarett, F. L. Kiechle, J. C. Parker, and S. L. Macaulay

Department of Pathology and Laboratory Medicine, University of Pennsylvania School of Medicine, Philadelphia, Pennsylvania 19104

Despite intensive investigation since the discovery of insulin 50 years ago, the immediate events following the binding of insulin to its receptor have remained obscure. The events that ultimately result in the alteration of various membrane and intracellular metabolic pathways must be initiated within the plasma membrane. Our laboratory developed a preparation of rat adipocyte plasma membranes which retained the components and organization necessary to respond to insulin. The data generated using this preparation suggested that the interaction of insulin with its receptor leads to the generation of a new family of mediators or second messengers from the plasma membrane. These messengers may mediate at least some of the short-term intracellular effects of the hormone on metabolic pathways.

SUBCELLULAR SYSTEMS

A highly enriched preparation of adipocyte plasma membranes (38,14) was originally used by Jarett and Smith (19) to demonstrate that the addition of concanavalin A or of physiological concentrations of insulin rapidly increased the hydrolysis of ATP. A slight modification (36) of this membrane preparation was used by Seals, McDonald and Jarett (53-55). These studies demonstrated that the addition of physiological concentrations of insulin to plasma membranes generated a material which activated mitochondrial pyruvate dehydrogenase. The addition of insulin to the plasma membrane preparation decreased phosphorylation of two phosphoproteins of molecular weight 120,000 and 42,000 daltons (53). The first phosphoprotein has yet to be identified. The second phosphoprotein proved to be the alpha subunit of pyruvate dehydrogenase, present as a result of mitochondrial contamination of the plasma membrane preparation (54,55). The addition of

purified mitochondria to the plasma membrane preparation in the presence of insulin decreased the phosphorylation of the alpha subunit
associated with stimulation of pyruvate dehydrogenase activity (52).
Concanavalin A and anti-insulin-receptor antibody also stimulated the
enzyme. All three ligands affected the enzyme only when plasma membranes were present. Thus, a mediator which was not a fragment of the
insulin molecule was generated from the plasma membrane.

Kiechle et al. (23) and Seals and Czech (49) further characterized
the material which was generated from adipocyte plasma membranes.
This material, released from the membranes, was obtained by treating
the plasma membranes with insulin for short time periods. The membranes were sedimented by centrifugation and the supernatant retained.
This supernatant material was characterized by assaying its ability to
stimulate pyruvate dehydrogenase in isolated mitochondria. Supernatant material from insulin-treated membranes stimulated pyruvate dehydrogenase more than supernatant from control membranes. The material
generated was acid stable and had a molecular weight of less than 3000
as estimated by Sephadex G-25 gel filtration. Repeated washing of the
membrane preparation depleted the membranes of mediator. Saltiel et
al. (47) demonstrated that a mediator of similar molecular weight can
be generated in a insulin-sensitive manner from liver plasma
membranes.

INTACT TISSUE STUDY

Any substance proposed to fulfill the role of an intracellular
mediator of insulin action must have a ubiquitous distribution.
Furthermore, the amount or activity of the material must be altered by
insulin in a manner consistent with the known effects of insulin on
that cell type. The following summarizes studies which have tested
these criteria.

Larner et al. (28) showed that insulin increased the activity or
quantity of a low molecular weight (1000-1500), acid stable material
from rabbit skeletal muscle assessed by increased activity of glycogen
synthase. This material also activated pyruvate dehydrogenase in
adipocyte mitochondria (18). Kiechle et al. (22) showed that insulin
treatment of rat adipocytes increased the amount or activity of a
similar acid stable, low molecular weight material as estimated by its
ability to stimulate pyruvate dehydrogenase. A similar material has
been generated in an insulin-sensitive manner from a hepatoma cell
line (H4-II-E-C3') (43). The material has also been found in extracts
of IM-9 lymphocytes. However, in contrast to the other tissues
tested, the IM-9 lymphocytes responded to insulin stimulation with a
reduction in the amount or activity of the material which was
generated (16). These results are consistent with evidence that these
cells bind insulin but have no biological response to insulin.

INSULIN-SENSITIVE ENZYME STUDIES

The proposal that the low molecular weight acid stable material
from various cell types functions as an intracellular messenger or

mediator of insulin action would be further substantiated if it were shown that it acts on various insulin-sensitive enzyme systems. Larner et al. (28) showed that the mediator from skeletal muscle activated glycogen synthase by inhibiting cyclic AMP dependent protein kinase and stimulating phosphoprotein phosphatase. This laboratory has used pyruvate dehydrogenase as the major biological assay for the mediator. The mechanism by which pyruvate dehydrogenase activity is regulated has been established (5). A series of studies by this laboratory was performed using the subcellular system of isolated mitochondria and plasma membranes (45), the partially purified mediator from adipocytes (22), muscle (18), hepatoma cells (43), adipocyte plasma membranes (23) and liver plasma membranes (15) to determine the mechanism by which the mediator activates pyruvate dehydrogenase. Each of these studies indicated that the increase in pyruvate dehydrogenase activity was attributable to activation of the pyruvate dehydrogenase phosphatase rather than to any alteration of the pyruvate dehydrogenase kinase, a cyclic AMP independent kinase. These studies have been reviewed recently (17). The mediator released from adipocyte plasma membranes, as well as that isolated from hepatoma cells, stimulated pyruvate dehydrogenase activity in mitochondria which demonstrated respiratory control and were morphologically intact (Parker, Kiechle and Jarett, unpublished observations).

The low Km cyclic AMP phosphodiesterase present in the microsomal fractions of hepatocytes (30) and adipocytes (31,33) is stimulated by insulin-treatment. Kiechle and Jarett (21) demonstrated that the mediator from adipocytes and adipocyte plasma membranes activated this microsomal enzyme when added directly to microsomal preparations. Parker et al. (43) showed a similar increase in adipocyte low Km cyclic AMP phosphodiesterase activity using mediator from hepatoma cells. The mediator from insulin-treated sources always stimulated the low Km cyclic AMP phosphodiesterase more than that from untreated sources. The mediator derived from various sources had no effect on adipocyte high Km cyclic AMP phosphodiesterase activity. This finding is consistent with the insulin insensitivity of this enzyme in intact cellular systems (33). McDonald et al. (37) reported that the mediator from adipocyte plasma membranes stimulated $[Ca^{++} - Mg^{++}]$ -ATPase activity and the Ca^{++} transport system of adipocyte plasma membranes.

EVIDENCE FOR A FAMILY OF MEDIATORS

Several direct and indirect lines of evidence are consistent with the proposal that the interaction of insulin with the plasma membrane generates more than one mediator. One explanation for the biphasic response of some tissues to insulin is that more than one mediator was being produced in response to insulin treatment. In these tissues increasing the concentration of insulin increased the amount of mediator generated to a maximum level. Higher insulin concentrations reduced the amount of mediator to control levels. A biphasic response to insulin was first described by Turakulov et al. (60) using an extract prepared from the cytosol of liver from insulin-treated and control rats. The response was assessed using Ca^{++} uptake by mitochondria. Larner et al. (28) showed that the mediator from muscle of insulin-treated rabbits stimulated glycogen synthase phosphatase in a biphasic manner. Seals and Jarett (52) reported that the direct addition of insulin, concanavalin A or anti-insulin receptor antibody to the adipocyte subcellular system composed of mitochondria and plasma membranes also produced this biphasic response curve as determined by activation of pyruvate dehydrogenase. Subsequently, Seals and Czech (50) demonstrated that the supernatant prepared from adipocyte plasma membranes incubated with increasing insulin concentrations produced a biphasic stimulation of pyruvate dehydrogenase when added to isolated mitochondria. Saltiel et al. (47,48) demonstrated the same phenomenon with liver membranes using adenylate cyclase and pyruvate dehydrogenase as assays for mediator activity.

Two studies have used chemical methods to demonstrate that at least two mediators exist. Chen et al. (3) have separated the skeletal muscle mediator into two fractions by electrophoresis. One increased the cyclic AMP dependent protein kinase and inhibited the glycogen synthase phosphoprotein phosphatase, while the other fraction inhibited the kinase and increased the phosphatase activity. Saltiel et al. (48) used ethanol extraction to separate the mediator obtained from liver membranes into two fractions. One fraction activated pyruvate dehydrogenase while the other inhibited that enzyme and adenylate cyclase. In view of these findings it is possible that insulin treatment of IM-9 lymphocytes stimulated generation of a mediator which inhibits pyruvate dehydrogenase. The studies with hepatoma cells were consistent with the proposal that insulin caused the generation of only the activating substance but not of the inhibitory substance in these cells. The inhibitory substance may be derived from the activating substance or they may be formed by independent pathways.

Other membrane signalling systems have been shown to generate mediators which appear to be similar to the insulin mediator. Beachy et al. (2) reported that the interaction of lectins with lymphocyte plasma membranes activated lymphocyte mitochondrial pyruvate dehydrogenase. Teyssot et al. (58,59) demonstrated that the addition of prolactin or insulin to membranes from lactating rabbit mammary tissue resulted in the production of a low molecular weight material. This mediator induced the transcription of the beta casein genes in mammary gland nuclei. A growth hormone fragment with insulin-like properties generated from liver plasma membranes an acid stable material of molecular weight less than 2000 (11,41). This mediator activated pyruvate dehydrogenase and acetyl CoA carboxylase. In contrast, when added to liver plasma membranes, a fragment of growth hormone with insulin-antagonistic activity produced a mediator that inhibited pyruvate dehydrogenase and acetyl CoA carboxylase. These studies suggest that this apparently new family of mediators may have a broad and significant role in biological processes which could help explain the mechanisms of action of many other hormones and factors whose mechanisms remain to be elucidated.

CHARACTERISTICS AND CHEMICAL NATURE OF THE MEDIATORS

Mediators isolated from various tissue sources have several common characteristics. The molecular weight of the material from adipocytes (22), skeletal muscle (28), liver plasma membranes (15,47), adipocyte plasma membranes (23), IM-9 lymphocytes (16), and hepatoma cells (43) appears to be between 1000 and 3000 on the basis of gel filtration chromatography. The estimate of the molecular weight was found to be dependent on the buffer used (43). The material from all sources seemed to be acid-stable and when determined, was found to have an isoelectric point of approximately pH 4.5 to 5. The mediator from adipocyte plasma membranes (50) and from hepatoma cells (43) has been shown to adsorb to anion exchange resin (Dowex AG1X8) and to elute at high salt concentrations.

The chemical structures of the mediators of insulin action are unknown at present. However, since the mediators can be derived from plasma membranes of both adipocyte and liver, they must be derived from membrane components. These components and some of their derivatives include proteins, glycoproteins, carbohydrates, phospholipids, fatty acids, lipopeptides, prostaglandins, and leukotrienes.

Initial studies suggested that the mediator was a peptide. This postulate was based on the observations that the mediator purified with a peak of absorbance at 230 nm and ninhydrin positivity (3,28). Our laboratory reported (22,23) that there was no correlation between the activity of the mediator and the amount of absorbance at 230 nm. This finding may be attributable to the impure nature of the material. Seals and Czech (49) used proteases, protease inhibitors and synthetic analogs as substrates for proteases to study the generation of the mediators from adipocyte plasma membranes. They interpreted their data to suggest that the material was a peptide. Their further studies demonstrated that the material was not generated by intact adipocytes in the presence of protease inhibitors and, therefore, must be generated by proteolytic action (51). Larner and coworkers (25,27) concluded that the mediator was generated by a proteolytic process. This conclusion was drawn from studies using trypsin and various protease inhibitors. However, there are other possible interpretations of these data. Recently DeHaen and colleagues (40) have shown that the effects of most proteolytic inhibitors of insulin action in fat cells can be attributed to the non-protease inhibitory properties of these inhibitors. Our laboratory has been unable to confirm that peptide bonds are a structural component necessary for the biological activity of the mediator. We have incubated the insulin mediator derived from adipocytes and from hepatoma cells from 1-24 hours with non-specific and specific proteolytic enzymes bound to Sepharose. When the bound enzymes were separated and the material was reassayed, little, if any, loss of activity was detected. Furthermore, dansylation had little or no effect on the activity of the mediator. In our laboratory the mediator, both in thin layer chromatographic and in high pressure liquid chromatographic systems, did not behave in a manner consistent with a simple peptide (Macaulay, Kiechle and Jarett, unpublished observations).

Larner et al. (27) have proposed a model which suggests that the proteolytic activity which generates the insulin mediators acts on the outside of the plasma membrane forming an oligoglycopeptide. They have proposed a model for internalizing this oligoglycopeptide which is based on the work of Cullis et al. (4). We, however, have been unable to establish that common sugar or aminosugar residues are structural components necessary for the biological activity of the mediator. In our hands, the mediator did not bind to any immobilized lectin-Sepharose column tested.

Our inability to implicate simple peptides and glycopeptides as a part of the mediator led us to consider phospholipids, their derivatives, or metabolites as potential mediators. The possible role of phospholipids and related compounds in biological regulation has become an area of increasing interest. Several major regulatory enzymes have been shown to be modulated in part by phospholipids. The recent description of a calcium-dependent protein kinase that requires phospholipid, predominantly phosphatidylserine, as a cofactor (20,57), suggests a direct relationship between phospholipids and phosphorylation (39). This enzyme has a wide tissue distribution (26,66) and occurs both in cytosolic and particulate fractions (26,65,66). Various hormones have been shown to alter phosphatidylinositol metabolism (8,10,46,63) and phospholipid methylation (12). Derivatives of phospholipid metabolism, such as prostaglandins and leukotrienes, are also known to induce rapid changes in biological regulation (6,56).

Some studies suggest that insulin affects the metabolism of phospholipids and/or their derivatives. Recently, Farese et al. (9) showed that insulin markedly stimulated the metabolism in adipocytes of several phospholipids including phosphatidylinositol and phosphatidylserine (personal communication). Walaas et al. (61) demonstrated that insulin stimulated the phosphorylation of a muscle sarcolemmal membrane proteolipid of molecular weight 3600. Wasner (62) described a second messenger, designated cyclic AMP antagonist, which stimulated phosphoprotein phosphatase and inhibited adenylate cyclase and protein kinases. This cyclic AMP antagonist was generated by insulin and by epinephrine through alpha adrenergic stimulation. The material had a molecular weight of approximately 500, required PGE_1 for its synthesis and possibly contained PGE_1 as a structural component.

We have investigated the possible role of phospholipids or related compounds as mediators of insulin action. Chloroform-methanol extraction followed by thin layer chromatography of the supernatant from adipocyte plasma membranes and the partially purified mediator from insulin-treated and control hepatoma cells showed the presence of 10 phospholipids (Macaulay, Kiechle, Jarett, unpublished observation). Aqueous dispersions of these phospholipids and others were added individually to pyruvate dehydrogenase (24) and low Km cyclic AMP phosphodiesterase assays (32). Phosphatidylserine stimulated and phosphatidylinositol-4'-phosphate (DPI) inhibited pyruvate dehydrogenase activity in a dose dependent manner from 1 µM to 800 µM with or without ATP. Eight other phospholipids had no effect upon, or slightly inhibited pyruvate dehydrogenase activity. The stimulation of pyruvate dehydrogenase activity by phosphatidylserine was reversed by DPI. The inhibition of pyruvate dehydrogenase activity by DPI was abolished by increasing the calcium concentration in the assay, which suggested that DPI complexed calcium. Sodium fluoride, a known pyruvate dehydrogenase phosphatase inhibitor, which blocked the ability of the mediator to stimulate pyruvate dehydrogenase, also inhibited the activation of the enzyme by phosphatidylserine. These findings demonstrated that the phospholipid worked through the phosphatase system, as does the mediator. Low Km cAMP phosphodiesterase from adipocyte microsomes was stimulated by 3 of 10 phospholipids tested, (phosphatidylglycerol > phosphatidylserine > lysophosphatidylcholine). The same 3 phospholipids activated the adipocyte plasma membrane enzyme but in the reverse order. Kinetic studies demonstrated the apparent V_{max} of both enzymes was increased in the same order as the stimulation of enzyme activity. These 3 phospholipids had no effect on the apparent Km for cAMP for either enzyme. The mediator prepared from hepatoma cells also stimulated the low Km cyclic AMP phosphodiesterase by increasing apparent V_{max} without altering apparent Km. DPI inhibited the low Km cAMP phosphodiesterase in a dose-dependent manner. Kinetic studies showed that DPI did not alter the apparent V_{max} of both enzymes but increased the apparent Km. No phospholipid tested altered the activity of the high Km cAMP phosphodiesterase from plasma membranes or microsomes. These results suggested a counterregulatory role for phosphatidylserine and DPI. Preliminary experiments with ^{32}P-labeled adipocytes and ^{32}P-labeled hepatoma cells have produced data which is consistent with this proposal (43).

More experimentation will be required to determine the relationship between phospholipid metabolism, the mediator and the mechanism of insulin action. Simple phospholipids, such as phosphatidylserine, have limited water solubility. However, the phospholipid could be released from the membrane as a proteolipid or a small lipopeptide. The phospholipids could also bind to specific cytoplasmic, heat stable, transfer proteins (1). These proteins facilitate transport of phospholipids to their sites of action. Aqueous dispersions of phosphatidylserine have been shown to affect the activity of a number of enzymes, including pyruvate dehydrogenase, low Km cyclic AMP phosphodiesterase, the calcium-dependent protein kinase (57), cyclic AMP dependent protein kinase (7), $[Ca^{++} - Mg^{++}]$-ATPase (42), high Km cyclic AMP phosphodiesterase (13) and adenylate cyclase (29).

CONCLUSIONS

The information described in this chapter reviews the evidence that the interaction of insulin with its receptor on the plasma membrane of various cell types causes the generation of a group of mediators from the plasma membrane. These mediators appear to account for many of the short term actions of insulin on numerous intracellular enzyme systems. The exact chemical structures of the mediators are unknown. The difficulty in identification and purification of these mediators suggests that they have some unusual chemical characteristics. Novel purification techniques may be required. Furthermore, all of the assay systems for the mediators are bioassays which are not consistently reproducible and which cannot determine the absolute quantities of mediator present. Thus, monitoring purification is difficult.

The mechanisms by which the mediators affect various enzyme systems may be complex and varied. The activation of glycogen synthase and pyruvate dehydrogenase by the mediator was originally interpreted to indicate that the mediator acted solely through phosphorylation reactions. In the glycogen synthase system, the mediator appeared to inhibit cyclic AMP dependent protein kinase and to activate the glycogen synthase phosphoprotein phosphatase. Experiments using mitochondrial preparations indicated that the mediator activated the phosphatase system in the pyruvate dehydrogenase complex and had no effect on the cyclic AMP independent protein kinase. These findings need to be substantiated by experiments utilizing purified pyruvate dehydrogenase phosphatase before it can be concluded that the mediator acts directly on the phosphatase. Alternatively, the mediator could

activate this phosphatase by altering the calcium distribution within
the mitochondria. Earlier work in this laboratory demonstrated that
insulin treatment of adipocytes caused redistribution of calcium in
the mitochondria (34). Since a number of other enzymes that are
insulin-sensitive are controlled by phosphorylation, it is possible
that the mediator could act on these enzymes by controlling phosphorylation. If phospholipids should prove to be involved in the
mechanism of insulin action, it is possible that they act, in part,
through the newly described phospholipid-sensitive, calcium-dependent
kinase. It has been proposed that alterations in calcium might be
important in the mediation of insulin action (5). It is possible that
the insulin mediator alters calcium distribution throughout the cell,
and, through this alteration of calcium, affects enzyme activities
directly, through calmodulin and/or through modulation of phosphorylation state. Insulin has been shown to alter the subcellular distribution of calcium in the adipocyte (34,35,36). The mechanism by which
insulin regulates the activity of low Km cAMP phosphodiesterase is not
clear. However, our data suggest that the mediator acts directly on
the enzyme since the enzyme, when partially purified, remains sensitive to the mediator (Macaulay, Kiechle and Jarett, unpublished observations).

The finding of this second messenger or mediator system for insulin
stimulates one to speculate on its clinical significance. The most
obvious potential applications would be in those states of insulin resistance with post-receptor defects, such as obesity and Type II diabetes. In these conditions there may be a defect in the generation or
degradation of the mediator. Approaching these questions will be
easier once the mediators are identified and quantitative assays are
developed. Perhaps a set of structural analogs to the mediators could
be developed as therapeutic agents. Such analogs might be used in
place of, or in addition to, insulin.

REFERENCES

1. Baronska, J. and Grabarek, Z. (1979): FEBS Lett., 104: 253-257.
2. Beachy, J.C., Goldman, D. and Czech, M.P. (1981): Proc. Nat.
   Acad. Sci. USA, 78: 6256-6260.
3. Chen, K., Galasko, G., Huang, L., Kellogg, J. and Larner, J.,
   (1980): Diabetes, 29: 659-661.
4. Cullis, P.R. and DeKruijff, B. (1979): Biochim. et Biophys.
   Acta, 559: 399-420.
5. Denton, R.M., Brownsey, R.W. and Belsham, G.J. (1981):
   Diabetologia, 21:347-362.
6. Dietze, G.J. (1982): Mol. Cell. Endoc., 25: 127-149.
7. Endo, T. and Hidaka, H. (1981): Arch. Biochem. Biophys., 211:
   108-112.
8. Exton, J.H. (1981): Mol. Cell. Endoc., 23: 233-264.
9. Farese, R.V., Larson, R.E. and Sabir, M.A. (1982): J. Biol.
   Chem., 257: 4042-4045.
10. Fourcans, B. and Jain, M.K. (1974): Adv. Lipid Res., 12:
    147-226.
11. Heng, D.L.F., Ng, F.M. and Bornstein, J. (1982): 12th Int. Cong.
    Biochemistry, Abst. 001-188:138.

12. Hirata, F. and Axelrod, J. (1980): Science, 209: 1082-1090.
13. Itano, T., Stano, R. and Penniston, J.T. (1981): Biochem. Int., 3: 379-383.
14. Jarett, L. (1974): In Methods in Enzymology, Vol. XXXI, Edited by S. Fleischer and L. Packer, pp. 60-71, Academic Press, New York.
15. Jarett, L. and Kiechle, F.L. (1981): In Current Views in Insulin Receptors, Edited by D. Andreani, R. DePirro, R. Lauro, J. Olefsky and J. Roth, pp. 245-253. Academic Press, London and New York.
16. Jarett, L., Kiechle, F.L., Popp, D.A., Kotagal, N. and Gavin, J.R., III, (1980): Biochem. Biophys. Res. Commun., 96: 735-741.
17. Jarett, L., Kiechle, F.L., Popp, D.A. and Kotagal, N. (1981): In Cold Spring Harbor Conferences on Cell Proliferation Vol. 8: Protein Phosphorylation, Edited by E.G. Krebs and O.M. Rosen, pp. 715-725, Cold Spring Harbor Laboratory Press.
18. Jarett, L. and Seals, J.R. (1979): Science, 206: 1407-1408.
19. Jarett, L. and Smith, R.M. (1974): J. Biol. Chem., 249: 5195-5199.
20. Kaibuchi, K., Takai, Y. and Nishizuka, Y. (1981): J. Biol. Chem., 256: 7146-7149.
21. Kiechle, F.L. and Jarett, L. (1981): FEBS Lett., 133: 279-281.
22. Kiechle, F.L., Jarett, L., Popp, D.A. and Kotagal, N. (1980): Diabetes, 29: 852-855.
23. Kiechle, F.L., Jarett, L., Popp, D.A. and Kotagal, N. (1981): J. Biol. Chem., 256: 2945-2951.
24. Kiechle, F.L., Strauss III, J.F., Tanaka, T. and Jarett, L. (1982): Federation Proceedings, 41:1082.
25. Kikuchi, K., Schwartz, C. Creacy, S. and Larner, J. (1981) Mol. and Cell. Biochem., 37: 125-130.
26. Kuo, J.F., Andersson, R.G.G., Wise, B.C., Mackerlova, L., Salomonsson, I., Brackett, N.L., Katoh, N., Shoji, M. and Wrenn, R.W. (1980): Proc. Nat. Acad. Sci. USA, 77: 7039-7043.
27. Larner, J., Cheng, K., Schwartz, C., Dubler, R., Creacy, S., Kikuchi, K., Tamura, S., Galasko, G., Pullin, C., and Katz, M. (1981): Mol. and Cell. Biochem., 40: 155-161.
28. Larner, J., Galasko, G., Cheng, K., DePaoli-Roach, A.A., Huang, L., Daggy, P. and Kellogg, J. (1979): Science, 206: 1408-1410.
29. Levey, G.S. (1973): Recent Prog. Horm. Res., 29: 361-386.
30. Loten, E.G., Assimacopoulos-Jeannet, F.D., Exton, J.H. and Park, C.R. (1978): J. Biol. Chem., 253: 746-757.
31. Loten, E.G., and Sneyd, J.G.T. (1970): Biochem. J., 120: 187-195.
32. Macaulay, S.L., Kiechle, F.L. and Jarett, L. (1982): Federation Proceedings, 41:1082.
33. Makino, H. and Kono, T. (1980): J. Biol. Chem., 255: 7850-7854.
34. McDonald, J.M., Bruns, D.E. and Jarett, L. (1976): Biochem. Biophys. Res. Commun., 71: 114-121.
35. McDonald, J.M., Bruns, D.E. and Jarett, L. (1976): Proc. Nat. Acad. Sci. USA, 73: 1542-1546, 1976.
36. McDonald, J.M., Bruns, D.E. and Jarett, L. (1978): J. Biol. Chem., 253: 3504-3508.
37. McDonald, J.M., Pershadsingh, H.A., Kiechle, F.L. and Jarett, L. (1981): Biochem. Biophys. Res. Commun., 100: 857-864.

38. McKeel, D.W. and Jarett, L. (1970): J. Cell. Biol., 44: 417-432.
39. Michell, B. (1981): Trends in Biochem. Sci., 6:VII.
40. Muchmore, D.B., Raess, B.U., Bergstrom, R.W. and DeHaen, L. (1982): Diabetes, (In Press).
41. Ng, F.M., Blaskett, E., Larsen-Disney, P. and Bornstein, J. (1982): 12th Int. Cong. Biochemistry, Abst. 001-187:138.
42. Niggli, V., Adunyah, E.S., Penniston, J.T., and Carafoli, E. (1981): J. Biol. Chem. 256: 395-401.
43. Parker, J.C., Kiechle, F.L. and Jarett, L. (1982): Arch. Biochem. Biophys., 215: 339-344.
44. Parker, J.C., Macaulay, S.L., Kiechle, F.L. and Jarett, L. (1982): Diabetes, 31 (Supplement 2): 29A.
45. Popp, D.A., Kiechle, F.L., Kotagal, N. and Jarett, L. (1980): J. Biol. Chem., 255: 7540-7543.
46. Putney, J.W., Jr. (1981): Life Science, 29: 1183-1194.
47. Saltiel, A., Jacobs, S. Siegel, M. and Cuatrecasas, P. (1981): Biochem. Biophys. Res. Commun., 102: 1041-1047.
48. Saltiel, A.R., Siegel, M.I., Jacobs, S. and Cuatrecasas, P. (1982): Proc. Nat. Acad. Sci. USA, 79: 3513-3517.
49. Seals, J.R. and Czech, M.P. (1980): J. Biol. Chem., 255: 6529-6531.
50. Seals, J.R. and Czech, M.P. (1981): J. Biol. Chem., 256: 2894-2899.
51. Seals, J.R. and Czech, M.P. (1982): Federation Proceedings (In Press).
52. Seals, J.R. and Jarett, L. (1980): Proc. Nat. Acad. Sci. USA, 77: 77-81.
53. Seals, J.R., McDonald, J.M. and Jarett, L. (1978): Biochem. Biophys. Res. Commun., 83: 1365-1372.
54. Seals, J.R., McDonald, J.M. and Jarett, L. (1979): J. Biol. Chem., 254: 6991-6996.
55. Seals, J.R., McDonald, J.M. and Jarett, L. (1979): J. Biol. Chem., 254: 6997-7005.
56. Siroir, P. and Borgeat, P. (1980): Int. J. Immunopharmac., 2: 281-293.
57. Takai, Y., Kishimoto, A., Iwasa, Y., Kawahara, Y., Mori, T. and Nishizuka, Y. (1979): J. Biol. Chem. 254: 3672-3695.
58. Teyssot, B., Djiane, J., Kelly, P.A. and Houdebine, L.M. (1982): Biol. Cell. 43: 81-88.
59. Teyssot, B. Houdebine, L.M. and Djiane, J. (1981): Proc. Nat. Acad. Sci. USA, 78: 6729-6733.
60. Turakulov, Y.K., Gainutdinov, M.K., Lavinaa, J.I. and Akhmatov, M.S. (1977): Rep. Acad. Sci. U.S.S.R., 234: 1471-1474.
61. Walaas, O., Sletten, K., Horn, R.S., Lystad, E., Adler, A. and Alertsen, Aa. R. (1981): FEBS Lett., 128: 137-141.
62. Wasner, H.K. (1981): FEBS Lett., 133: 260-264.
63. Williamson, J.R., Cogsen, R.H. and Hoek, J.B. (1981): Biochim. et Biophys. Acta., 639: 243-295.
64. Wise, B.C., Anderson, R.G.G., Mackerlova, L., Raynor, R.L., Solomonsson, I. and Kuo, J.F. (1981): Biochem. Biophys. Res. Commun., 99: 407-413.
65. Wrenn, R.W., Katoh, N. and Kuo, J.F. (1981): Biochem. Biophys. Acta., 676: 266-269.
66. Wrenn, R.W., Katoh, N., Wise, B.C. and Kuo, J.F. (1980): J. Biol. Chem., 255: 12042-12046.

The Adipocyte and Obesity: Cellular and
Molecular Mechanisms, edited by A. Angel,
C. H. Hollenberg, and D. A. K. Roncari.
Raven Press, New York © 1983.

Role of the Glucose Transport System in the Post-Receptor Defect of Non-Insulin Dependent Diabetes Mellitus and Reversibility of this Abnormality with Insulin Treatment

J. M. Olefsky, T. P. Ciaraldi, J. A. Scarlett, and O. G. Kolterman

*Department of Medicine, University of Colorado Health Sciences Center,
Denver, Colorado 80262; and Veterans Administration Hospital, Denver, Colorado 80222*

ABSTRACT

We have studied the insulin receptor linked glucose transport system in isolated adipocytes in an attempt to determine the mechanisms of the insulin resistance in subjects with impaired glucose tolerance and non-insulin dependent diabetes mellitus (NIDDM). In the subjects with impaired glucose tolerance, basal and maximal insulin stimulated 3-0-methyl glucose transport was normal, but rates of transport were decreased at all submaximal insulin levels. Thus, the dose response curves were shifted to the right indicative of decreased insulin sensitivity due to decreased insulin receptors. In the subjects with non-insulin dependent diabetes mellitus, not only were the dose response curves shifted to the right but there was also a marked decrease in basal and maximally insulin stimulated glucose transport. This indicates decreased insulin sensitivity as well as decreased insulin responsiveness consistent with a combination of receptor and post-receptor defects in insulin action. In all subjects the magnitude of the rightward shift in the glucose transport dose response curve was correlated with the reduction in adipocyte insulin receptors ($r = -.47$, $p < .02$). In the patients with NIDDM, the magnitude of the decrease in maximal glucose transport rate was well correlated to the level of fasting hyperglycemia. An excellent agreement existed between the in vitro studies of adipocyte glucose transport and in vivo glucose clamp studies of peripheral glucose metabolism. Thus, in subjects with impaired glucose tolerance, maximal in vivo insulin stimulated glucose disposal rates were normal, whereas maximal glucose disposal rates were markedly reduced in subjects with non-insulin dependent diabetes mellitus. Furthermore, a significant correlation was found between the maximal insulin stimulated rate of glucose transport in vitro and the maximal insulin stimulated rate of overall glucose disposal in vivo ($r = 0.49$, $p < .01$). In a subgroup of the Type II diabetic patients adipocyte glucose transport and in vivo insulin resistance were measured before and after a 14 day period of intensive insulin treatment, and both abnormalities were found to be ∿ 70% reversed.   In conclusion, 1) the insulin resistance of patients with impaired glucose tolerance appears to be due to decreased insulin receptors with no post-receptor defect in insulin action.   2) The insulin resistance of patients with NIDDM is due to a combination of receptor and post-receptor defects, and the magnitude of the post-receptor defect is greatest in the most hyperglycemic patients, 3) the post-receptor defect in insulin action in patients with NIDDM is related to a decrease in the intrinsic activity of the glucose transport effector system, and 4) the decrease in adipocyte glucose transport activity in Type II diabetes is largely reversable by intensive insulin therapy. This closely corresponds to the reversal by insulin therapy of the post-receptor defect expressed in vivo and provides further evidence that a cellular cause of the post-receptor defect in Type II diabetes is a decrease in glucose transport system activity in the major insulin target tissues.

INTRODUCTION

   Insulin resistance is a common characteristic of patients with impaired glucose tolerance (IGT) and Type II or non-insulin dependent diabetes mellitus (NIDDM)(23a,28). Subjects with IGT have mild insulin resistance while NIDDM subjects have more severe insulin resistance(23a, 28). The degree and frequency of this insulin resistance increases as carbohydrate intolerance worsens (23a,28).
   The weight of the evidence indicates that this insulin resistance is due to a defect in insulin action at the tissue level and not due to the presence of circulating antagonists (22a). The first step in insulin action at the tissue level involves binding to specific receptor sites on the plasma membrane, followed by initiation of a stimulus-response sequence which results in changes in the activity of certain effector systems (7). Alterations in any of these events could serve as a cause for insulin resistance. A pure decrease in insulin receptors would lead to a decrease in insulin action at low hormone concentration with normal effects seen at maximal concentrations (13,22a), assuming that sufficient receptors remain to exceed the spare receptor level (19,25). This would result in a right-ward shift of the dose response curve and is termed a decrease in insulin sensitivity(13,22a). A defect in a post binding step in insulin action should be manifested by a decrease in insulin effect at all insulin concentrations and this is termed a decrease in insulin responsiveness (13,22a). A combination of receptor and post-receptor defects would result in a dose response curve that was both right shifted and depressed at all hormone levels (13,15,22a).
   Previous studies of insulin binding to isolated adipocytes and circulating monocytes have shown that cells from subjects with impaired glucose tolerance or NIDDM have decreased numbers of insulin receptors (1,8,15,22a). In vivo studies have suggested that this decrease in insulin receptor number can account for the insulin resistance in patients with impaired glucose tolerance, but that a post-receptor defect is also present, and predominates, in subjects with Type II diabetes (16). However, the cellular mechanisms of the insulin resistance in patients with NIDDM have not been elucidated. In this report we have

utilized a recently developed assay for 3-0-methyl glucose transport in isolated human fat cells (3,4,5) to explore this question. The results in Type II diabetic patients (5) show a decrease in glucose transport activity which was well correlated in individual subjects to the magnitude of the post-receptor defect as assessed in vivo by the glucose clamp technique (5,16). This indicates that a defect in target tissue glucose transport activity is a cellular abnormality responsible, at least in part, for the post-receptor defect in NIDDM.

Since most Type II diabetic patients are both insulin resistant and insulin deficient, we also tested the hypothesis that the insulin resistance was a secondary abnormality by measuring in vivo insulin action before and after a period of intensive insulin therapy. The results showed that about 75% of the in vivo post-receptor defect, as assessed by the euglycemic glucose clamp method, could be reversed and that this corresponded to a similar reversal of the defect in glucose transport activity.

MATERIALS AND METHODS

Materials

Porcine monocomponent insulin was the kind gift of Dr. Ronald Chance of Eli Lilly and Co. (Indianapolis, IN.). 3-0-methyl-[1-^{14}C]glucose, L-[^{14}C]glucose and Na^{125}I were purchased from New England Nuclear (Boston, MA.), collagenase from Worthington Biochemical Corporation (Freehold, N.J.), bovine serum albumin (Fraction V) from Armour Pharmaceutical Company (Phoenix, AZ.), phloretin from Biochemical Laboratories Company (Redondo Beach, CA.) and silicone oil (viscosity = 125 centistokes, density = .99) from Union Carbide (New York, N.Y.).

Subjects

The study group consisted of 9 non-obese control subjects, 6 subjects with impaired glucose tolerance, and 19 subjects with Type II NIDDM as defined by the criteria of the National Diabetes Data Group (20). The clinical and metabolic features of the subjects are presented in Table 1. All subjects, after giving informed consent, were admitted to the

TABLE 1. Clinical and Metabolic Features of the Study Groups[a]

	n	Age	Relative Weight	Fasting Glucose (mg/100 ml)	Fasting Insulin (μU/ml)
Controls	7	46 ± 5	0.91 ± .03	87 ± 2	11 ± 1
Impaired Glucose Tolerance	6	45 ± 6	1.03 ± .11	101 ± 5	20 ± 5
Obese NIDDM	7	54 ± 4	1.31 ± .04	255 ± 30	33 ± 5
Lean NIDDM	12	56 ± 2	.95 ± .03	252 ± 17	19 ± 4

[a]Results are mean ± SEM

University of Colorado Clinical Research Center where they were placed on a weight maintenance (30 Kcal/kg) liquid formula diet and remained active to approximate their pre-hospital exercise level. None of the subjects had evidence of disease states, other than diabetes, or were ingesting agents known to affect carbohydrate or insulin metabolism. 5 of the Type II patients underwent a 2 week period of intensive insulin therapy after the initial studies, and were restudied after this period of insulin treatment.

Diet

After admission to the Clinical Research Center, all subjects were placed on a weight maintenance (30 Kcal/kg/day), constant caloric diet containing 45% carbohydrate, 40% fat and 15% protein. The diet was divided so that 1/5, 2/5, and 2/5 of the daily calories were given at 0800, 1200 and 1700 hours, respectively. During the period of insulin treatment, portions of the calories alloted to the 1200 and 1700 meals were taken as snacks at 1030, 1530, and 1930 to minimize the likelihood of the subjects experiencing hypoglycemic reactions with a subsequent surge in counter-regulatory hormones. No significant weight changes were noted during the study period.

Meal Tolerance Tests

Following an overnight fast, liquid formula meals, containing 45% carbohydrate, 40% fat and 15% protein, were given at 0800 (1/5 of daily calories) and 1200 (2/5 of daily calories). Serum samples for the measurement of glucose and insulin were obtained at 0800, 0900, 1000, 1100, 1200, 1300, 1400 and 1500 with the 0800 and 1200 hour samples being obtained just prior to the meals. As a measure of the degree of glycemic control, the integrated area under each subject's glucose curve during the meal tolerance test was calculated.

Preparation of Isolated Human Adipocytes

Adipose tissue was obtained from the lower abdominal region as was previously described (21). 1% xylocaine (lidocaine) was infiltrated in a square-field fashion and the biopsy obtained from the center. Tissue was obtained following a 14 h overnight fast. Isolated adipocytes were prepared by the method of Rodbell (30). Tissue was minced into polypropylene vials containing Krebs-Ringer bicarbonate buffer with collagenase (3 mg/ml) and albumin (40 mg/ml). The tissue was incubated for 70 minutes in a 37°C shaking water bath, and the cell suspension filtered through 250 μm nylon mesh. The cells were washed two times by centrifugation at 400 rpm for three minutes in a Krebs-Ringer phosphate (KRP) buffer containing 128mM NaCl, 5.2mM KCl, .62mM $CaCl_2$, 1.29mM $MgSO_4$, 1.29 mM KH_2PO_4, 4mM glucose and 5% bovine serum albumin, pH 7.4. Two additional washes were performed in the KRP-5% BSA buffer with no glucose and cells were diluted to a volume fraction of 0.3-0.5 in this same buffer. Adipocyte counts were performed according to a modification of Method III of Hirsch and Gallian (12). All data were normalized to a cell number of 2 X 10^5 cells.

3-0-Methyl Glucose Transport

Isolated fat cells in a volume of 400 μl ($\sim$ 1 X 10^6 cells/ml) were preincubated for sixty minutes at 37° in the absence or presence of the indicated concentrations of insulin. 3-0-methyl glucose transport was assayed as described previously (4,5). The substrate was placed in a 20 μl volume in 17 X 100 mm polypropylene test tubes. The reaction was started by the rapid addition of 50 μl of the concentrated cell suspension (50-70,000 cells). Transport was terminated after 10 sec by the addition of 11 ml of chilled 0.9% NaCl containing 0.3mM phloretin and 0.7% EtOH. Approximately 2 ml of silicone oil was layered over the phloretin mixture and tubes rapidly centrifuged (2000 X g for 15 sec) in a Heraeus Labofuge. The cells form a layer on the surface of the oil and can be collected by sweeping the oil with absorptive material (such as pieces of cotton pipe cleaner). The pipe cleaners with collected cells were then added to a liquid scintillation cocktail and the radioactivity determined. The amount of cell associated radioactivity due to diffusion and extracellular trapping of 3-0-methyl-[1-^{14}C]glucose was corrected for by performing parallel reactions where L-[^{14}C]glucose uptake was measured; the value for L-glucose uptake was subtracted from the total uptake of 3-0-methyl glucose to give the amount of specific transport. Transport studies were carried out for a reaction time of 10 sec at a substrate concentration of 15.8 μM (0.4 μCi). These conditions insure measurement of initial rates of transport since control studies demonstrated that the time course of uptake was linear for at least 1 minute (4).

Measurement of Insulin Binding

^{125}I-insulin was prepared by the chloramine T procedure as modified by Freychet et al. (9). For binding studies isolated fat cells were suspended in a buffer containing 35mM Tris, 120mM NaCl, 1.2mM $MgSO_4$, 2.5mM KCl, 1.2mM $CaCl_2$, 10mM glucose and 1% BSA, pH 7.6, and incubated with ^{125}I-insulin (0.2 ng/ml) and varying concentrations of unlabeled insulin in plastic vials for 90 min in a 24°C shaking water bath. Cells were separated from unbound hormone by the silicone oil microfuge flotation method described previously (21). All values are reported as % specific binding/2 X 10^5 cells.

RESULTS

In Vivo Studies

The metabolic characteristics of the study groups are summarized in Table 1. It can be seen that only the obese NIDDM subjects exceed normal ideal body weight. Fasting insulin levels were increased in the impaired glucose tolerance and NIDDM groups and this was most pronounced in the obese NIDDM subjects. In vivo glucose clamp studies showed that both NIDDM groups as well as the subjects with impaired glucose tolerance were insulin resistant (3). All of these study groups had decreased overall in vivo glucose disposal rates at submaximal insulin levels; at maximally effective insulin levels the glucose disposal rates were normalized in the subjects with impaired glucose tolerance but were still markedly depressed in both lean and obese NIDDM groups (Ref. 3 and Table 2).

In Vitro Glucose Transport

The in vitro insulin dose response curves for adipocyte 3-0-methyl glucose transport in normals, subjects with impaired glucose tolerance, and lean and obese patients with NIDDM are seen in Figure 1. In the

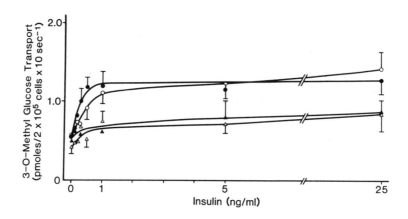

FIG. 1. Dose-response curves for insulin action on 3-0-methyl glucose transport in adipocytes from normals (●), subjects with impaired glucose tolerance (◐), lean subjects with non-insulin dependent diabetes mellitus (NIDDM, △) and obese subjects with NIDDM (▲). Adipocytes were preincubated for 60 min at 37° with the indicated insulin concentration and initial rates of 3-0-methyl glucose transport measured.

subjects with impaired glucose tolerance, both basal (0.59 ± .11 pmoles/ 2 X 10^5 cells X 10 sec^{-1}) and maximally insulin (25 ng/ml) stimulated (1.40 ± .26) glucose transport rates are normal (.55 ± .14 and 1.26 ± .15), while decreased glucose transport is seen at submaximal insulin concentrations (Fig. 1). Thus, insulin sensitivity is decreased and insulin responsiveness is normal, consistent with a pure decrease in insulin receptors and no post-receptor defect. In both lean and obese NIDDM groups, not only are the dose response curves shifted to the right, but there is also a marked decrease in both basal (.42 ± .09 and .49 ± .12, lean and obese, respectively) and maximal insulin stimulated (.84 ± .22 and .82 ± .21) rates of glucose transport. Thus, both decreased insulin sensitivity and decreased insulin responsiveness are demonstrated, consistent with both receptor and post-receptor defects.

These findings are comparable to what was observed in the in vivo multiple glucose clamp studies in these same patients (3).

Since the maximal rates of transport differ among the experimental groups, the functional form of the dose response curves can be better appreciated by plotting the data as a percent of the maximal insulin effect (Fig. 2). With this analysis the rightward shift in the curves from the impaired glucose tolerance and NIDDM groups can be clearly

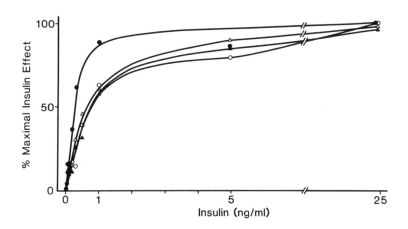

FIG. 2. Insulin stimulation of 3-0-methyl glucose transport in adipocytes isolated from normal (●), subjects with IGT (○), lean subjects with NIDDM (▲), and obese subjects with NIDDM (▲). Results from Figure 1 are plotted as a percent of the maximal insulin effect for each group.

seen and the 1/2 maximally effective insulin concentrations were 0.3, 0.85, 0.80, and 0.70 ng/ml for control subjects with impaired glucose tolerance, the obese NIDDM patients, and the lean NIDDM patients, respectively.

The rightward shift in the dose response curves is the predicted functional consequence of decreased insulin receptors, and we have previously reported decreased cellular insulin receptors in patients with impaired glucose tolerance and NIDDM (3). The potential causal relationship between decreased insulin receptors and the rightward shift in the in vitro glucose transport dose response curves, is supported by the data in Figure 3. With this analysis the half maximally stimulating insulin concentration and the level of adipocyte insulin receptors are plotted for each individual subject. As can be seen, the relationship between these two variables is such that the higher the EC_{50} (greater rightward shift) the lower the insulin binding ($r = -.47$, $p < .02$).

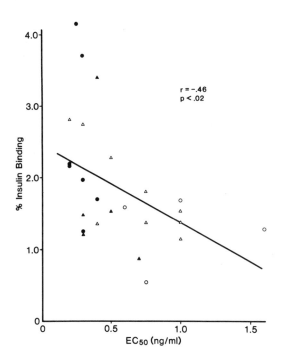

FIG. 3. Relationship between the half-maximally effective insulin concentration (EC_{50}) and the percent of ^{125}I-insulin bound (at .02 ng/ml) to isolated adipocytes from individual normal (●), impaired glucose tolerance (○), lean NIDDM (▲) and obese NIDDM (▲) subjects. Insulin binding was not available for all subjects in this study.

In Vivo - In Vitro Correlations

From the data in Figure 1, it is apparent that the in vitro adipocyte glucose transport data are quite consistent with the in vivo glucose disposal rates as measured by the glucose clamp technique. The details of this relationship can be better appreciated by directly comparing the in vivo and in vitro results in individual patients as presented in Table 2. This table presents the maximal insulin stimulated overall in vivo glucose disposal rates and maximal stimulated in vitro adipocyte 3-0-methyl glucose transport rates in the individual subjects. As can be seen, maximal absolute rates of in vivo glucose disposal and in vitro glucose transport are quite comparable in the normal and impaired glucose tolerance subjects whereas these values are markedly reduced in both NIDDM groups. The correlation between these two variables is presented in Figure 4 and a highly significant positive relationship ($r = .48$, $p < .01$) is present. This indicates that measure-

TABLE 2. Comparison of In Vivo and In Vitro Data

	Maximal Glucose Disposal Rate (mg/M^2/min)	Maximal Glucose Transport (pmoles/2 X 10^5) (Cells X 10 sec^{-1})
Normals		
Mean (± SEM)	399 ± 29	1.41 ± .18
Impaired Glucose Tolerance		
1	497	1.28
2	347	1.22
3	397	.87
4	294	1.33
5	347	1.35
6	481	2.14
Mean (± SEM)	394 ± 33	1.37 ± .17
Obese NIDDM		
7	121	1.09
8	133	1.48
9	151	.53
10	137	.43
11	207	.54
12	190	.60
13	223	1.05
Mean (± SEM)	166 ± 15	.82 ± .14
Lean NIDDM		
14	192	.65
15	396	1.41
16	124	1.55
17	104	.29
18	154	1.23
19	166	.86
20	287	.51
21	218	.83
22	248	.91
23	362	.51
24	123	.80
25	185	.25
Mean (± SEM)	205 ± 28	.82 ± .12

ment of the adipocyte glucose transport provides an accurate estimate of the overall capacity of insulin target tissues to dispose of glucose in vivo. The correlation between these two parameters is still significant when the values from the normals are not included in the calculation.

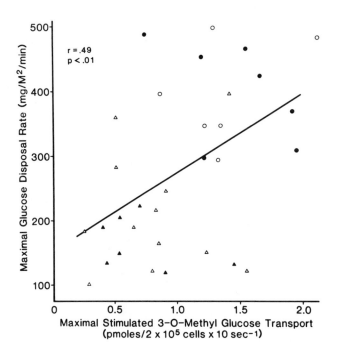

FIG. 4. Relationship between the maximal insulin
stimulated overall in vivo glucose disposal rate
($mg/M^2/min$), as measured by the euglycemic clamp
technique (3), and the maximally stimulated rate
of adipocyte 3-0-methyl glucose transport (pmole/
2×10^5 cells $\times$ 10 sec^{-1}) in individual control
(●), impaired glucose tolerance (◐), lean
NIDDM (▲) and obese NIDDM (▲) subjects.

The factors which chronically control the glucose transport system
are unknown, but two possibilities are the fasting serum insulin and
glucose levels. Accordingly the relationship between fasting plasma
insulin (Figure 5A) and glucose (Figure 5B) and maximally stimulated
3-0-methyl glucose transport are analyzed. No relationship exists between in vitro glucose transport rate and fasting insulin level whereas
a significant ($r = .^-58$, $p < .01$) inverse relationship exists with the
fasting glucose level.

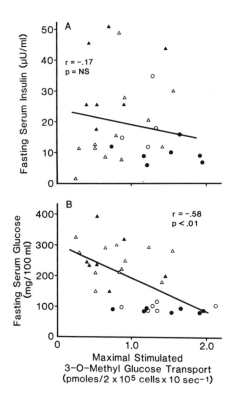

FIG. 5. Relationship between fasting serum insulin (A) or glucose (B) levels and maximally
stimulated rates of 3-0-methyl glucose transport
in individual normals (●), impaired glucose tolerance (○), lean NIDDM (▲), and obese NIDDM
(▲) subjects.

EFFECT OF TREATMENT ON REVERSAL OF INSULIN RESISTANCE

Effect of Treatment on Glycemic Control

Insulin treatment resulted in a decrease in the mean fasting serum
glucose from 292 ± 24 to 135 ± 29 mg/dl (p < .005) as measured on the
last day of the treatment protocol, and the mean integrated area under
the meal tolerance test glucose curve fell from 171,212 ± 20,403 to
72,408 ± 9,292 mg/min/dl.

Effect of Treatment on In Vivo Insulin Sensitivity

The individual maximal in vivo glucose disposal rates for the diabetic subjects before and after insulin treatment compared to values
in normal subjects are shown in Table 3. The maximal rate of insulin-

TABLE 3. Maximal In Vivo Rates of Insulin Stimulated Glucose Disposal
          (mg/M[2]/min) Before and After Insulin Therapy

Patient #[a]	Before	After
8	133	394
10	137	188
19	166	324
22	248	406
25	185	334
Mean ± SEM	174 ± 23	329 ± 39
Normals (mean ± SEM) 399 ± 29		

[a]Patient numbers refer to the same subjects as in Table 1.

stimulated glucose disposal was decreased by 63% compared to normal in
the diabetic subjects before treatment (177 ± 23 mg/M[2]/min vs 399 ± 21
mg/M[2]/min for the diabetic and normal subjects, respectively) indicating the presence of a severe post-receptor defect in insulin action
(13,16,25). Following 14 days of exogenous insulin treatment, the mean
maximal glucose disposal rate for the diabetic subjects was increased
by 85% from 177 ± 23 mg/M[2]/min to 329 ± 39 mg/M[2]/min (p < .005), indicating that this in vivo post-receptor defect was partially, although
not fully, reversed by insulin treatment (31).

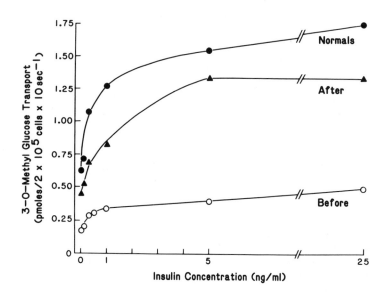

FIG. 6. Mean in vivo insulin dose response curves for 3-0-
methyl glucose transport before (◗) and after insulin
treatment (▲), and in normal subjects (●).

Effect of Treatment on In Vitro Adipocyte 3-0-Methyl Glucose Transport

The in vitro insulin dose response curves for adipocyte 3-0-methyl glucose transport in the diabetic subjects before and after treatment and in 7 normal subjects are shown in Figure 6. In the diabetic subjects prior to treatment transport activity was significantly lower than the normal subjects' values in the basal state and at all insulin concentrations studied. After 14 days of insulin therapy, glucose transport activity increased significantly in the basal state as well as at all insulin concentrations. Thus, basal and maximally insulin-stimulated values increased from 0.18 ± 0.05 to 0.45 ± 0.09; (p < .005), and from 0.50 ± 0.14 to 1.32 ± 0.30 pmoles/2 X 10^5 cells X 10^{-1} sec; (p < 0.025). Although the diabetics' maximal glucose transport activity after treatment (1.32 ± 0.30 pmoles/2 X 10^5 cells/10 sec) was still 24% decreased compared to the normal values ($1.74 \pm .32$ pmoles/2 X 10^5 cells/10 sec), this difference was not statistically significant. The changes in the rates of maximal glucose transport activity for each individual subject before and after the 14 day period of insulin therapy are shown in Figure 7. Each individual showed a significant increase with treatment.

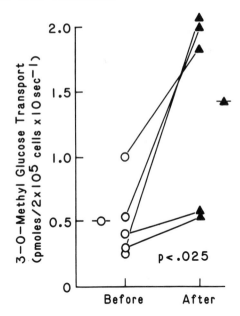

FIG. 7. Individual and mean maximal rates of in vitro adipocyte 3-0-methyl glucose transport before (●) and after (▲) insulin treatment. Cells were preincubated with an insulin concentration of 25 ng/ml.

Half-maximally effective insulin concentrations (EC_{50}) were also calculated from the insulin dose response curves for 3-0-methyl glucose transport. The mean EC_{50} for the diabetic subjects prior to treatment was 1.3 ng/ml, compared to 1.1 ng/ml after treatment and 0.4 ng/ml for the normal subjects. The diabetics' mean dose response curve was therefore shifted to the right compared to normal before insulin

treatment and remained right-shifted after treatment. This is consistent with the decreased insulin binding to adipocytes from Type II
diabetic subjects before (7,16,23a) or after (16) insulin therapy,
which has been shown previously.

In Vivo-In Vitro Correlation

From the data in Table 3 and Figures 6 and 7, it is apparent that
insulin therapy led to a quantitatively comparable mean increase in
maximal adipocyte 3-0-methyl glucose transport in vitro and maximal
overall glucose disposal rate in vivo, and that both of these variables
increased in each subject. The percent increase in maximal 3-0-methyl
glucose transport was highly correlated (r = 0.88, p < 0.05) to the percent increase in maximal in vivo glucose disposal rate in the individual subjects.

DISCUSSION

Insulin resistance and decreased cellular insulin receptors are important pathophysiologic features of impaired glucose tolerance and
NIDDM. However, due to the presence of spare (or excess) insulin receptors, the relationship between decreased insulin receptors and insulin resistance is not straightforward. The functional consequence of
a decrease in insulin receptors is a rightward shift in the insulin
biologic function dose response curve with no decrease in maximal insulin action, and this is termed a decrease in insulin sensitivity (7,
17). A post-receptor defect should lead to a proportionate reduction in
insulin action at all hormone concentrations, including maximally effective levels, and this is termed a decrease in insulin responsiveness.
Since the molecular mechanisms of insulin's cellular actions are not
well understood, it is possible that certain kinds of post-receptor defects could also result in a rightward shift in the dose response curve,
although in human obesity and NIDDM evidence against the proposition
has been presented (3,8). A combination of receptor and post-receptor
defects will lead to decreased insulin sensitivity and responsiveness
manifested by a rightward shift in the dose response curve and a decrease in maximal insulin action (15,17).
The degree of the insulin resistance is greater in patients with
NIDDM as compared to subjects with simple impaired glucose tolerance.
Despite this, the magnitude of the decrease in cellular insulin receptors is comparable in these two conditions, suggesting that additional
factors contribute to the insulin resistance in NIDDM. Recently, we
have presented direct evidence to support this contention (3). In
these studies, the multiple euglycemic glucose clamp technique was used
to construct the overall in vivo dose response curves in normals, patients with impaired glucose tolerance, and lean or obese patients
with NIDDM, by measuring peripheral glucose disposal at a variety of
plasma insulin levels. The results showed that in subjects with impaired glucose tolerance, the in vivo dose response curve was shifted
to the right with no change in maximal insulin action, indicating decreased insulin sensitivity due to decreased insulin receptors. In both
the lean and obese patients with NIDDM, the dose response curves were
not only shifted to the right, but also demonstrated a markedly reduced

maximal insulin effect, indicating decreased insulin responsiveness as well as decreased insulin sensitivity due to a combination of receptor and post-receptor defects in insulin action. The magnitude of the post-receptor defect was greatest in those patients with the greatest degree of fasting hyperglycemia, and in these patients the post-receptor defect was the predominant abnormality contributing to the insulin resistant state. The mechanisms of this post-receptor defect have not been elucidated, and in the current studies we have explored the possibility that this abnormality could be located at the level of the glucose transport system. We have measured basal and insulin stimulated glucose transport in adipocytes isolated from the subjects with impaired glucose tolerance and the lean and obese subjects with NIDDM who participated in the above described in vivo studies. The results have demonstrated a close correlation between the in vitro and in vivo results (Fig. 4). Thus, in subjects with impaired glucose tolerance the adipocyte 3-0-methyl glucose transport dose response curves were shifted to the right with no significant change in maximal insulin effect (Fig. 1). On the other hand, in the subjects with NIDDM, the dose response curves were shifted to the right, but in addition, a marked decrease in maximally insulin stimulated basal 3-0-methyl glucose transport was observed. Thus, as was seen in the in vivo studies, subjects with impaired glucose tolerance demonstrated decreased insulin sensitivity, whereas subjects with NIDDM demonstrated decreased insulin sensitivity and decreased insulin responsiveness. It seems likely that the findings in adipocytes are reflective of changes in other peripheral insulin target tissues since we also found a highly significant correlation between maximal insulin stimulated in vivo overall glucose disposal and maximal in vitro adipocyte glucose transport rates (Fig. 4).

In these studies it is important to consider the contribution of obesity to the metabolic abnormalities in NIDDM. We have previously shown that obese subjects with NIDDM are modestly more insulin resistant than lean NIDDM subjects, but that the lean NIDDM group was still markedly insulin resistant and demonstrated both receptor and post-receptor defects (3). In the current in vitro studies, we were unable to distinguish differences between the obese and lean NIDDM groups, as far as adipocyte glucose transport was concerned. However, it should be noted that the transport data were normalized on the basis of cell number rather than some aspect of cell size. Clearly, adipocytes from obese subjects are larger than cells from lean subjects, and if one expressed the data based on unit surface area, then basal and insulin stimulated glucose transport would be lower in the obese compared to the lean NIDDM groups. In this sense, obesity may indeed be an additional factor contributing to the cellular insulin resistance in this condition.

The mechanisms of the cellular defects observed in these patients are not elucidated by the present studies. In the patients with impaired glucose tolerance, decreased insulin receptor number appears to be the cause of the insulin resistance, but the reason for the loss of insulin receptors is still unknown. In the NIDDM subjects the combination of cellular defects adds a further degree of complexity. However, it is useful to note that the magnitude of the post-receptor defect is well correlated with the degree of hyperglycemia (Fig. 5B). Although the patients with NIDDM may display fasting hyperinsulinemia, they are uniformly hypoinsulinemic in response to glucose challenges and the magnitude of this defect in insulin secretion is greater as the degree of fasting hyperglycemia worsens (22a,23a,28). Thus, despite normal or elevated basal insulin levels, the 24 hour integrated plasma insulin levels may actually be low in these patients. With this formulation, insulin deficiency may contribute in some way to the generation of the post-receptor defect in the glucose transport system. Unfortunately, daylong insulin levels were not measured in these patients, but this concept would explain the lack of correlation between the post-receptor defect in glucose transport and the fasting insulin level (Fig. 5A). In other conditions, such as fasting (22b) and streptotozocin induced diabetes (24), insulin deficiency is correlated with a decrease in maximal glucose transport rates, suggesting the possibility that these factors may be causally related.

To pursue the possibility that absolute or relative insulin deficiency may primarily or secondarily lead to a post-receptor defect in the glucose transport system and in vivo insulin resistance, we carried out additional studies in which the effects of insulin replacement therapy on insulin resistance in Type II diabetes was assessed. The purpose behind this approach was to: 1) test the idea that the component of the insulin resistant state which was responsible for the post-receptor defect in insulin action could be reversed in Type II diabetics, and 2) to perturb the system in order to gain further insight into the relationship between in vivo insulin action and cellular glucose transport. We have recently reported that following a 14 day period of intensive insulin therapy the in vivo post-receptor defect in insulin action, as assessed by the multiple euglycemic glucose clamp technique approach, was largely ameliorated (31). Thus, following insulin therapy, maximal in vivo glucose disposal rates in insulin treated diabetic patients were approximately 80% of normal (as compared to 25% of normal in the pre-treated state).

As shown in Figures 6 and 7, we also find that a 14 day period of intensive insulin therapy reverses the post-receptor defect in adipocyte glucose transport activity. Thus, prior to insulin therapy the dose response curve for adipocyte glucose transport in cells from Type II diabetics was characterized by a marked decrease in basal and maximally insulin-stimulated rates of 3-0-methyl glucose uptake, along with a rightward shift in the dose response curve. After insulin therapy, basal and maximal insulin-stimulated rates of glucose transport are largely corrected to near normal levels. This corresponded quite well to the magnitude of the effect of insulin therapy to reverse the post-receptor defect in insulin action as measured in vivo (31). The adipocyte glucose transport dose response curve following therapy was still shifted to the right compared to normal, but this was consistent with the fact that adipocyte insulin receptors were still decreased (31). From these studies we suggest that the major mechanism for the post-receptor defect in Type II diabetes is a decrease in glucose transport system activity in insulin target tissues. Furthermore, we suggest that this post-receptor defect in insulin action is secondary to some aspect of the chronic hyperglycemic diabetic state. The evidence for this latter suggestion comes from the studies which show that insulin therapy reverses the in vivo expression of the post-receptor defect in insulin action as measured by the glucose clamp technique (31), and also reverses the post-receptor defect in adipocytes from these same patients.

In these studies we have used a decrease in maximally insulin-stimulated adipocyte glucose transport and maximally insulin stimulated in vivo rates of glucose disposal as measurements of post-receptor defects in insulin action. The reasoning behind this relates to the spare receptor concept of insulin action. It is well known that only a fraction of total cellular insulin receptors need to be occupied in order to elicit a maximal insulin biologic effect and thus the remaining receptors are considered spare (17). Of course, the proportion of spare recpetors depends upon which particular insulin action is being measured as well as the cell type studied. For stimulation of overall in vivo glucose disposal, evidence exists in man that approximately 60-70% of the receptors are spare (15). Thus, a decrease in insulin receptors can only lead to a decrease in maximal insulin action if the decrease in insulin receptors is so profound that more than the number of spare receptors have been lost. This is unlikely to be the case, since direct measurements of monocyte and adipocyte insulin receptors in Type II diabetes have demonstrated that despite the decrease in insulin binding, there are more than enough receptors left to generate a maximal biologic effect (16,23a,26). Consequently, at maximally effective insulin levels, the rate limiting step for overall insulin action on glucose disposal in vivo or glucose transport in vitro is distal to the insulin binding step. With this formulation, the defect in maximally insulin-stimulated overall in vivo glucose disposal rate reflects the magnitude of the post-receptor defect in insulin action in the major insulin target tissues. The in vitro studies of adipocyte glucose transport directly measure one specific post-receptor effector system, namely the glucose transport system, and the magnitude of the decrease in maximally stimulated 3-0-methyl glucose transport represents the magnitude of the post-receptor defect in this effector system.

We have used the adipocyte glucose transport system as an in vitro model because adipocytes are a convenient and easy to obtain insulin target tissue in man. However, it should be noted that adipose tissue accounts for only a small percentage of overall glucose consumption (2) and that the major insulin target tissue responsible for glucose disposal is muscle. Consequently, the conclusions drawn from these studies regarding the role of the glucose transport system are quantitatively valid only insofar as the adipocyte glucose transport system is reflective of overall glucose disposal, and in particular, muscle glucose transport. Although this point cannot be definitively proven, we believe that the available data support this contention. Firstly, in individual Type II diabetic patients, the defect in adipocyte glucose transport was well correlated to the magnitude of the defect in overall glucose disposal measured in vivo (5). This suggests the possibility that the defect in adipocyte glucose transport is relfective of the defect in overall glucose disposal in vivo, and therefore must be representative of the glucose transport system in the major glucose consuming tissue muscle. Secondly, in human obesity, a similar set of findings were observed: i.e., the post-receptor defect in overall in vivo glucose disposal was highly correlated to a similar defect in adipocyte glucose transport in individual subjects (4). Thus, in two common insulin resistant states, measurements of post-receptor defects in vivo correlated with the magnitude of defects in adipocyte glucose transport. Of course, correlation analysis simply shows associations of static measurements made at one point in time, and does not prove causality. In order to more closely approach a causal relationship, it is necessary to carry out a perturbation study, as in the current report. When the system was perturbed by insulin therapy, a marked reversal of the post-receptor defect measured in vivo was observed and was accompanied by a quantitatively similar reversal of the defect in adipocyte glucose transport. This provides additional evidence that the adipocyte glucose transport system provides an accurate model to assess overall glucose transport in the major glucose consuming tissues. Finally, a number of more direct studies have been conducted which demonstrate that changes in adipocyte glucose transport are paralleled by quantitatively similar changes in skeletal muscle glucose transport in a number of different pathophysiologic conditions in rodents (10,11, 18,19,24,29,32). We believe that the findings stated above provide a reasonable rationale to suggest that measurements of adipocyte glucose transport can be used as a model for glucose transport activity in other insulin target tissues. However, this formulation is clearly tentative and will require additional experimentation. This could take the form of additional manipulations or static measurements seeking relationships between in vivo glucose disposal rates and adipocyte glucose transport activity. Ideally, this hypothesis should be tested by directly measuring muscle glucose transport rates in man. Unfortunately, such studies are not currently technically or ethically feasible.

These studies do not tell us what feature of the diabetic state leads to the development of this post-receptor defect in insulin action. Since insulin treatment ameliorates the abnormality, it is possible that the post-receptor defect is secondary to insulin deficiency. On the other hand, a number of other metabolic abnormalities exist in Type II diabetes which may also contribute to this cellular defect. As one example, we have found that the magnitude of the post-receptor defect in vivo is closely correlated to the height of the fasting plasma glucose concentrations in individual subjects (16). Thus, perhaps hyperglycemia itself in some way mediates the cellular abnormality. Obviously, other possibilities exist which will require further study before more definitive statements can be made.

In summary, we have shown that the in vitro glucose transport dose response curve is shifted to the right with no change in maximal insulin action in patients with impaired glucose tolerance, consistent with a decrease in insulin receptors only. In patients with NIDDM, the dose response curves are shifted to the right and in addition a marked decrease in maximal insulin action was observed, consistent with the presence of both receptor and post-receptor defects. These in vitro results correlate quite well to in vivo dose response curves obtained in the same subjects. From this, we conclude that the post-receptor defect observed in many patients with NIDDM, is due to a defect in the intrinsic activity of the plasma membrane glucose transport carrier. Whether this is due to a decrease in the number of glucose carriers(14), or a decrease in the accessability of the carrier to the cell surface (6) cannot be determined by the present data. Regardless of the precise biochemical nature of this defect in glucose transport activity, our studies show that this abnormality is a secondary phenomenon and can be largely reversed by a 14 day period of intensive insulin therapy. Lastly, it should be pointed out that although these results indicate that the post-receptor defect in NIDDM is localized to the glucose transport system, this does not exclude further, more distal, post-receptor defects in insulin action located intracellularly. If such additional post-receptor defects exist they might assume physiologic importance under conditions in which glucose transport is not rate limiting for overall glucose metabolism.

ACKNOWLEDGEMENTS

This work was supported in part by funds from the Medical Research Service of the Veterans Administration, by grants AM 19905 and AM 21680 from the National Institutes of Health, by grant RR-00051 from the Clinical Research Center Branch of the National Institutes of Health, and by a grant from the KROC Foundation. Dr. Scarlett was the recipient of an Associate Investigator Award from the Veterans Administration and Dr. Kolterman was the recipient of a Clinical Investigator Award (AM 00580) from the National Institute of Arthritis, Metabolism, and Digestive Disease of the National Institutes of Health. The authors wish to thank the staff of the Clinical Research Center for the excellent nursing care provided to our patients, Miss Cathy Christian and Mrs. Joan Weyant for their technical assistance, and Mrs. Elizabeth Martinez for her excellent secretarial support in the preparation of this manuscript.

REFERENCES

1. Beck-Nielsen, H. (1978): Diabetes 27:1175-1181.
2. Bjorntorp, P., and Sjorstrom, L. (1978): Metabolism 27:1853-1860.
3. Ciaraldi, T.P., Kolterman, O.G., Siegel, J.A., and Olefsky, J.M. (1979): Am. J. Physiol. 236:E621-E625.
4. Ciaraldi, T.P., Kolterman, O.G., and Olefsky, J.M. (1981): J. Clin. Invest. 68:875-880.
5. Ciaraldi, T.P., Kolterman, O.G., Scarlett, J.A., Kao, M., and Olefsky, J.M. (1982): Diabetes (In press).
6. Cushman, S.W., and Wardzala, L.J. (1980): J. Biol. Chem. 255: 4758-4762.
7. Czech, M.P. (1977): Annu. Rev. Biochem. 46:359-384.
8. DeFronzo, R.A., Diebert, D., Hendler, R., Felig, P., and Soman, V. (1979): J. Clin. Invest. 63:939-946.
9. Freychet, P., Roth, J., and Neville, D.M., Jr. (1971): Biochem. Biophys. Res. Commun. 43:400-408.
10. Goodman, M.N., Berger, M., and Ruderman, N.D. (1974): Diabetes 23:881-888.
11. Grundleger, M.L., and Therren, S.W. (1982): Diabetes 31:232-237.
12. Hirsch, J., and Gallian, E. (1968): J. Lipid Res. 9:110-119.
13. Kahn, C.R. (1978): Metabolism 27:1893-1902.
14. Karnieli, E., Hissin, P.J., Simpson, I.A., Salans, L.B., and Cushman, S.W. (1981): J. Clin. Invest. 68:811-814.
15. Kolterman, O.G., Insel, J., Saekow, M., and Olefsky, J.M. (1980): J. Clin. Invest. 65:1272-1284.
16. Kolterman, O.G., Gray, R.S., Griffin, J., Burstein, P., Insel, J., Scarlett, J.A., and Olefsky, J.M. (1981): J. Clin. Invest. 68: 957-969.
17. Kono, T., and Barham, F.W. (1971): J. Biol. Chem. 246:6210-6216.

18. LeMarchand-Brustel, Y., and Freychet, P. (1979): J. Clin. Invest. 64:1505-1515.
19. Morgan, H.E., Cadenas, E., Regen, D.M., and Park, C.R. (1961): J. Biol. Chem. 236:262-268.
20. National Diabetes Data Group. (1979): Diabetes 28:1039-1057.
21. Olefsky, J.M., Jen, P., and Reaven, G.M. (1974): Diabetes 23: 565-571.
22a. Olefsky, J.M. (1976): Diabetes 25:1154-1165.
22b. Olefsky, J.M. (1976): J. Clin. Invest. 58:1950-1960.
23. Olefsky, J.M. and Reaven, G.M. (1977): Diabetes 26:650-688.
24. Olefsky, J.M. and Kobayashi, M. (1978): Metabolism 27:1917-1929.
25. Olefsky, J.M. (1981): Diabetes 30:148-162.
26. Olefsky, J.M., and Kolterman, O.G. (1981): Am. J. Med. 70:151-168.
27. Reaven, G.M., Bernstein, R., Davis, B., and Olefsky, J.M. (1976): Am. J. Med. 60:80-88.
28. Reaven, G.M. and Olefsky, J.M. (1978): Adv. Modern Nutri. Vol. II (Part I):229-266.
29. Riddeck, F.A., Jr., Feisler, D.M. and Kipnis, D.M. (1962): Diabetes 11:171-178.
30. Rodbell, M. (1964): J. Biol. Chem. 239:375-380.
31. Scarlett, J.A., Kolterman, O.G., Gray, R.S., Griffin, J., and Olefsky, J.M. (1982): Diabetes Care 5:353-363.
32. Susini, C., and Lavau, M. (1978): Diabetes 27:114-120.

The Adipocyte and Obesity: Cellular and Molecular Mechanisms, edited by A. Angel, C. H. Hollenberg, and D. A. K. Roncari. Raven Press, New York © 1983.

Mechanism of Insulin Resistant Glucose Transport in the Isolated Rat Adipose Cell

*Samuel W. Cushman, *Lawrence J. Wardzala, **Paul J. Hissin, †Eddy Karnieli, *Ian A. Simpson, and *Lester B. Salans

*Cellular Metabolism and Obesity Section, NIADDK, National Institutes of Health, Bethesda, Maryland 20205; **Department of Chemistry, Mount Sinai Hospital, New York, New York 10029; and †Metabolic Unit, Endocrine Institute, Rambam Medical Center, Haifa, Israel*

Insulin resistant glucose metabolism is frequently observed in man with high fat/low carbohydrate feeding, insulin-dependent diabetes mellitus, and obesity. In experimental animal models of these perturbed metabolic states, systemic insulin resistance is paralleled by a similar resistance to insulin's stimulatory action on glucose metabolism in adipose and muscle cells in vitro (5,11,14,15,17,18). A fundamental action of insulin in regulating glucose metabolism at the cellular level is its stimulation of glucose transport (1,7). Furthermore, insulin has recently been shown to stimulate glucose transport in rat adipose cells and diaphragm through a rapid, reversible, and insulin concentration-dependent translocation of glucose transport systems from a large intracellular pool to the plasma membrane (3,13,16,21-24). The intracellular pool of glucose transport systems is associated with a unique membrane species found in a low-density microsomal membrane fraction enriched in marker enzyme activities characteristic of membranous components of the Golgi apparatus. The present studies were undertaken to examine the role of this translocation in the insulin resistant glucose transport of the isolated adipose cell from the rat fed a high fat/low carbohydrate diet (9), the streptozotocin-induced diabetic rat model of insulin-dependent diabetes mellitus (12), and the aging male rat model of obesity (10).

METHODS

Ad libitum-fed, male Sprague-Dawley rats (CD strain) were used in all experiments. In studies of the effects of dietary composition (9), weanling rats were raised for 3 weeks on either a high carbohydrate/low fat (71%:9% by calories) or low carbohydrate/high fat (30%:50% by calories) diet. Protein (20% by calories) and caloric density were kept constant. Under these conditions, animals on the two diets consumed equal quantities of food, grew at the same rate, and had identical epididymal adipose cell sizes (0.100 μg of lipid/cell) (20). Post-prandial plasma glucose levels at the time of sacrifice were similar (147 mg/dl) whereas plasma insulin levels were somewhat higher in the former (26 μU/ml) than in the latter (16 μU/ml). In studies of the effects of insulin-dependent diabetes mellitus (12), 150-200 g rats were intraperitoneally injected with either 0.1 mM citrate buffer alone or 65 mg of streptozotocin/kg of body weight in 0.1 mM citrate buffer, and maintained for 7 days. During the maintenance period, the latter consumed 1.6-fold more standard chow, but grew more slowly, exhibited 4+ urine glucose levels, and had smaller epididymal adipose cell sizes (0.114 and 0.071 μg of lipid/cell, respectively). Post-prandial plasma glucose levels at the time of sacrifice were markedly elevated in the latter (477 mg/dl) compared to the former (145 mg/dl) whereas plasma insulin levels were similar (45 μU/ml). In studies of the effects of obesity (10), 180 g young, lean and 850 g old, obese animals were maintained for roughly 7 days on standard chow. The latter had approximately 12-fold larger epididymal adipose cell sizes than the former (0.080 and 0.935 μg of lipid/cell, respectively). Post-prandial plasma glucose levels at the time of sacrifice were similar (142 mg/dl) whereas plasma insulin levels were roughly 3-fold higher in the latter (68 μU/ml) than the former (26 μU/ml). All animals were sacrificed at approximately 8:00 a.m. by cervical dislocation and decapitation.

Isolated adipose cells were prepared from the whole epididymal fat pads by collagenase digestion (19). Adipose cell size and number were determined by the osmic acid fixation, Coulter Electronic Counter technique (2,8) in the pooled stock cell suspension. The isolated cells were then incubated at 37 C for 30 min in a glucose-free Krebs-Ringer-bicarbonate-HEPES buffer containing 10 mg of untreated bovine serum albumin/ml and 0 or 7.0 nM (1000 μU/ml) insulin. Samples of cells were removed and glucose transport activity was assayed by measuring the rate of transport of 0.1 mM 3-0-methylglucose at 37 C (6,13). The remaining cells were washed in a TRIS, EDTA, sucrose buffer and homogenized. Plasma and low-density microsomal membrane fractions were prepared by differential ultracentrifugation (3,13). The number of glucose transport systems in each membrane fraction was quantitated by measuring specific D-glucose-inhibitable cytochalasin B binding (13,23). The membrane species comprising each subcellular fraction and the reproducibility of the fractionation procedure were assessed by measuring the specific activities of the following marker enzymes: 5'-nucleotidase and isoproterenol-stimulated adenylate cyclase, characteristic of plasma membranes; rotenone-insensitive NADH-cytochrome c reductase and glucose-6-phosphate phosphatase, characteristic of endoplasmic reticulum; and UDP-galactose:N-acetylglucosamine galactosyltransferase, characteristic of the Golgi apparatus (3,13).

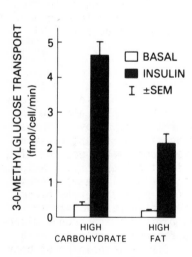

FIG. 1. Glucose transport activity in isolated adipose cells from rats fed a high carbohydrate or high fat diet.

RESULTS AND DISCUSSION

The insulin resistant glucose transport response of intact isolated adipose cells from rats fed a high fat/low carbohydrate diet compared to those fed a high carbohydrate/low fat diet (9) is illustrated in Figure 1. While the basal rate of 3-0-methylglucose transport is not statistically significantly influenced by

dietary composition, the stimulatory action of insulin on glucose transport activity is diminished by 51% by high fat feeding.   Figure 2 illustrates the corresponding effects of dietary composition on the numbers
of glucose transport systems in the plasma and low-density microsomal
membrane fractions prepared from these same basal and maximally insulin-
stimulated cells.   In the basal state, dietary composition does not
influence the number of glucose transport systems/mg of membrane protein

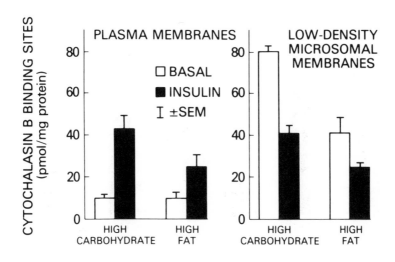

FIG. 2.   Distribution of glucose transport systems between subcellular
membrane fractions of isolated adipose cells from rats fed a high carbohydrate or high fat diet.

in the plasma membrane fraction.   However, high fat, relative to high
carbohydrate, feeding is accompanied by a 48% decrease in the basal
number of glucose transport systems/mg of membrane protein in the low-
density microsomal membrane fraction.

In response to insulin, on the other hand, high fat feeding is accompanied by a 53% reduction in the number of glucose transport systems
appearing in the plasma membrane fraction and a concommitant 59% reduction in the number of glucose transport systems disappearing from the
low-density microsomal membrane fraction.   The effects of dietary composition on glucose transport activity in the intact cells (Fig 1) closely
correlate with those on the number of glucose transport systems in the
plasma membrane fraction (Fig 2).   Under the experimental conditions employed here, altered dietary composition is not associated with changes
either in insulin binding to its specific receptors or in the sensitivity
of the cells' transport and metabolic responses to insulin (20).   Thus,
insulin resistant glucose transport in isolated rat adipose cells with
high fat/low carbohydrate feeding, compared to high carbohydrate/low fat
feeding, appears to be the consequence of 1) a depletion of glucose
transport systems in the intracellular pool in the basal state, and 2) a
corresponding reduction in the translocation of glucose transport

systems from this intracellular pool to the plasma membrane in response
to insulin.

Figures 3 and 4, and 5 and 6 illustrate the similar results obtained
in the streptozotocin-induced diabetic rat model of insulin-dependent
diabetes mellitus (12) and the aged male rat model of obesity (10), respectively. However, the former is accompanied by a 38% decrease in
adipose cell size, and the latter, by an approximately 12-fold increase
in adipose cell size (volume when expressed as μg of lipid/cell). The

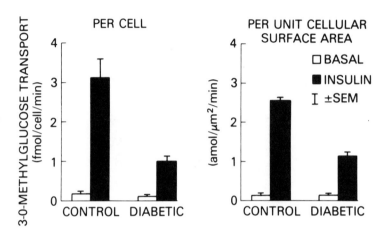

FIG. 3.   Glucose transport activity in isolated adipose cells from control and streptozotocin diabetic rats.

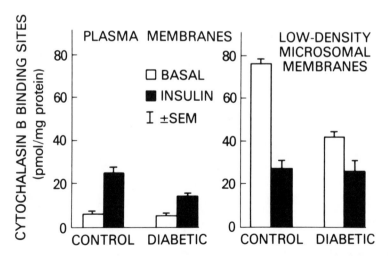

FIG. 4.   Distribution of glucose transport systems between subcellular
membrane fractions of isolated adipose cells from control and streptozotocin diabetic rats.

modestly decreased basal glucose transport activity/cell in the streptozotocin-induced diabetic rat and markedly increased basal glucose transport activity/cell in the aged, obese rat both disappear when expressed
per unit of cellular surface area (Figs 3 and 5, respectively), corresponding to the constant basal numbers of glucose transport systems/mg
of membrane protein in the plasma membrane fraction (Figs 4 and 6, respectively). Moreover, the diminished stimulatory effects of insulin on
glucose transport in the intact cells of both the streptozotocin-induced
diabetic and aged, obese rats are more readily demonstrable when glucose

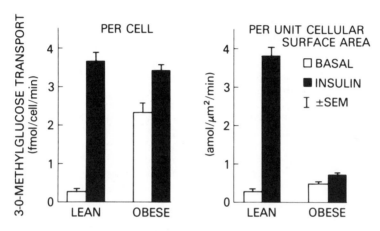

FIG. 5. Glucose transport activity in small isolated adipose cells from
young, lean rats and large isolated adipose cells from aged, obese rats.

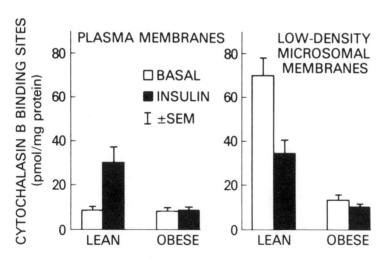

FIG. 6. Distribution of glucose transport systems between subcellular
membrane fractions of small isolated adipose cells from young, lean
rats and large isolated adipose cells from aged, obese rats.

transport activity is expressed per unit of cellular surface area than per cell (Figs 3 and 5, respectively). These effects directly correlate with the decreased basal numbers of glucose transport systems/mg of membrane protein in the low-density microsomal membrane fraction and correspondingly reduced translocations of glucose transport systems from the intracellular pool to the plasma membrane (Figs 4 and 6, respectively). Both the plasma and low-density microsomal membrane fractions are recovered from the original homogenate in proportion to the surface area of the starting intact cells. In addition, while the specific activities of the marker enzymes are altered to varying degrees among the various metabolic states examined here, the membrane species comprising each subcellular fraction are not altered. Insulin does not influence the subcellular distribution of marker enzyme activities under any of the conditions studied. Streptozotocin-induced diabetes in the rat has been reported to be associated with an increase in insulin binding to isolated adipose cells and an increase in the sensitivity of the cells' transport and metabolic responses to insulin (14,15). The aged, obese rat has also been reported to be associated with an increase in insulin binding/cell, but unchanged insulin binding/unit of cellular surface area (4) and an unchanged sensitivity to insulin (10).

Thus, insulin resistant glucose transport in the isolated adipose cell of the rat fed a high fat/low carbohydrate diet, the streptozotocin-induced diabetic rat model of insulin-dependent diabetes mellitus, and the aged male rat model of obesity can be explained by a reduction in the number of glucose transport systems appearing in the plasma membrane in response to insulin. This reduction appears to reflect a depletion of glucose transport systems in the intracellular pool which is the source of those glucose transport systems translocated to the plasma membrane. In none of these perturbed metabolic states can the resistance of the isolated adipose cell to insulin at the glucose transport level be explained by alterations in insulin binding or the cell's sensitivity to insulin. Indeed, the present results suggest that the mechanism through which insulin initiates the the translocation process remains completely intact. While the factors influencing, and the mechanisms regulating, the size of the intracellular pool of glucose transport systems have not yet been established, the development of insulin resistant glucose transport may represent an adaptative process through which substrate and/or metabolite fluxes control the synthesis and degradation of specific proteins. Although the adipose tissue mass probably contributes in a minor way only to total glucose utilization in the intact organism, the mechanism of insulin resistant glucose transport in the adipose cell may very well reflect the operation of a similar mechanism in muscle. The major contribution of muscle to systemic glucose homeostasis is well established. However, the role of glucose transport as the rate limiting step in glucose metabolism _in vivo_ remains to be established.

ACKNOWLEDGMENTS

The authors wish to thank Mary Jane Zarnowski and Dena R. Yver for their expert technical assistance during this work, and Joy Glotfelty for her typing of the manuscript. These investigations were supported in part by a research grant from The Kroc Foundation.

REFERENCES

1. Crofford, O.B., and Renold, A.E. (1965): J. Biol. Chem., 240:3237-3244.
2. Cushman, S.W, and Salans, L.B. (1978): J. Lipid Res., 19:269-273.
3. Cushman, S.W., and Wardzala, L.J. (1980): J. Biol. Chem., 255:4758-4762.
4. Cushman, S.W., Noda, D., and Salans, L.B. (1981): Am. J. Physiol., 240:E166-E174.
5. Czech, M.P. (1976): J. Clin. Invest., 57:1523-1532.
6. Foley, J.E., Cushman, S.W., and Salans, L.B. (1978): Am. J. Physiol., 234:E112-E119.
7. Foley, J.E., Cushman, S.W., and Salans, L.B. (1980): Am. J. Physiol., 238:E180-E185.
8. Hirsch, J., and Gallian, E. (1968): J. Lipid Res., 9:110-119.
9. Hissin, P.J., Karnieli, E., Simpson, I.A., Salans, L.B., and Cushman, S.W. (1982): Diabetes 31:589-592.
10. Hissin, P.J., Foley, J.E., Wardzala, L.J., Karnieli, E., Simpson, I.A., Salans, L.B., and Cushman, S.W. (1982): J. Clin. Invest., 70:in press.
11. Ip, C., Tepperman, H.M., DeWitt, J., and Tepperman, J. (1977): Horm. Metab. Res., 9:218-222.
12. Karnieli, E., Hissin, P.J., Simpson, I.A., Salans, L.B., and Cushman, S.W. (1981): J. Clin. Invest., 68:811-814.
13. Karnieli, E., Zarnowski, M.J., Hissin, P.J., Simpson, I.A., Salans, L.B., and Cushman, S.W. (1981): J. Biol. Chem., 256:4772-4777.
14. Kasuga, M., Akanuma, Y., Iwamoto, Y., and Kosaka, K. (1978): Am. J. Physiol., 235:E175-E182.
15. Kobayashi, M., and Olefsky, J.M. (1979): Diabetes, 28:87-95.
16. Kono, T., Suzuki, K., Dansey, L.E., Robinson, F.W., and Blevins, T.L. (1981): J. Biol. Chem., 256:6400-6407.
17. Olefsky, J.M. (1976): J. Clin. Invest., 57:842-851.
18. Olefsky, J.M. (1978): Endocrinology, 103:2253-2263.
19. Rodbell, M. (1964): J. Biol. Chem., 239:375-380.
20. Salans, L.B., Foley, J.E., Wardzala, L.J., and Cushman, S.W. (1981): Am. J. Physiol., 240:E175-E183.
21. Suzuki, K., and Kono, T. (1980): Proc. Natl. Acad. Sci. U.S.A., 77:2542-2545.
22. Wardzala, L.J., and Jeanrenaud, B. (1981): J. Biol. Chem., 256:7090-7093.
23. Wardzala, L.J., Cushman, S.W., and Salans, L.B. (1978): J. Biol. Chem., 253:8002-8005.
24. Wheeler, T.J., Simpson, I.A., Sogin, D.C., Hinkle, P.C., and Cushman, S.W. (1982): Biochem. Biophys. Res. Commun., 105:89-95.

The Adipocyte and Obesity: Cellular and Molecular Mechanisms, edited by A. Angel, C. H. Hollenberg, and D. A. K. Roncari. Raven Press, New York © 1983.

The Native Insulin Receptor of Adipocytes Exists in Three Partially Reduced Forms

Cecil C. Yip and Margaret L. Moule

Banting and Best Department of Medical Research, University of Toronto, Toronto, M5G 1L6 Canada

The characterization of the structure of the insulin receptor has been hampered by the reversibility of the hormone-receptor interaction. During the past years, we (4,6) have successfully applied the technique of photoaffinity labelling to link insulin covalently to its receptor. The success of this approach has been based on the synthesis of photo-reactive insulin derivatives, $N^{\alpha B1}$-monoazidobenzoyl-insulin (B_1MABI) and $N^{\epsilon B29}$-monoazidobenzoyl-insulin ($B_{29}MABI$) which have been fully characterized with respect to the location of the photoreactive group, light-sensitivity, ability to crosslink upon photolysis, and biological and receptor binding activity. We first used isolated plasma membrane fractions from different tissues as the source of insulin receptors. Photoaffinity labelling of isolated plasma membrane fractions demonstrated that the insulin receptor was composed of at least two different kinds of glycoprotein subunits of approximately 130K and 90K dalton in molecular-weight which are linked by disulfide bonds. These two types of receptor subunits are detected in all tissues tested except in brain where only a 115K band has been demonstrated (7).

We have since applied this photoaffinity labelling technique to study the insulin receptor on intact cells, specifically on isolated rat adipocytes. Experimental conditions and results of this study have recently been published (8). Briefly, intact adipocytes were isolated from the epidydimal fat pads of the rat by collagenase digestion. The adipocytes were then incubated with either radioiodinated B_1MABI or B_{29}-MABI in the dark at 18 C for 30 minutes. At the end of the incubation period, the cells were exposed to the appropriate light source for 20-30 seconds. Plasma membrane fraction was then prepared from the cells, solubilized in sodium dodecylsulfate (SDS), reduced with dithiothreitol (DTT) and analyzed by SDS-polyacrylamide gel electrophoresis and radio-autography. The results of this study showed that B_1MABI labelled specifically a 130K and a 40K subunits and that $B_{29}MABI$ labelled in addition a 90K subunit (Figure 1, in-set). The major difference between the use of isolated plasma membranes and isolated intact cells is the labelling of the additional 40K subunit when intact cells were used. We have exhaustively eliminated the possibility that the 40K subunit might be a degradative product of either the 130K or the 90K subunit.

We have further established that the 40K subunits labelled by the two
different photoreactive insulins were different. Thus we (8) have proposed that the insulin receptor of 300K is composed of one 130K, one 90K
and two 40K subunits linked by disulfide bonds. Figure 1 diagram-
matically depicts the proposed receptor model, taking into consideration
the known structure of monomeric insulin, the structural requirements
for biological and receptor binding activity and the location of the
photoreactive groups on the two insulin derivatives. Thus in this model
of the insulin receptor, the 130K subunit is presented as the subunit
intimately interacting with the putative receptor binding region on the
carboxyl terminal sequence of the B-chain (2). As well, the role of the
carboxyl terminus of the A-chain (A-21) (5) and the amino terminal
region of the B-chain (3) in the binding of insulin to its receptor is
shown as direct interaction with the 130K subunit. This proposed subunit structure of the insulin receptor is different from the symmetrical
subunit structure postulated by Czech and coworkers (1) using chemical
bifunctional crosslinker.

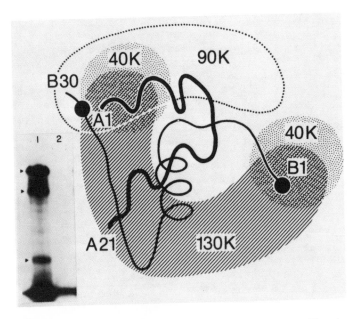

FIG. 1. Proposed model of the 300K insulin receptor. The A and B
chains of insulin are represented by the heavy and light lines respectively, according to Pullen et al. (2). The black dots indicate the
positions (B1 and B29) where the photoreactive azidobenzoyl group is
attached to insulin. The 130K, 90K and 40K subunits are indicated.
In-set:Lane 1. Radioautograph of SDS-PAGE of reduced plasma membranes
from cells photoaffinity labelled with $B_{29}MABI$. The 130K, 90K and 40K
bands are indicated. Lane 2. Same as Lane 1 except an excess of native
insulin was added to the incubation medium.

The 300K receptor is apparently one of three receptor species present on the cell surface. Figure 2, lane 1, shows that three high molecular-weight receptor species were specifically photolabelled by either one of the two photoreactive insulins. The molecular-weights of these three species are estimated to be about 380K, 300K and 230K. Each one of these receptor species is apparently composed of a complement of the three types of subunits since reduction of the individual receptor species gave rise to 130K, 90K and 40K subunits. These observations suggest that the 380K, 300K and 230K receptor species are the native un-reduced forms of the insulin receptors and they are likely related to each other. This relationship is demonstrated by the observation that, after photolabelling, exposure of the cells to sulfhydryl reagent such as N-ethylmaleimide or p-chloromercuriphenylsulfonate resulted in the quantitative conversion of the 230K and 300K forms to the 380K species (Figure 2, lane 2). This conversion was dependent on the concentration of the sulfhydryl reagent in that partial conversion was obtained at low reagent concentration whereas conversion was inhibited at high concentration of the reagent. These data suggest that sulfhydryl groups of different reactivity or accessibility to the reagent play a role in the formation of these three receptor species. These observations are best explained by proposing that the native insulin receptors are of one molecular size of 380K but exist in three partially reduced/oxidized forms in which one or two of the subunits being totally reduced remain associated with the receptor complex but are dissociated in the presence of SDS yielding the 380K, 300K and 230K receptor species. Low concentration of sulfhydryl reagent might have inhibited a factor or factor(s) regulating the partial reduction of the receptor thus allowing the re-oxidation of those subunits. Alkylation of sulfhydryl groups on the reduced subunits occurs at high concentration of reagent thus preventing re-oxidation. The activity of such a factor or factors may in turn be controlled by the metabolic state of the cell or tissue. The relative presence of these three partially reduced receptor forms could well be related to cellular or tissue sensitivity to insulin.

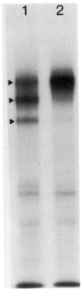

FIG. 2. Lane 1: Radioautograph of gradient SDS-PAGE analysis of unreduced plasma membranes from cells photoaffinity labelled with B_{29}MABI. The 380K, 300K and 230K receptor species are as marked.
Lane 2: Same as Lane 1 except that p-chloromercuri-phenylsulfonate (0.3 mM) was added to the homo-genization buffer used for the preparation of plasma membranes.

REFERENCES

1. Massague,J., Pilch,P.F., and Czech,M.P. (1980): Proc. Natl. Acad. Sci. USA, 77:7137-7141.

2. Pullen,R.A., Lindsay,D.G., Wood,S.P., Tickle,I.J., Blundell,T.L., Wollmer,A., Krail,G., Brandenburg,D., Zahn,H., Gliemann,J., and Gammeltoft,S. (1976): Nature, 259:369-373.

3. Yeung,C.W.T., Moule,M.L., and Yip,C.C. (1979): J. Biol. Chem., 254:9453-9457.

4. Yeung,C.W.T., Moule,M.L., and Yip,C.C. (1980): Biochemistry, 19:2196-2203.

5. Yip,C.C., and Moule,M.L. (1976): Can. J. Biochem., 54:866-871.

6. Yip,C.C., Moule,M.L., and Yeung,C.W.T. (1980): Biochemistry, 19:70-76.

7. Yip,C.C., Yeung,C.W.T., and Moule,M.L. (1980): Biochem. Biophys. Res. Commun., 96:1671-1678.

8. Yip,C.C., Moule,M.L., and Yeung,C.W.T. (1982): Biochemistry, 21:2940-2945.

ACKNOWLEDGEMENT

This work was supported by the Medical Research Council (Canada) and the C.H. Best Foundation. We thank Miss K. Kokolic for her technical assistance.

The Adipocyte and Obesity: Cellular and Molecular Mechanisms, edited by A. Angel, C. H. Hollenberg, and D. A. K. Roncari. Raven Press, New York © 1983.

Lipoprotein Lipase

Thomas Olivecrona and Gunilla Bengtsson

Department of Physiological Chemistry, University of Umea, S-901 87 Umea, Sweden

The major route for lipid acquisition by the adipose tissue is through uptake from circulating lipoproteins. In the lipoprotein this lipid is triglyceride. It is also triglyceride when deposited in the adipocyte. However, it can not be transported from the lipoprotein to the cell as triglyceride. The transfer requires a temporary degradation of the triglycerides to more polar lipids; fatty acids and monoglycerides (45). This degradation is effected by lipoprotein lipase, which thus can be viewed as a transport catalyst. Its activity is hormonally controlled and rises and falls with the energy balance, determining the flow of lipid into the adipose tissue (17) much as the state of the glucose transporter determines the flow of carbohydrate into the tissue (34,46). The role of lipoprotein lipase as a transport catalyst may not be confined to triglyceride transport. Scow et al. (41) have reported that lipoprotein lipase action causes uptake of cholesterol and of phospholipids by the lactating mammary gland. The Steins and their collaborators have recently presented evidence that lipoprotein lipase causes uptake of cholesteryl esters into a variety of cells (27).

Two types of lipoproteins take part in the transport of lipids to the adipose tissue; chylomicrons carrying lipids from the intestine and very low density lipoproteins (VLDL) carrying lipids from the liver. Through the action of lipoprotein lipase most of the triglycerides and some of the phospholipids are removed from the particles which are degraded to cholesteryl ester rich "core remnants" (19). During this process the surface becomes redundant and parts of it are shed from the particles as "surface remnants". Some of the remnants, e.g. the chylomicron core remnants rapidly disappear from the circulation, but most of the remnants stay in the circulation where they are transformed into low density lipoproteins (LDL) and high density lipoproteins (HDL) (19). Thus, the major lipoproteins in plasma are either substrates for or products of lipoprotein lipase action. In the normal individual the number of substrate particles (i.e. chylomicrons and VLDL) is relatively low, whereas the number of product particles is high (LDL and HDL) indicating that the lipoprotein lipase system is working efficiently. In patients deficient in the enzyme there is a massive accumulation of substrate particles and low concentrations of product particles (26).

MOLECULAR PROPERTIES

Lipoprotein lipases have been isolated from several species, but most of the structural work has been carried out with the enzyme from bovine milk. The subunit of this enzyme has a molecular weight of 41,700 (36) and contains 8% carbohydrate (32). The isoelectric point is about 9 (1) so that the enzyme is positively charged at physiological pH. The active form of the enzyme is a dimer (7,32). The subunits are probably

identical; no separation has been achieved and there is only a single
N-terminal residue, aspartic acid (unpublished). The enzyme can be
cleaved in its middle by trypsin (7). This suggests that it is organized
into two separately folded domains. The "nicked" enzyme is catalytically
active and also retains its other properties, although some are modified
(7). Lipoprotein lipase is sparingly soluble and only marginally stable
in buffer solution. This has hampered detailed studies on the enzyme
molecule and its interactions.

Lipoprotein lipases similar to the bovine enzyme have been isolated
from several species (25,37,48), but there are also reports of lipoprotein lipases with significantly lesser molecular sizes and with somewhat
different kinetic properties (16,24). There must be a fairly close relationship between lipoprotein lipases from different tissues since they
show immunological crossreactivity (40,48). We reported several years
ago that antisera raised against the bovine enzyme can completely inhibit
lipoprotein lipase activity in human post-heparin plasma (30). More
recently we have been able to raise more widely crossreacting antisera
which also recognize lipoprotein lipases from rats, mice and guinea pigs.

Studies on the lipoprotein lipase molecule have revealed a number of
interesting interactions. To some of these we can ascribe physiological
functions. The enzyme binds strongly to heparin (35). This affinity is
the basis for most current isolation procedures. We shall see later in
the talk that the heparin binding site on the enzyme may interact in vivo
with heparan sulfate at the capillary endothelium. The enzyme binds
rapidly and reversibly to emulsion droplets (4), liposomes (44) and other
interfaces (33). This reflects the way in which the enzyme acts; before
it can hydrolyze the lipids it must adsorb to the lipid-water interface.
The enzyme forms soluble complexes with fatty acids and with some deter-
gents (3). Fatty acids are the enzyme's main product and their binding
to the enzyme may bring about the strong product inhibition which is
characteristic for lipoprotein lipase (5). It is a well-known fact that
the enzyme's action is accelerated by serum components. In human serum
this property has been shown to reside in apolipoprotein CII; other
species have analogous activator proteins (17,45).

KINETIC PROPERTIES

Lipoprotein lipases have rather low specificity for the chemical
structure of the substrate. The active site is probably similar to that
on several other lipases, for instance pancreatic lipase. The two
properties which distinguish lipoprotein lipase from other lipases are
its stimulation by specific activator proteins and its strong inhibition
by lipolytic products.

When lipoprotein lipase had been purified it could be shown that it
had catalytic activity also in the absence of activator protein (18,22).
Thus, the activator is not required for catalysis. What it does is to
restore the activity under some conditions when the enzyme itself can
not function effectively (Fig. 1) (4). The fact that humans who suffer
a genetic deficiency of apolipoprotein CII have massive hypertriglyceridemia (10) demonstrate that for lipoprotein metabolism in vivo the activator protein is of crucial importance. Studies with model emulsions
have demonstrated two ways in which the activator protein promotes the
enzyme's action. When incubated with a triglyceride-phospholipid
emulsion (Intralipid) the enzyme was found to bind virtually completely
to the lipid droplets whether or not there was activator protein in the

system (Table 1) (4). The rate of hydrolysis was, however, about 6 times higher in the presence than in the absence of activator (Fig. 1). In this type of system the activator must affect enzyme molecules which are already bound to the lipid droplets, making them catalytically more efficient. For this effect, it is not necessary that the activator protein itself binds to the lipid droplets, as demonstrated by studies using synthetic fragments of apolipoprotein CII (12,45). Further support for the concept was derived from experiments in which the enzyme was cleaved in its middle by mild tryptic digestion (7). The "nicked" molecule retained its overall physicochemical properties although there was a small change in circular dichroism indicating loss of helical structure (36). The "nicked" enzyme had very low activity against Intralipid (Fig. 2), although it bound to the lipid droplets. In contrast, the catalytic activity against soluble substrates was unchanged (7). Our interpretation is as follows: for effective catalysis it is not enough that the lipid binding part of lipoprotein lipase binds to the interface, but the active site region must also become properly oriented with respect to the interface. This orientation can be partially achieved by the native enzyme

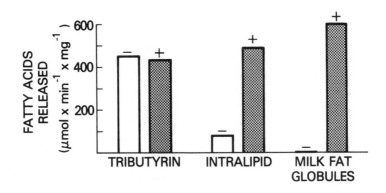

FIG. 1. Effect of apolipoprotein CII on the activity of lipoprotein lipase against three different triglyceride emulsions. The incubations were carried out at pH 8.5, 25°C with lipoprotein lipase purified from bovine milk. Data on tributyrin are from ref. 39, data on Intralipid are from ref. 4. For hydrolysis of milk fat globules, bovine milk was heated for 15 min at 65°C to inactivate the endogenous lipase. To 0.7 ml of this milk was added 0.3 ml bovine serum albumin (30 mg/ml) in 0.5 M Tris-Cl buffer, with (+) or without (-) apolipoprotein CII (final concentration 8 μg/ml), and the reaction was started by addition of the purified lipase. Note that the activity with CII present was similar in all three systems. With tributyrin as substrate the same high activity was obtained also without CII, but with the other two substrates the activity was depressed.

but virtually not at all by the cleaved enzyme. The proteolytic cleavage presumably results in a more flexible molecule, and may well interfere with the cooperation between the lipid-binding region and the active site region. A plausible role for the activator protein is to bring the enzyme into the proper orientation; this effect becomes more marked with the cleaved enzyme (Fig. 2).

With bovine milk fat globules as the substrate we get a different picture. We use milk as a convenient source of biologically packaged triglycerides with no activator protein, i.e., as a model for CII-deficient chylomicrons. In this system the enzyme does not bind to the lipid droplets (Table 1), and there is virtually no hydrolysis (Fig. 1). Addition of activator protein causes binding of the enzyme (Table 1), and rapid hydrolysis ensues (Fig. 1). That the activator can promote binding of the lipase to lipid droplets has been directly demonstrated by Posner (38).

We do not think these are two distinct mechanisms, but rather that they are two aspects of the same underlying phenomenon - a protein--protein interaction between the enzyme and the activator. The first situation, when the enzyme binds but has low activity in the absence of activator illustrates that the enzyme at the interface can exist in at

TABLE 1.   Effect of apolipoprotein CII on the binding of lipoprotein lipase to lipid droplets.

Substrate	Apolipoprotein CII	^{125}I-lipoprotein lipase in top phase (%)	Lipase activity in top phase (%)
Intralipid	-	92	70
"	+	85	72
Milk fat globules	-	< 1	< 1
"	+	16	12

1 ml heat-inactivated bovine milk or 1 ml 0.15M NaCl containing triglyceride-rich particles from Intralipid (6 mg triglyceride) was mixed with 0.45 ml bovine serum albumin (100 mg/ml in 0.5 M Tris-Cl buffer pH 8.0) with or without human apolipoprotein CII (8 µg). 150 mg sucrose was dissolved in each sample. A trace amount of ^{125}I-labeled lipoprotein lipase (15,000 cpm, 30 ng) and 1.5 µg unlabeled lipoprotein lipase was added. Then 1 ml of sample was layered under 4 ml 0.15 M NaCl, 10 mM Tris-Cl ph 8.0 containing 1 mg bovine serum albumin/ml. The tubes were centrifuged 25,000 rpm for 20 min at 15°C in a Beckman SW 50.1 rotor. The top layer (1 ml) containing a thin lipid cake was recovered after slicing the tubes. The fat cake was resuspended and aliquots taken for determination of ^{125}I-radioactivity and of lipoprotein lipase activity. The radioactivity is expressed as percent of the total radioactivity in the tube. The lipase activity is expressed as percent of that added. See Fig. 1 for the activity expressed by lipoprotein lipase against Intralipid and against milk fat globules. Note that with Intralipid there is binding of the lipase to the fat droplets and enzyme activity in the absence of activator, but with the fat globules there is virtually no binding and no activity. Here, the activator is required for binding and activity.

least two conformational states which differ in catalytic efficiency. The activator probably acts by preferential binding to the catalytically most effective state, thus driving the equilibrium in its favour. In the other situation when the enzyme itself is virtually unable to bind to the interface, it is apparent that formation of a complex with an activator molecule bound to the interface can add sufficient energy to accomplish binding of the enzyme.

While we are beginning to get some insight into the molecular mechanism by which the activator promotes enzyme activity, we do not know what the biological function is. It appears unlikely that the level of activator in normal individuals serves to modulate enzyme activity; there is usually an excess of activator (20). We find the observation that the enzyme alone is virtually unable to attack milk fat globules (Fig. 1) interesting. This suggests that the need for activator protein is a safety mechanism built into the lipoprotein lipase system. The enzyme should not attack tissue lipids such as those within adipocytes or in milk fat globules, but its activity should be restricted to its proper substrate, the plasma lipoproteins.

Another aspect of enzyme control is the product inhibition (42). Some inhibition by lipolytic products is seen with most lipases. This is because forward and back reactions, i.e. hydrolysis and esterification

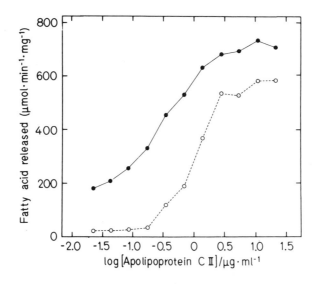

FIG. 2. Dose-response curve for the activation of native and of trypsin-treated lipoprotein lipase by apolipoprotein CII. Data from ref. (7). (●) native and (O) trypsin-treated lipoprotein lipase. The substrate was Intralipid pretreated with phospholipase A_2. The activities without CII were not significantly different from those showed for the lowest dose. Note that the activity of the trypsin-treated enzyme was much lower than that of the native enzyme, but the activity could be restored by CII.

approach an equilibrium (9). However, the inhibition is particularly
marked for lipoprotein lipases indicating that additional factors contribute (5). Two such factors have been identified, namely that fatty
acids abolish the lipolysis promoting effects of the activator protein
(2,5) and that fatty acids displace the lipase into solution (5), presumably through formation of soluble enzyme-fatty acid complexes. The
strong product inhibition may serve as a feed-back control of the entire
transport process. If, during degradation of a lipoprotein at the endothelium, the capacity of the tissue to utilize the fatty acids is
exceeded, lipolysis immediately slows down, and the particle dissociates
from the enzyme and goes back into the circulation.

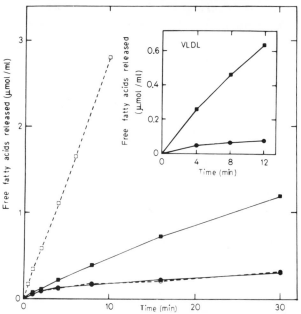

FIG. 3. Lack of effect of apolipoprotein CII when there is no fatty
acid acceptor in the system. Data from ref. 5. The substrate was a
phospholipid stabilized emulsion of triolein. (□) CII and albumin,
(■) albumin but no CII, (O) CII but no albumin, (●) no CII or
albumin. The insert shows an experiment with human VLDL as substrate
(■) with albumin. (●) no albumin. Note that with albumin present,
CII caused an about 5-fold stimulation of hydrolysis, but without
albumin there was no effect.

ACTION ON LIPOPROTEINS

In man the major transport of triglycerides to the adipose tissue
probably occurs with the chylomicrons. Let us consider the actual events
involved in this triglyceride transport. A chylomicron contains several
million molecules triglyceride and has a residence time in the circulation of less than 10 min (29). During this time at least 90% of the triglycerides are hydrolyzed. That such rapid hydrolysis can in fact take
place has been directly demonstrated in vitro with rat chylomicrons and
lipoprotein lipase (42). Assuming that the clearing of a typical
chylomicron requires 6×10^6 hydrolytic events in 10 min, we can

calculate that 15 lipase molecules must act continuously on the particle (the turnover number of the enzyme is about 650 sec^{-1}). Since the particle spends much of its time in the circulating blood the number of lipase molecules which act on the particle during the time it is at the endothelium must in fact be higher. Expriments with model emulsions have shown that an individual lipase-particle interaction is relatively short--lived (unpublished). However, interaction with several lipase molecules attached to the endothelium should have a cooperative effect and result in a more long-lived interaction. It may well be that a large chylomicron which interacts with perhaps 20 or 30 lipase molecules remains at the endothelium until the reaction is terminated by product inhibition or until the particle is reduced in size and its composition/ surface structure is sufficiently changed (19) to break the interaction.

Consider instead a VLDL. Such a particle typically contains less than 15,000 triglyceride molecules; they could be hydrolyzed by a single lipase molecule in less than one min. That triglycerides in human VLDL can in fact be hydrolyzed by lipoprotein lipase at this rate had been directly demonstrated (4). One min is much less than the residence time for VLDL particles in the circulation, which in man is several hours (19). Thus, in contrast to a chylomicron, a VLDL probably spends only a short fraction of its life-time in contact with lipoprotein lipase at the endothelium. The degradation can easily be accomplished by several short--lived interactions with a single lipase molecule. In vivo studies have shown a precursor-product relationship between circulating large and small VLDL particles (19). This suggests that the metabolism occurs as a series of interactions of the particles with lipoprotein lipase at the endothelium. After any given interaction, a particle depleted of some of its triglycerides is released back into the blood stream. This particle will then interact again with the enzyme at another site, until it is finally depleted of most of its triglycerides.

LIPOPROTEIN LIPASE AT THE ENDOTHELIUM

Some years ago we proposed that lipoprotein lipase is attached to the capillary endothelium via a membrane associated polyanion, probably heparan sulphate (35). This proposal was based on the demonstration in model systems that the enzyme has an affinity for this polysaccharide (6) and on considerations of the known properties of the enzyme at the endothelium. The hypothesis has since received support from several other groups who have studied binding of lipoprotein lipase to cultured endothelial cells (11,15,43). These studies have demonstrated that the binding can be virtually abolished by treating the cells with enzymes which degrade heparan sulphate. Furthermore, it has been directly demonstrated that the enzyme is catalytically active and can interact with apolipoprotein CII while it is bound to heparin (8). The hypothesis is attractive since it can reconcile the known functional properties of the enzyme at the endothelium with the known molecular properties of purified lipoprotein lipase. It provides a ready explanation for the release of the lipase into the circulation by heparin; heparin is a stronger ligand than heparan sulphate (6). The model allows the enzyme to bind to the lipoprotein with its lipid binding part, yet remain firmly anchored to the endothelium via the electrostatic interaction with heparan sulphate. The model is also in accord with two other observations, namely that the kinetic properties of the enzyme at the endothelium are similar to those for the soluble enzyme (23) and that

only a small fraction of the enzyme is carried into the circulating blood
with the partially lipolyzed lipoprotein particles (21). It is of
interest to consider also how the substrate lipoprotein interacts with
the endothelium. The endothelial cells are covered by a layer of polysaccharide chains extending from cell-associated glycoproteins and glyco-
lipids, the so called glycocalyx. Small water-soluble molecules can
relatively easily diffuse through this layer. However, the situation is
different for lipoprotein particles. Their initial interaction must be
with the polysaccharide chains. Chylomicrons and VLDL themselves can
bind to heparan sulphate and other acid polysaccharides (31). In this
perspective it appears logical that lipoprotein lipase is placed within
the glycocalyx. The lipoprotein may travel through the vascular bed with
frequent short-lived interactions with polysaccharides on the endothelial
cells looking for sites where there is also lipase. Here the particles
stay longer and go through hydrolysis.

METABOLISM OF LIPOPROTEIN LIPASE

There is much evidence to demonstrate that the active lipase at the
endothelium is rapidly turned over, but the mechanism for this is not
known. In the rat half-lives as short as 30 min have been reported (13).
The most obvious possibility would be that the enzyme is degraded by the
endothelial cells. However, studies with cultured endothelial cells have
emphasized that the enzyme is relatively stable; there is no evidence for
rapid degradation (11,15,43). This leaves us with two other possibilities; that the enzyme is detached into the circulating blood or that the
enzyme is taken up and degraded by other cells in the tissue.

To explore the first possibility we injected labeled lipase intravenously. This lipase rapidly disappeared from the circulating blood
with a half-life of about 1 min (47). Most of it was taken up by the
liver. Heparin markedly retarded the removal of the enzyme from the
circulation, thus explaining why a high and persistant enzyme activity is
found in post-heparin plasma. The nature and properties of the receptor
mediating the hepatic uptake of lipoprotein lipase is presently not known.
However, it is clear that if lipoprotein lipase becomes dislodged from
the endothelium into the circulating blood it will rapidly and efficiently be taken up by the liver. Whether this is a normal route of enzyme
metabolism or is a safety mechanism to clear the blood from any lipase
that may accidentally come loose in the blood is not known. ^{125}I-labeled
The Steins and their collaborators have demonstrated that
lipoprotein lipase interacts with various cells in culture by being
bound to their cellular surface, internalized and degraded (14,28). This
process was particularly rapid and extensive in heart cells and in preadipocytes (14), cells which are known to produce lipoprotein lipase.
This suggests that transport of the lipase may occur in both directions,
i.e not only from the lipase-producing cells to the endothelium, but also
from the endothelium back to the cells. This process can be viewed as
analogous to the recirculation of membrane receptors within a cell, but
for lipoprotein lipase the process may also involve transfer between
cells. Insulin affects glucose transport in the adipocyte by shifting
the glucose transporter from intracellular membranes to the plasma membrane (34,46). In a similar manner, hormones could affect lipid transport
to the adipocyte by shifting the lipase recycling system towards the
endothelium.

Acknowledgements. The work reported from the authors' own laboratory was supported by the Swedish Medical Research Council (13x-727). Thomas Olivecrona is presently a Visiting Scientist at the National Institutes of Health, Bethesda, Md., USA. We thank Mrs. Dorothy Connolly for preparing the manuscript.

REFERENCES

1. Bengtsson, G., and Olivecrona, T. (1977): In: Electrofocusing and Isotachophoresis, edited by B.J. Radola and D. Graesslin, pp. 189-195. de Gruyter, Berlin.
2. Bengtsson, G. and Olivecrona, T. (1979): FEBS Lett., 106:345-348.
3. Bengtsson, G., and Olivecrona, T. (1979): Biochim. Biophys. Acta, 575:471-474.
4. Bengtsson, G., and Olivecrona, T. (1980): Eur. J. Biochem., 106:549-555.
5. Bengtsson, G., and Olivecrona, T. (1980): Eur. J. Biochem., 106:557-562.
6. Bengtsson, G., Olivecrona, T., Höök, M., Riesenfeld, J. and Lindahl, U. (1980): Biochem. J., 189:625-633.
7. Bengtsson, G., and Olivecrona, T. (1981): Eur. J. Biochem., 113:547-554.
8. Bengtsson, G., and Olivecrona, T. (1981): FEBS Lett., 128:9-12.
9. Borgström, B. (1964): J. Lipid Res., 5:522-531.
10. Breckenridge, W.C., Little, J.A., Steiner, G., Chow, A., and Poapst, (1978): N. Engl. J. Med., 298:1265-1273.
11. Brown, W.V., Wang-Iverson, P., and Paterniti, J.R. (1981): In: Chemistry and Biology of Heparin, edited by R.L. Lundblad, W.V. Brown, K.G. Mann, and H.R. Roberts, pp. 175-185. North Holland, New York.
12. Catapano, A.L., Kinnunen, P.K.J., Breckenridge, W.C., Gotto, A.M., Jackson, R.L., Little, J.A., Smith, L.C., and Sparrow, J.T. (1979): Biochem. Biophys. Res. Commun., 89:951-957.
13. Chajek, T., Stein, O., and Stein, Y. (1978): Biochim. Biophys. Acta, 528:456-465.
14. Chajek-Shaul, T., Friedman, G., Stein, O., Olivecrona, T., and Stein, Y. (1982): Biochim. Biophys. Acta (in press).
15. Cheng, C-F., Oosta, G.M., Bensadoun, A., and Rosenberg, R.D. (1981): J. Biol. Chem. 256:12893-12898.
16. Chung, J., and Scanu, A.M. (1977): J. Biol. Chem., 252:4202-4209.
17. Cryer, A. (1981): Int. J. Biochem., 13:525-541.
18. Egelrud, T., and Olivecrona, T. (1973): Biochim. Biophys. Acta, 306:115-127.
19. Eisenberg, S. (1979): In: Progr. Biochem. Pharmacol., edited by S. Eisenberg, pp. 139-165. Karger, Basel.
20. Erkelens, D.W., Brunzell, J.D., and Bierman, E.L. (1979): Metabolism, 28:495-501.
21. Felts, J.M., Itakura, H., and Crane, T.R. (1975): Biochem. Biophys. Res. Commun., 66:1467-1475.
22. Fielding, C.J. (1970): Biochim. Biophys. Acta, 206:109-117.
23. Fielding, C.J., and Higgins, J.M. (1974): Biochemistry, 13:4324-4330.
24. Fielding, P.E., Shore, V.G., and Fielding, C.J. (1974): Biochemistry, 13:4318-4323.

25. Fielding, P.E., Shore, V.G., and Fielding, C.J. (1977): Biochemistry, 16:1896-1900.
26. Fredrickson, D.S., Goldstein, J.L., and Brown, M.S. (1978): In: The Metabolic Basis of Inherited Disease, edited by J.B. Wyngaarden and D.S. Fredrickson, pp. 604-655. McGraw Hill, New York.
27. Friedman, G., Chajek-Shaul, T., Stein, O., Olivecrona, T., and Stein, Y. (1981): Biochim. Biophys. Acta, 666:156-164.
28. Friedman, G., Chajek-Shaul, T., Olivecrona, T., Stein, O., and Stein, Y. (1982): Biochim. Biophys. Acta, 711:114-122.
29. Grundy, S.M., and Mok, H.Y.I. (1976): Metabolism, 25:1225-1239.
30. Hernell, O., Egelrud, T., and Olivecrona, T. (1975): Biochim. Biophys. Acta, 381:233-241.
31. Iverius, P-H. (1972): J. Biol. Chem., 247:2607-2613.
32. Iverius, P-H., and Östlund-Lindquist, A-M. (1976): J. Biol. Chem., 251:7791-7795.
33. Jackson, R.L., Pattus, F., and deHaas, G. (1980): Biochemistry, 19:373-378.
34. Karnieli, E., Zarnowski, M.J., Hissin, P.J., Simpson, I.A., Salans, L.B., and Cushman, S.W. (1981): J. Biol. Chem., 256: 4772-4777.
35. Olivecrona, T., Bengtsson, G., Marklund, S-E., Lindahl, U., and Höök, M. (1977): Fed. Proc., 36:60-65.
36. Olivecrona, T., Bengtsson, G., and Osborne, J.C. (1982): Eur. J. Biochem., (in press).
37. Östlund-Lindquist, A-M. (1979): Biochem. J., 179:555-559.
38. Posner, I. (1980): Acta Cient. Venezolana, 31:318-323.
39. Rapp, D., and Olivecrona, T. (1978): Eur. J. Biochem., 91:379-385.
40. Schotz, M.C., Twu, J.S., Pedersen, M.E., Chen, C.H., Garfinkel, A.S., and Borensztain, J. (1977): Biochim. Biophys. Acta, 489:217-227.
41. Scow, R.O., Chernick, S.S., and Fleck, T.R. (1977): Biochim. Biophys. Acta, 487:297-306.
42. Scow, R.O., and Olivecrona, T. (1977): Biochim. Biophys. Acta, 487:472-486.
43. Shimada, K., Gill, P-J., Silbert, J.E., Douglas, W.H.J., and Fanburg, B.L. (1981): J. Clin. Invest., 68:995-1002.
44. Shirai, K., Matsuoka, N., and Jackson, R.L. (1981): Biochim. Biophys. Acta, 665:504-510.
45. Smith, L.C., and Scow, R.O. (1979): In: Progr. Biochem. Pharmacol, edited by S. Eisenberg, vol. 15, pp. 109-138. Karger, Basel.
46. Suzuki, K., and Kono, T. (1980): Proc. Natl. Acad. Sci., USA, 77:2542-2545.
47. Wallinder, L., Bengtsson, G., and Olivecrona, T. (1979): Biochim. Biophys. Acta, 575:166-173.
48. Wallinder, L., Bengtsson, G., and Olivecrona, T. (1982): Biochim. Biophys. Acta, 711:107-113.

The Adipocyte and Obesity: Cellular and Molecular Mechanisms, edited by A. Angel, C. H. Hollenberg, and D. A. K. Roncari. Raven Press, New York © 1983.

Hormonal Control of Rat Adipose Tissue Lipoprotein Lipase Activity

Donald S. Robinson, Susan M. Parkin, Brian K. Speake and John A. Little

Department of Biochemistry, University of Leeds, Leeds, LS2 9JT England

Lipoprotein lipase determines the rate of removal of triacylglycerol fatty acids from the bloodstream by the extrahepatic tissues and also, through tissue-specific variations in its activity, controls the sites of their tissue uptake (21). Several such variations in activity have been reported in response to alterations in physiological conditions and of particular interest in the context of the present meeting is the rise in the activity of the adipose tissue enzyme that is associated with the obese state in man and in experimental animals. Such an increase could be determined, directly or indirectly, by hormonal action and in this paper we, therefore, summarize our recent studies on the hormonal regulation of the activity of the enzyme in rat adipose tissue.

The activity of lipoprotein lipase in adipose tissue *in vivo* is high in the fed state and falls on starvation. In previous work we have shown that the low activity in adipose tissue from starved rats increases progressively towards the fed level when the intact tissue is incubated in appropriate media *in vitro* and several hormonal effects on this increase have been observed (22). Of particular interest are the effects of insulin and glucocorticoids in promoting the increase by protein synthesis-dependent mechanisms (1,2). In addition, the protein-synthesis independent activation of the enzyme that occurs in the presence of glucose and certain other sugars is prevented or reversed by catecholamines (1,20).

The synthesis of lipoprotein lipase in adipose tissue occurs in the fat cell component of the tissue. Thereafter it is secreted and transported, by an unknown pathway and mechanism, to the luminal surfaces of the endothelial cells lining the blood capillaries where it is probably bound by heparin-like proteoglycans and where *in vivo* it exerts its action on the triacylglycerols of circulating chylomicrons and very low density lipoproteins (18,22,23,24). At the time of its removal from the animal, or following its incubation in a particular medium *in vitro*, therefore, the tissue will contain lipoprotein lipase in a number of intracellular compartments within the fat cell, as well as at various extracellular sites. In such circumstances, the total activity of the enzyme measured in the tissue will not only represent the sum of the individual activities at these various locations but will also reflect the dynamic balance of hormonal and non-hormonal effects being exerted on the synthesis/degradation and the activation/inactivation of the enzyme.

In the light of the foregoing considerations, we have formulated a working hypothesis for the hormonal control of adipose tissue lipoprotein lipase as shown in Fig. 1 (1). This involves:

a) control of the synthesis of pro-enzyme within the fat cell by glucocorticoids, insulin and probably other hormones

b) post-translational modification of the pro-enzyme by a glucose-dependent process that is associated with an increase in its specific activity

c) inactivation that is catecholamine-mediated and that occurs before secretion from the fat cell and transport to the enzyme's functional site at the endothelial cell surface.

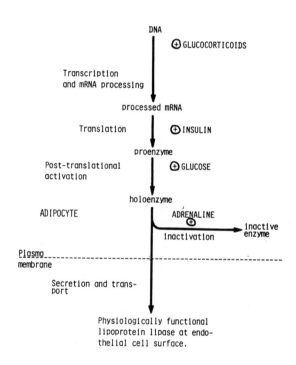

FIG. 1., Scheme for synthesis, secretion and control of lipoprotein lipase in adipose tissue.

The scheme in Fig. 1 clearly does not exclude the possibility of additional sites and mechanisms of control of the enzyme's activity. For example, it is known that in fed rats the adipose tissue enzyme *in vivo* has a rapid rate of turnover since its activity falls following the injection of cycloheximide with a half-life of less than 1 h (22). This rapid decline may be related to the marked instability of the enzyme that has been observed under a variety of conditions *in vitro*. Alterations in the stability of the enzyme in particular cellular or extracellular compartments could, therefore, also play a role in the regulation of the enzyme's functional activity.

PURIFICATION AND IDENTIFICATION OF RAT ADIPOSE TISSUE LIPOPROTEIN LIPASE

Antibodies to lipoprotein lipase have been raised against the enzyme in a variety of tissues and animals. However, in our own work we have not been successful in attempts to raise antibodies to the enzyme in rat adipose tissue. In these circumstances, we have been obliged in further studies on the control of the activity of lipoprotein lipase to utilize preparations of the rat adipose tissue enzyme that have been extracted from the delipidated tissue, purified by affinity chromatography on heparin-Sepharose and subsequently analysed by SDS/polyacrylamide-gel electrophoresis. Purification of lipoprotein lipase by its adsorption on heparin-Sepharose columns and its subsequent elution with concentrations of NaCl greater than 1 M has been widely used in work on the enzyme from other sources (see, for example, 3,7,9,10,26). However, it should be noted that the reported subunit molecular weight of the major polypeptide component shown by SDS/gel electrophoresis to be present in such eluates after heparin-Sepharose chromatography has varied between 55 000 and 74 000. Moreover, it has been recently reported that lipoprotein lipase preparations purified from post-heparin plasma by such procedures are heavily contaminated by anti-thrombin (19), which behaves similarly to lipoprotein lipase on heparin-Sepharose chromatography and which has a subunit molecular weight of about 65 000 (12).

When rat adipose tissue lipoprotein lipase, purified by heparin-Sepharose chromatography, was examined by SDS/polyacrylamide-gel electrophoresis, two major bands corresponding to polypeptides with molecular weights of 62 000 and 56 000, were routinely observed (Fig. 2a). The following studies were carried out to determine which of these two bands represented lipoprotein lipase.

(a) There is immunological evidence (11) that the decline in rat adipose tissue lipoprotein lipase that occurs on starvation is due to a fall in the amount of enzyme protein present in the tissue. Fig. 2b shows that only the intensity of staining of the 56 000 molecular weight polypeptide band on SDS/polyacrylamide-gel electrophoresis is reduced in starved animals.

(b) Östlund-Lindqvist & Boberg (19) employed heparin-Sepharose columns prepared with fractionated heparin that had a low affinity for anti-thrombin to prepare anti-thrombin-free lipoprotein lipase from post-heparin plasma. When rat adipose tissue lipoprotein lipase was applied to such columns and eluted with 2 M-NaCl, SDS/polyacrylamide-gel electrophoresis of the 2 M-NaCl eluate showed the presence of only a single major polypeptide band of 56 000 molecular weight (Fig. 2c).

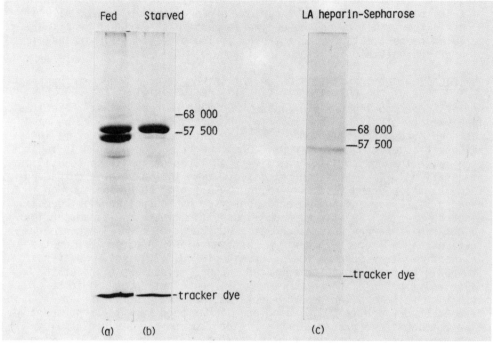

FIG. 2., SDS/polyacrylamide-gel electrophoresis of lipoprotein lipase
Acetone/ether-dried preparations of rat epididymal adipose tissue were
extracted in 5 mM-sodium barbital, pH 7.5,containing 20% glycerol and
0.1% Triton X-100. The extract was applied to a heparin-Sepharose 4B
column equilibrated with 5 mM-sodium barbital, pH 7.5, containing 20%
glycerol. The column was washed with the equilibration buffer and then
with the same buffer containing 0.7 M-NaCl. Finally, lipoprotein lipase
was eluted in a single peak with the equilibration buffer containing
2 M-NaCl. Fractions of the eluate containing the enzyme were dialysed
against 5 mM-NH_4HCO_3, pH 8.0,and freeze dried. The freeze-dried protein
was dissolved in 50 mM-Tris/HCl, pH 6.7, containing SDS (1%), mercapto-
ethanol (1%) and glycerol (10%), and analysed by SDS/polyacrylamide-gel
electrophoresis. Parallel separations of bovine serum albumin (mol. wt.
68 000) and bovine liver catalase (mol. wt. 57 500) were carried out and
the position of these marker proteins is shown. Lane (a): enzyme from
glucose-fed rats, 30 μg protein load. Lane (b): enzyme from 48 h-starved
rats from the same batch as used in (a), 18 μg protein load. Lane (c):
enzyme from glucose-fed rats but fractionated on heparin-Sepharose
columns prepared using heparin with a low affinity for anti-thrombin,
5 μg protein load.

(c) Lipoprotein lipase is inhibited completely by 1 mM-diisopropyl phosphofluoridate (DFP) (4), presumably by covalent interaction with a serine group at the active site of the enzyme. Heparin-Sepharose purified preparations of the enzyme from the adipose tissue of both fed and starved rats were, therefore, exposed to ^{3}H-labelled DFP and then analysed by SDS/polyacrylamide-gel electrophoresis. In both preparations, most of the radioactivity was associated with the polypeptide band of 56 000 apparent molecular weight, present only in the preparation from fed rats, rather than with the 62 000 molecular weight band (results not shown). Moreover, the ratio of the counts in the 56 000 molecular weight band in the two preparations was approximately the same (5:1) as that of the enzyme activities in the two original tissue extracts.

The foregoing experiments lead us to conclude that adipose tissue lipoprotein lipase is represented by the polypeptide band of 56 000 molecular weight, while that of 62 000 molecular weight represents contaminating anti-thrombin.

HORMONAL EFFECTS ON SYNTHESIS

In order to investigate the specificity of the effects of insulin and of glucocorticoids on the synthesis of lipoprotein lipase we have compared the rates of incorporation of radioactively-labelled leucine into total adipose tissue protein and into the presumed lipoprotein lipase polypeptide of 56 000 molecular weight, separated after heparin-Sepharose chromatography and SDS/polyacrylamide-gel electrophoresis. In these experiments intact adipose tissue from starved rats was incubated at 37°C in a medium containing salts, amino acids and glucose in the presence or absence of additional insulin and/or dexamethasone.

The results in Fig.3 and Table 1 show that, in the presence of insulin, incorporations of radioactivity into total adipose protein and into the '56 000' polypeptide are stimulated to approximately equivalent extents. However, when both insulin and dexamethasone are present, there is an additional and specific stimulation of incorporation into the '56 000' polypeptide. By comparison with the known effects of insulin and glucocorticoids in other tissues, these results may be interpreted as suggesting that dexamethasone specifically stimulates the transcription of the lipoprotein lipase gene but that insulin's effect is due to its non-specific stimulation of total mRNA translation. Consistent with this is the finding that the stimulation of labelled-leucine incorporation into the polypeptide band of 56 000 molecular weight in the presence of insulin and dexamethasone together was greatest after a lag period of about three hours; whereas the stimulation by insulin alone of incorporation into both total adipose tissue protein and into the '56 000' polypeptide was evident within two hours (results not shown). Further studies are evidently necessary to extend these findings. In particular, to exclude the possibility that the results may be due, at least in part, to hormonal effects on the degradation of the enzyme.

CATECHOLAMINE EFFECTS ON INACTIVATION

Previous studies have shown that the rise in the lipoprotein lipase activity of adipose tissue from starved rats during incubation in the presence of insulin is prevented when catecholamines are also present

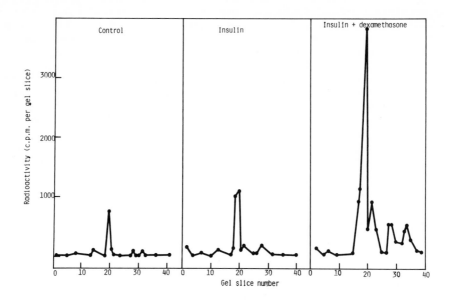

FIG. 3., Hormonal effects on lipoprotein lipase synthesis. Groups of 8 epididymal fat bodies from 24 h-starved rats were incubated for 6 h at 37°C. The incubation medium (20 ml)consisted of Krebs-Henseleit bicarb- onate buffer,pH7.4,under CO_2/O_2(19:1) supplemented with glucose (10 mM) and an amino acid mixture containing L-[4,5-^{3}H]leucine (250 μCi).Insulin (2 m-i.u./ml) and dexamethasone (400 nM) were present where indicated. Radio-labelled lipoprotein lipase was purified and analysed by SDS/poly- acrylamide-gel electrophoresis as described in Fig.2. The distribution of radioactivity was determined by scintillation counting of gel slices (0.2 cm) after their solubilization in H_2O_2. In each case the major peaks of radioactivity coincided with the position of the polypeptide band of 56 000 molecular weight.

TABLE 1. Effects of insulin and dexamethasone on the synthesis of total adipose tissue protein and lipoprotein lipase[a]

Hormone present	Fold increase in incorporation over that in incubations without hormones	
	Total protein	Lipoprotein lipase
Insulin	1.6 ± 0.12	2.5 ± 0.67
Insulin + dexamethasone	1.3 ± 0.23	5.0 ± 1.8

[a]Four experiments were carried out as described in the legend to Fig.3. Additionally incorporation of radioactivity into total adipose tissue protein was determined. Insulin and dexamethasone were present as indicated. The values are means ± S.D.

in the medium (22). Moreover, even when protein synthesis is inhibited
by cycloheximide, the activation of the enzyme,which still occurs under
such circumstances during incubations in the presence of glucose, is prevented or reversed when adrenaline is also present. These effects of
adrenaline are rapid and are potentiated by theophylline, a phosphodiesterase inhibitor, and are mimicked by dibutyrylcyclic AMP and by isoproterenol, a β agonist (1,2 and Fig.4). However, previous attempts to
demonstrate a direct role of cyclic AMP-dependent protein kinase in the
regulation of the enzyme have been unsuccessful (25). Moreover, in more
recent studies we have exposed the heparin-Sepharose purified enzyme,as
well as the enzyme in aqueous homogenates and in delipidated preparations
of adipose tissue, to catalytic sub-unit of cAMP-dependent protein kinase
under a variety of conditions in the presence of ATP without obtaining
any convincing evidence for a direct effect of the kinase on the enzyme's
activity.

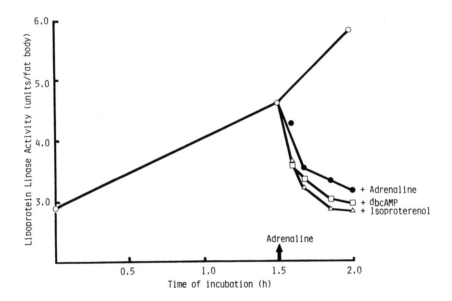

FIG. 4., Inactivation of lipoprotein lipase. Groups of 4 epididymal fat
bodies from 24 h-starved rats were incubated at 25°C. The incubation
medium (10 ml) was as in Fig.3 except that bovine serum albumin (2%) and
cycloheximide (36 μM) were present and insulin and dexamethasone were
omitted (○). After 1.5 h, adrenaline, (10 μM)(●), isoproterenol, (10 μM),
(△) or dibutrylcylic AMP, (1 mM), (□) were added as indicated. Lipoprotein lipase was determined in acetone/ether-dried preparations of the
fat bodies and medium combined at the times shown.

   In the above circumstances two other possible explanations for the
action of catecholamines may be considered. One is that the activation of
adipose tissue mobilizing lipase by the induced rise in cyclic AMP leads
to increased intracellular triacylglycerol hydrolysis and a consequent
rise in the cellular free fatty acid (FFA) concentration. Nikkilä &
Pykalistö (14) first proposed that such an increase might lead to the
inactivation of lipoprotein lipase and in support of this view they
noted that nicotinic acid, which inhibits the activation of mobilizing

lipase by adrenaline, brings about a rise in adipose tissue lipoprotein lipase activity as it lowers the intracellular FFA concentration (15). More recently adenosine has been reported to have similar effects (16). Such findings do not positively identify FFA as the agents responsible for the cyclic AMP-mediated effects of adrenaline. However, we have recently found that, in experiments similar to those reported in Fig.4, the addition of palmitic acid (2 mM) to the incubation medium can mimic the inactivating effect of adrenaline on lipoprotein lipase under appropriate conditions (results not shown).

The second possibility for the cyclic AMP-mediated inactivation of lipoprotein lipase that we have considered derives from the finding that the fusion of intracellular vesicles with lysosomes is stimulated by a rise in cyclic AMP concentration (5,13). In the light of this, we have carried out experiments to explore the effects of inhibitors of lysosomal activity on the adrenaline-mediated inactivation of the enzyme. Three such inhibitors, ammonia, methylamine and ethylamine, have been found to partially or wholly prevent such inactivation: see Fig.5 for the effect of ammonia. This is consistent with a stimulation of lysosomal activity by adrenaline which could bring about a diversion to the lysosomes of vesicles that were normally carrying lipoprotein lipase *en route* to secretion from the fat cell. If this were so, however, and the enzyme was then degraded by peptidase action, it might be expected that the lysosomal peptidase inhibitor, leupeptin, would mimic the effects of ammonia. In fact, as the results in Fig.5 also show, this is not the case and it appears, therefore, that lysosomal proteolytic activity is probably not involved. One interpretation of the findings would be that it is simply the low pH of the lysosomes, which would be raised in the presence of ammonia, methylamine and ethylamine (6,17), that is responsible for the inactivation of the enzyme. Experiments to test this, and to explore the further possibility that a rise in intracellular FFA may promote lysosomal fusion, are in progress.

SUMMARY

Evidence is presented that preparations of rat adipose tissue lipoprotein lipase purified by heparin-Sepharose chromatography are contaminated with anti-thrombin but that the enzyme protein band can be identified following SDS/polyacrylamide-gel electrophoresis.

Synthesis of the enzyme, as measured by the incorporation of radioactively-labelled amino acids, is increased during incubations of adipose tissue from starved animals in the presence of insulin but the stimulation is similar to that of total adipose tissue protein synthesis. On the other hand, in the presence of insulin and dexamethasone together, there is a much more marked and specific increase in lipoprotein lipase synthesis.

The mechanism of action of catecholamines in inactivating adipose tissue lipoprotein lipase remains unknown, as indeed does the physiological significance of such inactivation (see, for example, 8). Present evidence is consistent with the effect being mediated by cyclic AMP, either through an induced rise in the fat cell FFA concentration or by promoting the fusion of lysosomes with intracellular vesicles carrying lipoprotein lipase *en route* to secretion from the fat cell.

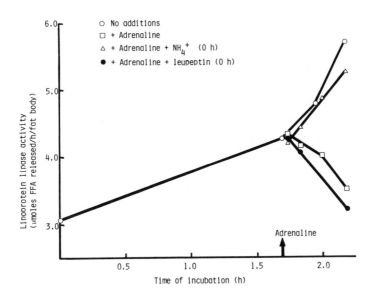

FIG. 5., Effects of NH_4Cl and leupeptin on the inactivation of lipoprotein lipase by adrenaline. Groups of epididymal fat bodies were incubated
as in Fig. 4 (○). In some incubations, NH_4Cl (10 mM) or leupeptin
(100 μg/ml) were present from 0 h. At 1.7 h, adrenaline (10 μM) was added
to media containing NH_4Cl (△), leupeptin (●) or to media containing
neither (□). Lipoprotein lipase was determined in acetone/ether-dried
preparations of the fat bodies and media combined at the times shown.

REFERENCES

1. Ashby, P., Bennett, D.P., Spencer, I.M. & Robinson, D.S. (1978):
   Biochem. J. 176:865-872.
2. Ashby, P. & Robinson, D.S. (1980): Biochem. J., 188:185-192.
3. Bensadoun, A. Ehnholm, C., Steinberg, D. & Brown, W.V. (1974):
   J. biol. Chem., 249:2220-2227.
4. Chung, J. & Scanu, A.M. (1977): J. biol. Chem., 252:4202-4209.
5. Crystal, R.G., Berg, R.A., Rennard, S.I. & Moss, J. (1982):
   Biochem. Soc. Trans., 9:89P.
6. DeDuve, C., De Barsy, T., Poole, B., Trouet, A., Tulkens, P. & van
   Hoof, F. (1974): Biochem. Pharmacol., 23:2495:2531.
7. Egelrud, T. & Olivecrona, T. (1972): J.biol. Chem., 247:6212-6217.
8. Hansson, P., Holmin, T. & Nilsson-Ehle, P. (1981): Biochem. biophys.
   Res. Comm., 103:1254-1257.
9. Huttunen, J.K., Ehnholm, C., Kinnunen, P.K.J. & Nikkilä, E.A. (1975):
   Clin. Chim. Acta, 64:335-347.
10. Iverius, P-H. & Östlund-Lindqvist, A-M. (1976): J. biol. Chem.,
    251:7791-7795.
11. Jansen, H., Garfinkel, A.S., Twu, J-S., Nikazy, J. & Schotz, M.C.
    (1978): Biochim. biophys. Acta, 150:342-351.

12. Miller-Andersson, M., Borg, H. & Andersson, L-O. (1974): Thrombosis Res., 49:667-693.
13. Mooney, R.A. & Lane, M.D. (1981): J. biol. Chem., 256:11724-11733.
14. Nikkilä, E.A. & Pykalistö, O. (1968): Biochim. biophys. Acta, 152: 421-423.
15. Nikkilä, E.A. & Pykalistö, O. (1968): Life Sciences, 7:1303-1309.
16. Ohisalo, J., Strandberg, H., Kostiainen , E., Kuusi, T. & Ehnholm, C. (1981): FEBS Lett., 132:121-123.
17. Ohkuma, S. & Poole, B. (1978): Proc. Nat. Acad. Sci., 75:3327-3331.
18. Olivecrona, T., Bengtsson, G., Marklund, S-E., Lindahl, U. & Höök,M. (1977): Fed. Proc., 36:60-65.
19. Östlund-Lindqvist, A-M. & Boberg, J. (1977): FEBS Lett., 83:231-236.
20. Parkin, S.M., Walker, K., Ashby, P. & Robinson, D.S. (1980):Biochem. J., 188:193-199.
21. Robinson, D.S. (1970): Compr. Biochem., 18:51-116.
22. Robinson, D.S. & Wing, D.R. (1971): Biochem. Soc. Symp., 33:123-135.
23. Schotz, M.C., Stewart, J.E., Garfinkel, A.S., Whelan, C.F., Baker,N., Cohen, K., Hensley, T.J. & Jacobson, M. (1969): In: Drugs affecting Lipid Metabolism, edited by W.L. Holmes, L.A. Carlson & R. Paoletti, pp 161-183. Plenum Press, New York.
24. Scow, R.O., Blanchette-Mackie, E.J. & Smith, L.C. (1976): Circ. Res., 39:149-162.
25. Steinberg, D. & Khoo, J.C. (1977): Fed. Proc., 36:1986-1990.
26. Twu, J-S, Garfinkel, A.S. & Schotz, M.C. (1975): Atherosclerosis, 22:463-472.

ACKNOWLEDGEMENTS

We thank Mrs Diane Bennett, Mr. Andrew Leadbeatter and Mr. Christopher Parkinson for their excellent assistance. The work was supported by a grant from the Medical Research Council. J.A.L. was the holder of a Medical Research Council studentship.

The Adipocyte and Obesity: Cellular and Molecular Mechanisms, edited by A. Angel, C. H. Hollenberg, and D. A. K. Roncari. Raven Press, New York © 1983.

Abnormal Triglyceride Clearance Secondary to Familial Apolipoprotein C-II Deficiency

*W. Carl Breckenridge, **J. A. Little, †P. Alaupovic, ‡D. Cox, §F. T. Lindgren, and §§A. Kuksis

*Department of Biochemistry, Dalhousie University, Halifax, Nova Scotia; **The Lipid Research Clinic Project and Department of Medicine, University of Toronto, and St. Michael's Hospital, Toronto, Canada; †Laboratory of Lipid and Lipoprotein Studies, Oklahoma Medical Research Foundation, Oklahoma City, Oklahoma 73104; ‡Research Institute, Hospital for Sick Children, Toronto, Ontario, Canada; §Donner Laboratory, University of California, Berkeley, California; §§Banting and Best Department of Medical Research, University of Toronto, Toronto; and The Departments of Paediatrics and Medical Genetics, University of Toronto, Toronto, Ontario, Canada*

Plasma lipoproteins provide at least two important functions. They represent the major mechanism for the transport of energy in the form of triglyceride from sites of synthesis in the intestine or liver to sites of energy use or storage in muscle or adipose tissue. The lipoproteins are important also in the delivery of cholesterol and phospholipid to cells and in some instances may also serve to remove cholesterol from peripheral tissues. These functions are accomplished as a result of important physiochemical properties of lipids and apolipoproteins as well as a variety of enzymes and cell surface receptors which interact with lipoproteins in the plasma compartment or extracellular space. Specific apoproteins act as modulators of enzyme activity or as recognition sites for the receptors. The major enzymes which are important in metabolism and modification of lipoproteins are lipoprotein lipase, hepatic lipase and lecithin cholesterol acyl transferase. Present knowledge of lipoprotein metabolism (8) indicates that nascent triglyceride rich lipoproteins are released from the intestine primarily as chylomicrons, containing apolipoproteins B and A-I, and from the liver as very low density lipoproteins containing primarily apo B and E and some C. Nascent discoidal HDL containing apo A-I and E and can also be detected from organ perfusates which contain an inhibitor of LCAT. During the release of triglyceride rich lipoproteins apo C is acquired. In vitro studies established that this acquisition was probably an important process in converting the lipoprotein to a suitable substrate for lipoprotein lipase since apolipoprotein C-II was found to decrease the apparent Km of purified lipoprotein lipase for triglyceride emulsions (7).

As a result of the activity of lipoprotein lipase the lipoprotein triglyceride is catabolized and some redundant surface constituents are believed to be transferred to HDL (15). Although the surface material was considered initially to contain primarily unesterified cholesterol, phosphatidyl choline and apolipoprotein C more recent studies of the catabolism of human VLDL by perfused rat heart suggest that most of the apo C-II, and C-III and E are transferred as sperical cholesteryl ester containing lipoproteins (18). The vesicles which are formed in this system are rich in cholesterol and phospholipid but extremely poor in apolipoprotein (17). Once formed these vesicles, which resemble Lp X, are not incorporated into HDL. Thus the incorporation of unesterified cholesterol and phospholipid into HDL may only occur under conditions of an excess of phospholipid relative to cholesterol. Lipoprotein lipase and hepatic lipase both possess phospholipase activity. Although phospholipase activity of lipoprotein lipase will cleave phospholipids of triglyceride rich lipoproteins (14) hepatic lipase may function as a phospholipase toward HDL_2 phospholipids (13). The triglyceridase activity of hepatic lipase appears to be directed towards the triglycerides of intermediate density lipoprotein, low density lipoprotein and high density lipoprotein (14). Recent in vivo evidence in subjects with familial hepatic lipase deficiency (4) suggests that hepatic lipase may play an important role in the catabolism of HDL and IDL since these lipoproteins accumulate in hepatic lipase deficiency.

LCAT in association with a subfraction of HDL is responsible for the conversion of unesterified cholesterol to cholesterol ester and phosphatidyl choline to lysophosphatidyl choline (1). The cholesterol ester can be tranferred from a HDL to other lipoproteins via cholesteryl ester transfer protein while the lysophosphatidyl choline can be bound by albumin. Thus the cholesterol and phospholipid required in the packaging of neutral lipids can be converted to a core constituent during metabolism.

A number of metabolic defects associated with lipoprotein metabolism have demonstrated, in vivo, the importance of the biochemical mechanisms that have been elucidated with in vitro studies. The importance of apolipoprotein C-II, lipoprotein lipase and hepatic lipase for normal triglyceride and lipoprotein metabolism will be discussed in this chapter.

Familial Apolipoprotein C-II Deficiency

The first case of familial apolipoprotein C-II deficiency was reported in 1978 (1,6). Subsequently three other kindreds were reported in Japan (22), Italy (5) and England (12). In the kindred studied at Toronto a total of 14 homozygotes and 23 obligate heterozygotes have been identified (2,10). The homozygotes all have severe hypertriglyceridemia and hyperchylomicronemia with triglyceride concentrations ranging from 550 to 5200 mg/dl and cholesterol from 100-

500 mg/dl. The heterozygotes have triglycerides in the high normal range for age and sex matched normal subjects. The homozygotes have no xanthomata despite the high triglyceride levels. Anemia is present in 9 of 14 homozygotes. None of the homozygotes has premature atherosclerosis. The obligate heterozygotes have no consistent clinical complications. The kindred thus serves as a large group of subjects who can be studied for the effects of a reduction, of apolipoprotein C-II on plasma lipoprotein structure and metabolism.

Apolipoprotein and Lipoproteins in Apolipoprotein C-II Deficiency.

Studies of apolipoprotein C-II concentrations in these subjects have been completed using an estimation of the biological activity of apo C-II by activation of skim milk lipoprotein lipase (2), an estimation of the relative amount of apo C-II/III in VLDL (2) and by immunochemical quantitation (3). Homozygotes were characterized by an inability to activate skim milk lipoprotein lipase, by the absence of apo C-II by polyacrylamide gel electrophoresis (Figure 1) and by the absence of immunoassayable apolipoprotein C-II (Table I). The obligate heterozygotes had a lower value for the activation assay, the ratio of apo C-II/C-III (Figure 1) and the estimate of absolute mass of apo C-II (Table II) compared to normal subjects. It is noteworthy that there was significant overlap of the estimates for apo C-II in the obligate heterozygotes with those of the normal subjects. In the homozygotes the plasma levels of several other apolipoproteins were very characteristic for this familial disorder. The concentrations of apo A-I and apo A-II were reduced to 50-60% of normal values. There was a reduction also in the levels of apo B although the concentration of this apolipoprotein was more variable than apo A-I or A-II. On the other hand, both apo C-III and apo E were elevated 2- to 3- fold in 9 of 11 patients. The mean levels of all the above apolipoproteins were very significantly different from those of normal controls. Obligate heterozygotes possessed normal levels of apolipoprotein A-II, B, C-III and E with a slight tendency for low values of apo A-I in association with low HDL cholesterol.

These alterations of apolipoprotein composition were associated with very dramatic alterations in the quantity and composition of lipoproteins in the homozygotes. As has been reported previously (2,6) for this kindred as well as other kindreds (5,12,22) chylomicron levels were extremely high (1550-6000 mg/dl total chylomicrons mass). In contrast VLDL was only moderately elevated. Low density lipoprotein (12-28 mg/dl) and high density lipoprotein (4-26 mg/dl) were extremely low. The marked alterations are shown in the lipoprotein mass profiles for analytical ultracentrifugation (Figure 2). Thus HDL and LDL mass were greatly reduced in concentration in comparison to normal subjects. However two groups of profiles emerged from the various homozygotes. In one group essentially no HDL_2 was observed and the HDL_3 concentration was low. In a second group HDL_3 was markedly reduced but the HDL_2 fraction was visible. In the latter instance there were proportionally greater amounts of intermediate density lipoprotein. These differences appear to be a reflection of the amount of hepatic lipase activity in these subjects as described below. The lipoprotein levels in heterozygotes were normal except for HDL (21-61 mg/dl) which tended to be low in a large proportion of the heterozygotes (2,10).

The composition of the lipoproteins revealed some important characteristics (Table II). Chylomicrons were found to contain only about 80% of mass as triglyceride. The unesterified cholesterol phospholipid molar ratio was approximately 0.95 + 0.05. This is an extremely high value in comparison to reports (16) for this ratio in nascent chylomicrons (0.3-0.4). However the high ratio does correspond well to reports of the estimates of this ratio for chylomicron remnants (16). The particles are also relatively rich in cholesterol ester. The protein content (4%) is comprised of relatively large proportions of apolipoprotein E (Figure 1) in relation to apolipoprotein C-III. The presence of significant amounts of these apolipoproteins in the chylomicron fractions clearly account for the marked elevation of these apolipoproteins in plasma (Table I). On the basis of animal studies it has been estimated that most apolipoprotein E is synthesized in the liver (20). However apo E can transfer to chylomicrons and accumulate in chylomicron remnants (1). Thus the composition of the chylomicrons would suggest that they may be partially catabolized product.

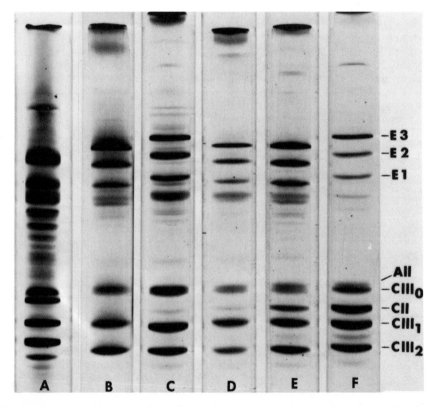

Figure 1. Isoelectric focusing of Apolipoproteins. A is chylomicrons and B, C and D are VLDL from homozygotes for apolipoprotein C-II deficiency; E is from a heterozygote; F is VLDL from a normal subject.

Table I

Apolipoproteins Concentrations in Familial Apolipoprotein C-II Deficiency

Subjects	Activation[a] Units	VLDL[b] CII/CIII	Apolipoproteins mg/dl					
			C-II	C-III	A-I	A-II	B	E
Homozygotes(11)	N.D.[c]	N.D.[c]	N.D.[c]	21.9+ +8.3	70.2+ +12.4	24.4+ +6.5	59.0+ +25.6	22.5+ +8.0
Heterozygotes(9)	18.6* +2.8 (14-22)	0.16* + 0.04 (0.09-21)	1.8* +0.5 (1.2-2.7)	7.6 +1.7	106.5 15.1	60.0	100.3 +26.2	11.4
Normal[d]	25.0 +7.8 (20-45)	0.27 +0.04 (0.22-0.35)	2.9 +0.9	8.2 +2.0	134.0 +27.0	66.0 +15.2	98.4 +26.5	11.3 +4.0

a Ability of plasma to stimulate the release of fatty acid from triolein by skim milk lipoprotein lipase. Values are in arbitrary units related to a reference serum.

b Ratio of the optical densities of Apo C-II and ApoC-III determined from isoelectric focusing of apolipoproteins of VLDL.

c N.D. not detectable.

d Normal subjects (male + female n=117) sampled in the Oklahoma Medical Research Foundation for immunoassay apolipoprotein concentrations. Normal adults were sampled in Toronto for estimates of activation (n=57) and VLDL ApoC-II/ApoC-III (n=37). Values in parentheses indicate range of values.

*Significantly different from normals by student's test (p<0.01).

+Wilcoxon 2 sample test; p<0.0001.

Table II
Lipoprotein Composition of Homozygotes for apo CII Deficiency

	Chylo[a]	VLDL		LDL		HDL	
	HZ	HZ	N	HZ	N	HZ	N
			weight %				
UC	3.2+0.4	4.7+0.8	5.5+0.9	5.0+1.9	8.6+0.6	1.7+0.4	2.2+0.2
CE	8.9+1.6	8.4+2.7	11.8+1.0	*17.8+3.5	41.6+0.9	*11.1+3.8	19.8+1.1
T6	77.5+3.7	64.2+3.4	55.5+3.1	*33.6+5.8	6.1+0.7	*15.2+1.7	3.5+0.6
PL	6.6+0.5	15.2+2.0	18.2+1.0	15.4+2.3	22.8+1.0	17.6+8.2	26.8+3.2
Prot	4.0+2.6	7.6+2.4	9.1+1.1	28.1+2.9	21.3+0.8	54.6+9.9	47.5+2.8

[a] Lipids analyzed by gas liquid chromatography, UC, unesterified cholesterol; CE, chol-esteryl esters, T6, triglycerides; PL, phospholipids; Prot, Protein.

*Significantly different from normal (p<0.01).

Very low density lipoprotein lipid compostion was relatively similar to normal VLDL. The apoprotein composition (Figure 1) was normal except for the absence of apo C-II. Low density lipoproteins contained abnormally high amounts of triglyceride and lower amounts of cholesterol ester in comparison to normal low density lipoprotein. Finally HDL was enriched in triglyceride at the expense of cholesteryl ester. The protein content of HDL was higher than normal due to the extreme reduction of HDL_2 in some subjects. Phospholipid content was also reduced compared to normal. The protein content of HDL was comprised of essentially only apo A-I and A-II as estimated by isoelectric focusing gels and the distribution of apolipoproteins between the HDL and the LDL plus VLDL fractions (3). Thus the composition studies of the lipoproteins are consistent with present concepts of normal lipolytic processes where by LDL and HDL represent lipolytic products of triglyceride rich lipoproteins. HDL is extremely low and contains essentially only apoprotein A-I, A-II and a relative deficiency of phospholipid. Both LDL and HDL are enriched in triglyceride possibly due to the severe hypertriglyceridemia or to low levels of hepatic lipase, as described below.

Post Heparin Lipolytic Activity

The original proband in this kindred possessed very low post heparin lipolytic activity which could be stimulated by the addition of plasma or apolipoprotein C-II (1). It was apparent that the individual had essentially normal or slightly elevated levels of lipoprotein lipase which was inactive. The activity could be increased considerably by the addition of apolipoprotein C-II. However the other post heparin lipolytic enzyme, hepatic lipase, was extremely low. Yamamura et al (22) also reported low hepatic lipase activity for their subjects while Miller et al (12) noted normal hepatic lipase activity. Further studies of post heparin lipolytic activity in 8 of the 14 homozygotes indicate that they have inactive lipoprotein lipase activity. While five have low hepatic lipase, three have activities which are in the normal range. Figure 2 shows the analytical ultracentrifugation profiles of two homozygotes. The subjects with low hepatic lipase possess more HDL_2 and IDL than the individual with essentially normal hepatic lipase. Four subjects are compared in Table III for lipoprotein levels and hepatic lipase activity. It can be seen that there is an inverse relationship between HDL or IDL and hepatic lipase activity. Thus it would appear that hepatic lipase activity may also influence HDL and IDL levels in these subjects as has been reported for a deficiency of this enzyme (4). Klose et al (9) have suggested that the low hepatic lipase activity maybe secondary to the pancreatitis found in the proband in this kindred. An examination of the clinical features of these subjects in Table III indicates that all of them have a history of pancreatitis.

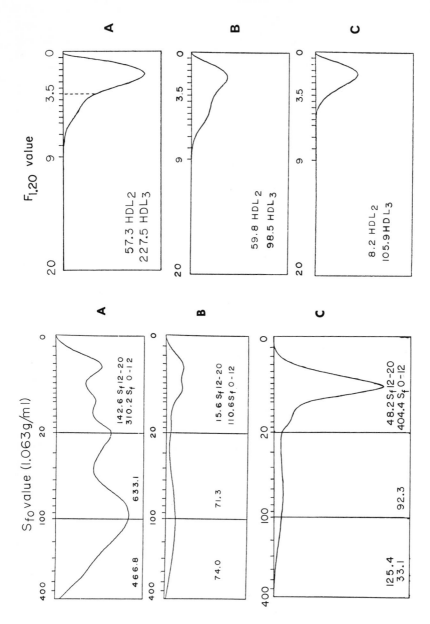

Figure 2. Analytical Ultracentrifugation at density 1.063 g/ml showing a normal subject (C) and two homozygotes for apolipoprotein C-II deficiency (A and B); and at density 1.21 g/ml showing a normal subject (A) and two homozygotes (B and C).

Table III
Hepatic Lipase Activity and Lipoproteins
in Homozygotes for Apolipoprotein C-II Deficiency

Subject	Hepatic Lipase[a]	Lipoproteins[b]			
		IDL	LDL	HDL$_2$	HDL$_3$
	μeq FFA/ml/h	mg/dl			
F059(F)	3.1	143	310	60	98
E027(M)	6.6	24	108	35	70
E061(M)	9.9	14	81	39	108
E085(M)	18.6	22	137	159	
E084(M)	33.2	16	111	8	106
[b]Normal(M)	26.4	32	369	57	228
(F)		17	288	145	237

[a] Assayed as described elsewhere.
[b] Separate by analytical ultracentrifugation.
[c] Hepatic Lipase on 10 subjects at Toronto. Lipoprotein concentration from Modesto Study, California.

Lipoprotein Metabolism Following Administration of Apo C-II.

Treatment of familial apolipoprotein C-II deficiency allows the possibility to study the clearance of triglyceride rich lipoprotein following the administration of apolipoprotein C-II through plasma transfusion. Under current concepts of lipoprotein metabolism it would be expected that the chylomicrons and VLDL catabolism might be associated with an increase in the concentrations of LDL and HDL. A number of studies have been conducted in this manner. The original proband in our kindred received plasma transfusions or infusions of apo VLDL (1,10). In both instances there was a rapid drop in plasma triglyceride and chylomicrons. We did not detect a significant increment in HDL lipids. In a similar study by Miller et al (12) a plasma transfusion resulted in a small increase in HDL mass detected by analytical ultracentrifugation. In our studies it is possible that the chylomicron remnants may have been rapidly removed with a slight amount of lipolysis. Studies (21) in animal models suggest that the recognition of chylomicrons remnants by the liver is related to the relative proportion of apo E and C-II in the remnant. In the present kindred the chylomicrons are extremely rich in apo E (Figure 1). The addition of apo C-II may allow a slight increase in lipolysis and the loss of sufficient apo C-III to result in recognition and rapid removal of the remnant with very little transfer of phospholipid or cholesterol to HDL. It must be stressed that all the lipoprotein fractions in these subjects tend to show a deficiency in phospholipid compared to lipoproteins from normal individuals. The triglyceride rich particles also show an extremely high ratio of unesterified cholesterol to phospholipid. There is reasonable evidence to suggest that the generation of excess surface material in the form of phospholipid may be important in augmenting HDL mass (15). This process may not occur in the short term experiments with the homozygote due to the relative deficiency of phospholipid. In preliminary studies of the lipolysis of chylomicrons by perfused rat heart we have found that the transfer of apo C-II to these lipoproteins from normal HDL is accompanied by a significant transfer of phospholipid to the chylomicrons (unpublished observations).

Recent studies (11) of the lipolysis of apo C-II deficient VLDL showed that the apparent Km of lipoprotein lipase with apo C-II deficient VLDL decreased from 7.8 to 1.0 when the lipoprotein was saturated with apolipoprotein C-II. There was no change in Vmax. Therefore apo C-II appears to enhance the interaction of the lipoprotein with the enzyme. Thus it could be envisaged that plasma chylomicron levels might increase until the rate of catabolism via lipoprotein lipase would be comparable to the rate of production of lipoprotein. This may help to explain the tendency for the chylomicron composition to resemble partially catabolized chylomicrons.

Does the marked limitation in the ability to catabolize triglyceride influence the capacity of the individual to maintain adipose tissue mass? Data on ponderal and quetelet indices suggest no major changes in the homozygotes. The proband and one other homozygotes who had severe malabsorption associated with pancreatitis possessed very little adipose tissue mass. Six female homozygotes had ponderal indices equal to values for the normal population (41.67 + 1.99 vs 41.12 + 2.55). Six male homozygotes tended to have ponderal indices which were higher than the normal mean (42.07 + 1.99 vs 40.60 + 2.19), but these differences were not significant. Differences in the quetelet index were not significant also. Thus the marked hypertriglyceridemia and low activity of lipoprotein lipase do not appear to influence adipose tissue mass provided adequate nutrition is maintained.

Acknowledgements. The research was supported in part by NIH NHLBI NO1-HV2-29017-L; HL-23181, The Ontario Heart Foundation and the Nova Scotia Heart Foundation.

References

1. Breckenridge, W.C., Little, J.A., Steiner, G., Chow, A., and Poapst, M., (1978): N. Engl. J. Med., 298 1265-1273.
2. Breckenridge, W.C., Cox, D., and Little, J.A., (1980): Atherosclerosis V 675-679 Springer Verlag, New York.
3. Breckenridge, W.C., Alaupovic, P., Cox, D.W., and Little, J.A. (1982): Atherosclerosis (in press).
4. Breckenridge, W.C., Little, J.A., Alaupovic, P., Wang, C.S., Kuksis, A., Kakis, A., Lindgren, F.T., and Gardiner, G. (1982): Atherosclerosis (in press).
5. Capuros, A., Pace, L., Bonomo, L., Catapano, A., Schiliro, G., LaRosa, M., Assman, G., (1980): Lancet 1: 268.
6. Cox, D.W., Breckenridge, W.C., Little, J.A., (1978): Inheritance of apolipoprotein C-II deficiency with hypertriglyceridemia and pancreatis, N. Engl. J. Med., 299: 1420.

7. Fielding, C.J. (1973): Biochim. Biophys. Acta. 316: 66-75.
8. Havel, R.J. (1982) In Symposium on Lipid Disorders. The Medical Clinics of North America, edited by R.J. Havel, W.B. Saunders Co. Philadelphia Vol. 66, pp 319-332.
9. Klose, G., Augustin, J., Greten, H. (1978): N. Engl. J. Med. 299 553.
10. Little, J.A., Cox, D.W., Breckenridge, W.C., McGuire, V.M., (1980): Atherosclerosis V , pp. 671-675, Springer Verlag, New York.
11. Matsuoka, N., Shirai, K., Johnson, J.D., Kashyap, M.L., Srivastava, L.S., Yamamura, T., Yamamoto, A., Saito, Y., Kumazai, and Jackson, R.L. (1981): Metabolism 30: 818-824.
12. Miller, N.E., Rao, S.N., Alaupovic, P., Noble, N., Slack, J., Brunzell, J.D., Lewis, B., (1981) Eur. J. Clin. Invest., 11, 69-76.
13. Musliner, T.A., Herbert, P.A. and Kingston, M.J. (1979): Biochim. Biophys. Acta. 575: 277-288.
14. Nicoll, A. and Lewis, B. (1980): Eur. J. Clin. Invest. 10: 487-495.
15. Patsch, J.R., Gotto, Jr., A.M., Olivecrona, T and Eisenberg, S. (1978): Proc. Natl. Acad. Sci. U.S.A. 75: 4519-4523.
16. Redgrave, T.G. and Small, D.M. (1979): J. Clin. Invest. 64: 162-171.
17. Tam, S.P. and Breckenridge, W.C. (1981): Circ., 64: 162-171.
18. Tam, S.P, Dory, L., and Rubenstein, D. (1981): J. Lipid Res., 22: 641-651.
19. Van Tol, A., Ven Gent, T., and Jansen, H. (1980): Biochem. Biophys. Res. Comm. 94: 101-108.
20. Wa, A.L. and Windmueller, H.G. (1979): J. Biol. Chem., 254: 7316-7322.
21. Windler, E., Chao, Y.S., and Havel, R.J. (1980): J. Biol. Chem. 255: 8303-8307.
22. Yamamura, T., Sud, H., Ishikawa, K., Yamamoto, A., (1979): Atherosclerosis 34: 53-65.

The Adipocyte and Obesity: Cellular and Molecular Mechanisms, edited by A. Angel, C. H. Hollenberg, and D. A. K. Roncari. Raven Press, New York © 1983.

Contribution of Adipose Tissue to the Clearance of Chylomicrons from Plasma

J. Borensztajn and T. J. Kotlar

Department of Pathology, Northwestern University Medical School, Chicago, Illinois 60611

The central role which lipoprotein lipase (LPL) plays in the removal of triacylglycerol (TG) rich lipoproteins (chylomicrons and very low density lipoproteins) from circulation has been amply documented (1, 8, 10). Two observations in particular have contributed to conclusively demonstrate the importance of LPL: 1) In experimental animals in whom LPL activity is inhibited in vivo by the injection of anti-LPL antibody, TG-rich lipoproteins accumulate in circulation (6). 2) Individuals that lack apo C-II, a required cofactor for the catalytic action of LPL, develop severe hypertriglyceridemia (see paper by Breckenridge in this volume).

LPL regulates the first of two phases which comprise the process of clearance of TG-rich lipoproteins from circulation. This initial phase involves the hydrolysis of most of the TG core of the lipoproteins, a process that takes place on the luminal surface of capillary endothelial cells of extrahepatic tissue. The unesterified fatty acids generated as a result of this hydrolysis are taken up by adipocytes for storage or are oxidized or stored by various other tissues. As a result of the hydrolysis of the lipoprotein TG the particles are reduced in size, selectively lose some of their surface constituents (phospholipids and apoproteins C and A) conserving, however, their cholesterol content as well as other apoproteins (B and E). These partially degraded lipoproteins (remnants) are then taken up by the liver in the final step of clearance from circulation of the TG-rich lipoproteins (9).

LPL is widely distributed in extrahepatic tissues. In starved animals LPL is particularly active in skeletal muscle (red fiber type) (4,7,11). It is in fact generally assumed that in starved animals when the rate of influx of TG-rich lipoproteins into the circulation is relatively low skeletal muscle LPL is responsible for initiating the TG-rich lipoproteins clearance process. In fed animals when the rate of influx of TG-rich lipoproteins into the circulation may be very high, the skeletal muscle LPL activity declines. In contrast, adipose tissue LPL activity which is very low during starvation markedly increases in the immediate post prandial period. In this condition the clearance of TG-rich lipoproteins from circulation has been generally assumed to occur mainly through the action of adipose tissue LPL (10). Indeed, defects in adipose tissue LPL activity have frequently been sought to explain the origin of hypertriglyceridemias (1). However, the evidence demonstrating a positive correlation between the development of hyper-triglyceridemias and decreased levels of LPL activity in the adipose tissue of man and experimental animals has been inconclusive (1). Adipose tissue LPL activity, as measured by available methods (e.g. homogenates of fresh or defatted tissue; elution of LPL from tissues by heparin) almost certainly includes activity which is not physiolog-ically functional, i.e. not involved in the hydrolysis of circulating TG on the capillary's endothelial surface. The difficulty in measuring this physiologically functional enzyme may account for the failure to establish a clear link between defects in the clearance of plasma TG and adipose tissue LPL levels. In this study we re-examined the role of adipose tissue LPL in the process of plasma TG clearance. Specifi-cally we examined the effect of the increase in the adipose tissue LPL activity from fasted to fed levels on the clearance of plasma TG.

METHODS

Male Sprague-Dawley rats (200-240 g) were used. All procedures used in this study have been previously described: preparation of H^3-choles-terol labelled chylomicrons (2); measurement of adipose tissue and muscle LPL activity (3); hepatic uptake of chylomicron remnants (2); plasma TG levels (5).

RESULTS

Effect of Insulin on Adipose Tissue LPL Activity

In most physiological conditions changes in adipose tissue LPL activity are accompanied by changes, usually in the opposite direction, in muscle LPL activity (1). Thus under normal conditions the effects of changes in adipose tissue LPL activity alone on the rate of clear-ance of chylomicrons from circulation cannot be properly assessed. To circumvent this problem we took advantage of the observation that insulin can stimulate adipose tissue LPL activity without affecting the muscle LPL activity (3). In Table 1 are shown the results of an experi-ment which confirms and extends these observations.

TABLE 1.   Effect of Insulin on Adipose Tissue and Muscle LPL Activity[a]

	Adipose Tissue	Soleus Muscle	Heart
- Insulin	31 ± 7 (20)	22 ± 8 (20)	112 ± 14 (18)
+ Insulin	132 ± 35 (18)	26 ± 8 (20)	133 ± 15 (12)

[a]All rats were starved for 18 hours and killed 3 hours after insulin injection (0.4 U/kg). Results are expressed as μMols FFA released/hr/ gram tissue (Mean ± S.D.).

When starved rats were injected with insulin the adipose tissue LPL activity increased 4-fold whereas cardiac and soleus muscles LPL activ-ity remained unchanged.

Chylomicron Clearance in Control and Insulin-Treated Rats

During the degradation of chylomicrons to remnants the cholesterol content of the particle is largely conserved (9). As the remnant is taken up by the liver as a unit, the amount of chylomicron cholesterol taken up by the liver can be used as a measure of chylomicron clearance from circulation. In Figure 1 are shown the results of an experiment in which starved rats or starved rats previously injected with insulin, were injected intravenously with H^3-cholesterol labelled chylomicrons and the incorporation of the label by the liver measured at different time intervals.

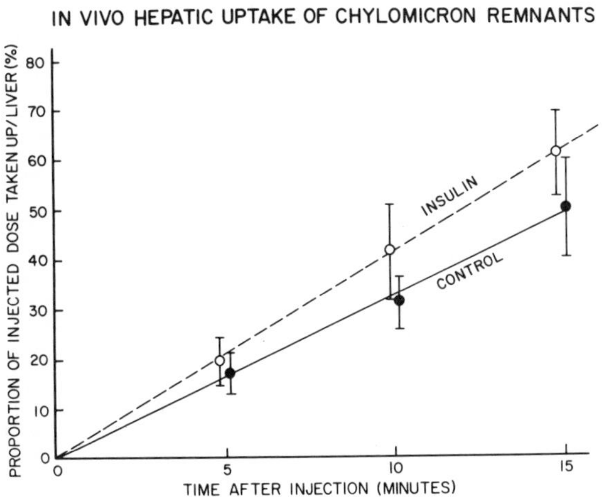

IN VIVO HEPATIC UPTAKE OF CHYLOMICRON REMNANTS

FIGURE 1. Rats starved for 18 hours were injected I.P. with saline or insulin (0.4 U/kg). Three hours later they were injected I.V. with H^3-cholesterol labelled chylomicrons (200 µg cholesterol/rat) and the label incorporated into the liver measured as previously described (2). Each point represents the average of 4 livers.

It is apparent that the amount of label incorporated into the livers of the insulin-injected animals at 5, 10 and 15 minutes was not significantly different from that of control rats.

The above results indicate that in the insulin-treated rats the large increase in total adipose tissue LPL activity was not accompanied by a corresponding significant increase in the rate of chylomicron clearance from circulation. However, in this study clearance was measured as a function of the rate of uptake of H^3-cholesterol remnants by the liver. It became necessary therefore to establish that under the experimental conditions used the capacity of the liver to take up remnants was not saturated by the amounts of remnants formed in the vascular space. In Figure 2 are shown the results of an experiment in which rats were injected simultaneously with H^3-cholesterol labelled chylomicrons and heparin. Heparin causes LPL as well as other lipases to be released into circulation and remnants are therefore generated at a much faster rate than in animals not injected with heparin (9).

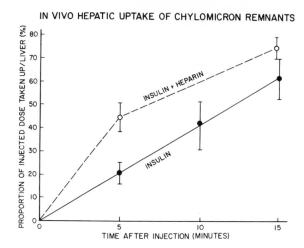

IN VIVO HEPATIC UPTAKE OF CHYLOMICRON REMNANTS

FIGURE 2.   Conditions were as described in Figure 1. Where indicated
rats were also injected I.V. with 100 units of heparin.

The results in Figure 2 show that in the heparin-injected animals
about 45% of the injected H^3-cholesterol was incorporated by the liver
within 5 minutes of injection compared to only 18% in the control rats.
Thus the capacity of the liver to take up H^3-cholesterol labelled remnants greatly exceeded the rates at which remnants were being generated
in the insulin-treated rats.

Effect of Insulin on Plasma Triglyceride Concentration

The effect of insulin treatment on the influx of triglycerides in
circulation was also examined. This was necessary to rule out the
possibility that unlabelled TG-rich lipoproteins competed with the injected labelled chylomicrons for degradation by LPL. The formation of
unlabelled remnants would result in the underestimation of the amounts
of H^3-cholesterol labelled remnants taken up by the liver. The amount
of triglycerides secreted in the circulation was determined using Triton
WR-1339 (12). Control rats and rats that had been injected with insulin
3 hours previously were bled (about 0.5 ml) from a tail vein and then
injected with 1 ml of a 10% solution of Triton WR-1339. After 15 minutes blood samples were again collected from the tail vein. The TG
concentrations in the plasma of control and insulin-treated rats measured before and 15 minutes after the injection of Triton were respectively: 47.6±11; 46.4±7.5 and 81.8±22; 73.5±20.7 mg/100 ml of plasma
(mean ± S.D.; n = 6). Thus insulin had no significant effect on the
influx of triglycerides into the circulation.

Chylomicron Clearance in Fasted and Glucose-fed Rats

The results in Figure 1 can be interpreted to mean that muscle LPL is
primarily responsible for the clearance of TG from the plasma even in
conditions when the adipose tissue LPL activity is high. It was of
interest therefore to examine the clearance of chylomicrons from the

plasma under conditions in which muscle LPL activity is low. For this purpose starved rats were fed 3 ml of a 60% glucose solution. Three hours later when the soleus muscle LPL activity had declined from 60±7 to 23±6 units and the adipose tissue activity had increased from 38±6 to 130±12 units (mean ± S.D.; n = 5) the animals were injected with H³-cholesterol labelled chylomicrons. The results in Figure 3 show that clearance of chylomicrons from the plasma of glucose fed rats was not significantly different than that of the fasted rats.

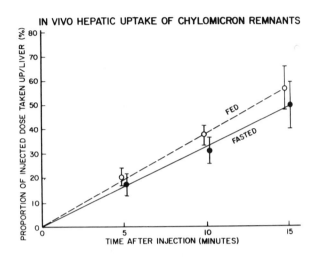

IN VIVO HEPATIC UPTAKE OF CHYLOMICRON REMNANTS

FIGURE 3.   Rats starved for 18 hours were fed 3 ml of a 60% glucose solution. Three hours later they were injected with H³-cholesterol labelled chylomicrons as described in Figure 1.

DISCUSSION

Clearance of chylomicrons from circulation is mediated by LPL present on the surface of endotheial cells. It is well-established that only a portion of a tissue's LPL activity is located on the endothelial surface, where it is physiologically functional. Thus, any interpretation of the effects of changes in the tissue LPL activity on clearance of TG requires knowledge of the changes which occur in the functional fraction. Since with the methods presently available, the functional LPL activity in adipose tissue and skeletal muscle cannot be properly determined, in the present study we took the opposite approach. We attempted to gain knowledge about the functional enzyme in the tissues by examining the clearance of chylomicrons from the plasma. Our findings that there is no significant difference in the clearance of chylomicrons of fed and fasted rats (Fig. 3) can be interpreted to mean that feeding produces reciprocal and equivalent changes in the functional fraction of muscle and adipose tissue LPL so that in the fasted animal clearance is mediated mainly by the muscle LPL and in the fed animal by adipose tissue LPL. To assess the role of adipose tissue alone in the clearance of chylomicrons from circulation, we used rats injected with insulin to increase the adipose tissue LPL to fed levels without affecting muscle LPL activity. The rate of clearance of chylomicrons in insulin-injected rats was no greater than control rats despite a 4-fold increase in adipose tissue LPL (Fig. 1). This finding can be interpreted to mean that the rise in adipose tissue LPL mediated by exogenous insulin occurs primarily in the nonfunctional fraction. If insulin-injected rats can be used as a valid model for the effect of feeding on adipose tissue LPL, then the increase observed in adipose tissue LPL which occurs after glucose feeding is also primarily in the nonfunctional fraction. If this conclusion is correct, then an alternate interpretation is required to explain the similarity in clearance rates in fed and fasted animals. It is possible that in fed as well as fasted animals clearance of chylomicrons from circulation is mediated mainly by skeletal muscle. This would require that the decrease in skeletal muscle LPL activity which occurs post prandially is predominantly in the nonfunctional fraction.

Defects in clearance of plasma TG have been thought to be associated with low adipose tissue LPL activity. If the latter interpretation of our results is correct, then it is more likely that such defects are to be found associated with skeletal muscle LPL.

REFERENCES

1. Borensztajn, J. (1979): In: The Biochemistry of Atherosclerosis, edited by A.M. Scanu, R.W. Wissler and G.S. Getz, pp. 231-245. Marcel Dekker, New York.

2. Borensztajn, J. and Kotlar, T.J. (1981): Biochem. J. 200:547-553.

3. Borensztajn, J., Samols, D.R. and Rubenstein, A.H. (1972): Am. J. Physiol. 233:271-1275.

4. Borensztajn, J. Rone, M.S., Babirak, S.P., McGarr, J.A. and Oscai, L.B. (1975): Am. J. Physiol. 229:394-397.

5. Fletcher, M.J. (1968): Clin. Chim. Acta 22:393-397.

6. Kompiang, I.P., Bensadoun, A. and Yang, M.W.W. (1976): J. Lipid Res. 17:498-505.

7. Linder, C., Chernick, S.S., Fleck, T.R. and Scow, R.O. (1976): Am. J. Physiol. 231:860-864.

8. Nilsson-Ehle, P., Garfinkel, A.S. and Schotz, M.C. (1980): Am. Rev. Biochem. 49:667-693.

9. Redgrave, T.G. (1970): J. Clin. Invest. 49:465-471.

10. Robinson, D.S. (1970): In: Comprehensive Biochemistry, edited by M. Florkin and E.H. Stotz, pp. 51-116. Elsevier, New York.

11. Tan, M.H., Sata, T. and Havel, R.J. (1977): J. Lipid Res. 18:363-370.

12. Otway, S. and Robinson, D.S. (1967): J. Physiol. 170:309-319.

The Adipocyte and Obesity: Cellular and Molecular Mechanisms, edited by A. Angel, C. H. Hollenberg, and D. A. K. Roncari. Raven Press, New York © 1983.

Control of Triglyceride Synthesis

David N. Brindley and Nigel Lawson

Department of Biochemistry, University of Nottingham Medical School, Queen's Medical Centre, Nottingham, NG7 2UH England

To understand the changes in metabolism that can lead to the excessive deposition of fat in adipose tissue, it is necessary to consider not only the adipocyte, but also the relation of adipose tissue metabolism to that in liver and muscle. A large proportion of the fatty acids that are stored in adipose tissue are transported to it from the liver. They could have been synthesized de novo, derived from the diet, or they could be obtained from the blood following lipolysis in adipose tissue itself. The liver can oxidise these fatty acids, or incorporate them into triacylglycerols (triglycerides) to be released into the blood in very low density lipoproteins (VLDL). It is therefore important to determine a) how the liver is able to control fatty acid esterification relative to β-oxidation, and b) whether muscle or adipose tissue will take up the fatty acids from VLDL-triacylglycerols in different physiological conditions. This article will be concerned with how changes in the effective concentrations of insulin relative to glucagon, catecholamines, corticotropin and glucocorticoids determine the rates of fatty acid metabolism and triacylglycerol synthesis.

CONTROL OF FATTY ACID METABOLISM IN LIVER

One of the major factors that regulates the rate of fatty acid synthesis in the liver is the insulin/glucagon ratio. This helps to control the supply of substrates and cofactors by glycolysis and the pentose phosphate pathway, and the activity of acetyl-CoA carboxylase. Thus high concentrations of insulin relative to glucagon favour the synthesis of malonyl-CoA and the production of fatty acids. In these conditions high concentrations of glucocorticoids can further enhance fatty acid synthesis (11,19). The rate of β-oxidation behaves reciprocally to that of fatty acid biosynthesis. One of the major regulators for this relationship is the concentration of malonyl-CoA (26). This compound inhibits carnitine palmitoyltransferase and thereby decreases the entry of fatty acids into β-oxidation (Fig. 1). The rate of glycerolipid synthesis does not bear any simple relationship to that of β-oxidation and fatty acid biosynthesis. This is because the fatty acids that are esterified are derived from

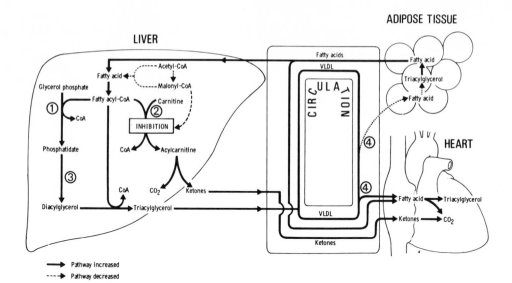

FIG. 1. <u>Fatty acid metabolism in ketotic diabetes or severe stress</u>
    The direction of fatty acid metabolism is shown in conditions where
the concentration of insulin is low relative to that of glucagon,
catecholamines, corticotropin and glucocorticoids.   The enzyme
activities are indicated by 1) GPAT; 2) carnitine palmitoyltransferase;
3) PAP and 4) LPL. This figure is reproduced with the permission of
Clin. Sci. (6).

synthesis <u>de novo</u>, and also from the diet or from lipolysis in adipose
tissue. Furthermore, the pathway of esterification is involved in the
synthesis of phospholipids as well as triacylglycerols.
    The rate at which fatty acids are oxidized will influence the rate
of esterification since there is competition for acyl-CoA esters
between these pathways. However, the rate of oxidation does not always
change reciprocally to that of triacylglycerol synthesis.   In some
stress conditions both oxidation and triacylglycerol synthesis can
increase in response to large increases in fatty acid supply from
adipose tissue (6). The partitioning of fatty acids between oxidation
and glycerolipid synthesis is partly regulated by changes in malonyl-
CoA concentrations that control carnitine palmitoyltransferase, and
partly by changes in the activities of the acyltransferases that
incorporate fatty acids into glycerolipids. There are three different
acyltransferases that initiate the production of phosphatidate (for
details, see ref.20): a) GPAT* located in the endoplasmic reticulum
which can esterify dihydroxyacetone phosphate in addition to glycerol
phosphate; b) a specific GPAT located in the mitochondrial outer
membrane and (c) a specific DHAPAT which is thought to be mainly
peroxisomal (see ref. 20).

----

*Abbreviations. DGAT = diacylglycerol acyltransferase (EC 2.3.1.20);
DHAPAT = dihydroxyacetone phosphate acyltransferse (EC 2.3.1.42); GPAT
= glycerol phosphate acyltransferase (EC 2.3.1.15); LPL = lipoprotein
lipase (EC 3.1.1.34);   PAP = phosphatidate phosphohydrolase (EC
3.1.3.4).

Decreases in the activity of microsomal GPAT from rat liver have been reported after starvation by some (24,42,48), but not by all authors (2,12,44). Microsomal GPAT activity is also not decreased in diabetes (1,43). Two mechanisms have been proposed to explain the modification of the microsomal GPAT activity: a) the accumulation of Ca^{2+} in the endoplasmic reticulum (39,40) and b) the phosphorylation of GPAT (33) although this work was from adipose tissue. Mitochondrial GPAT is decreased more than the microsomal activity in starvation (2,42) and diabetes (1), and the former activity may be controlled by insulin (1,4). The mitochondrial GPAT has lower Km values for glycerol phosphate (32), and acyl-CoA esters (2,46) than the microsomal activity. This should mean that fatty acid esterification is favoured in mitochondria, especially at low substrate concentrations. The mitochondrial GPAT is well situated to compete with carnitine acyltransferase and to regulate the partitioning of fatty acids beteen oxidation and esterification. However, although about 50% of the GPAT activity in rat liver is mitochondrial there is no obvious pathway for metabolizing the bulk of the phosphatidate that can be synthesized. Phosphatidate can be converted to cardiolipin in mitochondria, but this synthesis is relatively low compared with the total fatty acid flux. PAP does exist in mitochondria, but it is widely believed that the rate of conversion of diacylglycerol to phosphatidylcholine or to triacylglycerol is low, or non-existent in these organelles.

The fate of the phosphatidate that could be synthesized in mitochondria is therefore obscure. One possibility is its conversion back to glycerol phosphate. A phosphatidate deacylase system is present in the microsomal, soluble (41) and mitochondrial (27) fractions of rat liver. Alternatively, the phosphatidate or lysophosphatidate that is produced in mitochondria might be transported to the endoplasmic reticulum. There is no direct evidence for this mechanism, but a number of heat stable proteins that stimulate triacylglycerol synthesis have recently been characterized (36). It was suggested that these might promote the inter- and intramembrane transport of hydrophobic precursors in lipid synthesis (36).

The role of the "peroxisomal" DHAPAT is also obscure. It is known that up to 60% of the glycerolipids synthesized in vitro from glycerol by whole cell preparations of liver can arise by direct acylation of dihydroxyacetone phosphate (25). However, the physiological importance of this route is not yet known. The peroxisomal DHAPAT could also help to regulate the balance between esterification and β-oxidation (35). However, it is not clearly established that the lysophosphatidate that can be synthesized in peroxisomes can significantly contribute to the production of triacylglycerols and phosphatidylcholine. Their major site of synthesis is the endoplasmic reticulum. The GPAT in these membranes can esterify dihydroxyacetone phosphate, but this is thought not to be a major reaction in vivo because of the kinetic properties of this GPAT, and the relatively low concentrations of dihydroxyacetone phosphate relative to glycerol phosphate (38).

One of the major factors that controls esterification is the supply of substrates. The decrease in esterification that is observed in starvation is particularly apparent when this supply is low e.g. in hepatocytes that have been depleted of glycogen (9). However, in vivo, the transport of fatty acids from adipose tissue to the liver increases in starvation and diabetes, and the hepatic concentration of acyl-CoA esters and glycerol phosphate may also increase (26,48). If the supply of fatty acids to the liver satisfies the basal requirement for oxidation, then some of the excess are sequestered as triacylglycerols. This removes the potentially toxic effects of the fatty acids and their acyl—CoA esters, and it regenerates CoA. The total enzymic capacity to synthesize triacylglycerol (measured after inhibiting oxidation) is not decreased in starvation (9,17,26), or after treating hepatocytes with glucagon (10). The microsomal GPAT which has relatively high Km values for its substrates and which changes little in activity in starvation and diabetes, may be responsible for the retention of this capacity to synthesize phosphatidate in these conditions.

Glucocorticoids may produce small increases in the activities of the mitochondrial and microsomal GPAT (2,3,20). However, the major effect of these hormones are on PAP. Glucocorticoids stimulate its synthesis in perfused liver (23), and in isolated hepatocytes (18,22). Stimulations in PAP activity are observed at 10^{-7} to 10^{-6} M corticosterone (Fig. 2) which is within the normal physiological range found in the rat (18). Insulin antagonises these effects of corticosterone, but in the absence of added glucocorticoid it has little effect (Fig. 2). These results explain in diabetes why a) the high PAP activity (30,43,45); b) the fatty liver; and c) the hypertriglyceridaemia can be decreased by insulin therapy (30,45). PAP activities are also increased in the livers of genetically obese (ob/ob) mice (13), and this can be understood in relation to the high corticosterone concentrations in the blood of these animals (15).

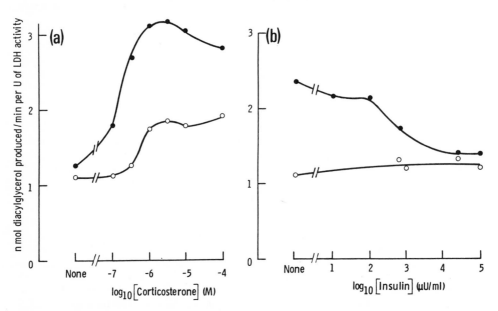

FIG. 2. Effects of corticosterone and insulin on the activity of PAP in isolated rat hepatocytes

Hepatocytes were incubated for 6 h with various concentrations of corticosterone and in the presence (O), or absence (●) of 20 mU of insulin per ml (a). In (b) the incubations contained various concentrations of insulin in the absence (O), or in the presence (●) of 10^{-5} M corticosterone. This figure is reproduced with permission of FEBS Letters (22).

The role of DGAT in controlling triacylglycerol synthesis is controversial. It is at a branch-point which could regulate the rates of synthesis of phosphatidylethanolamine, phosphatidylcholine and triacylglycerol, and it is the only enzyme unique to triacylglycerol synthesis. When hepatocytes were incubated with glucagon there was a decrease in DGAT activity without altering choline phosphotransferase activity (14). This could explain the preferential decrease in triacylglycerol synthesis relative to the synthesis of phosphatidylethanolamine and phosphatidylcholine. However, this decrease has to be reconciled with the observation that phosphatidylcholine synthesis is inhibited by cyclic-AMP analogues (34). In addition, the enzymic capacity for triacylglycerol synthesis is maintained even when the ratio of insulin to glucagon is low and cyclic-AMP concentrations are high (see above). It should also be noted that DGAT activity is increased in ketotic diabetes (30,47) and it is normal in mildly ketotic diabetes (43).

Insulin and glucocorticoids both appear to be important in stimulating triacylglycerol synthesis in the liver, but by different mechanisms. When insulin concentrations are high, fatty acid synthesis increases and these acids are largely incorporated into triacylglycerols and secreted as VLDL. High glucocorticoid concentrations may further facilitate the synthesis of fatty acids and triacylglycerols. Low concentrations of insulin relative to glucagon promote the oxidation of fatty acids and decrease fatty acid synthesis. If in these conditions the hepatic availabilities of glycerophosphate and acyl-CoA esters are low then the acids that are esterified are preferentially incorporated into phospholipids. However, when the supply of fatty acids from adipose tissue exceeds the basal requirement for oxidation and phospholipid synthesis, the fatty acids are then incorporated into triacylglycerols. This is facilitated by the increased capacity of PAP that is induced by glucocorticoids. This change can be seen in a wide variety of stress and toxic conditions. The increased rate of triacylglycerol synthesis can result in a fatty liver and an increased synthesis of VLDL (6,7). The uptake and further metabolism of fatty acids from the triacylglycerols of VLDL by muscle and adipose tissue also depends upon the balance of insulin and glucocorticoid concentrations.

CONTROL OF FATTY ACID METABOLISM IN MUSCLE TISSUE

The VLDL that are released by the liver when insulin concentrations are low are preferentially metabolized by heart and skeletal muscle. This is because the LPL activity of these tissues is increased by glucocorticoids, although other "stress" hormones may also be involved (8). High insulin concentrations are not required to maintain the LPL activity. Thus in many conditions there appears to be a reciprocal relationship between LPL activity in muscle tissue and adipose tissue (Fig. 1). This is seen in starvation, diabetes and in severe stress (8). A similar effect can sometimes be seen when animals are fed diets rich in fat rather than starch (8,21). High fat diets can produce insulin-insensitivity and the increase in muscle LPL activity relative to that in adipose tissue may result from this (21).

This control of LPL activity in muscle by glucocorticoids ensures the supply of energy in periods of metabolic stress when insulin concentrations are low. The fatty acids that are taken up are destined for β-oxidation, but they may be stored temporarily as triacylglycerols. This is reflected in the fatty infiltration that can accompany diabetes (29) and high fat feeding (16). The fatty changes in diabetes are accompanied by increases in the activities of the enzymes responsible for triacylglycerol synthesis. However, it is not entirely clear whether this specifically involves GPAT (31) or PAP (29). The direct action of glucocorticoids in producing such alterations is not yet established, but it is tempting to predict that they should do so. Glucocorticoids have been implicated in having a permissive effect in facilitating the lipolysis of endogenous triacylglycerol in the heart (16). The increased capacity to esterify fatty acids in muscle tissue that occurs in "stress" conditions enables the muscle tissue to store energy. Furthermore, it also helps to regulate the concentrations of fatty acids and acyl-CoA esters in muscle when lipolysis in adipose tissue is high. This has a protective function, since high fatty acid concentrations are toxic to myocardial activity (16).

CONTROL OF FATTY ACID METABOLISM IN ADIPOSE TISSUE

The control of fatty acid metabolism in adipose tissue is more easily understood than that in liver since adipose tissue specifically stores fatty acids when energy supplies are readily available, and it releases them when energy is needed. Insulin stimulates the uptake of glucose by adipocytes and this substrate is used for fatty acid synthesis and to provide the glycerol backbone of triacylglycerol. Furthermore, insulin increases the LPL activity of adipose tissue thus facilitating the uptake of fatty acids derived from chylomicrons or VLDL (8). High concentrations of glucocorticoids can complement the action of insulin in increasing LPL activities (8). Thus, at the time when fatty acid synthesis in the liver is stimulated, the enzymic apparatus of adipose tissue adapts so that it can receive and store energy.

Conversely, when insulin concentrations are low the activity of LPL falls and fatty acids are released from adipose tissue because of the activation of the hormone sensitive lipase (Fig. 1). These fatty acids are oxidized by heart, skeletal muscle and liver. Additionally, as discussed above, the liver may secrete some of the fatty acids back into the circulation in VLDL. The decrease in LPL activities in adipose tissue helps to minimise its metabolism of VLDL. The activities of the enzymes responsible for the esterification of fatty acids may also be decreased in times of metabolic stress. This could reduce not only the re-esterification of fatty acids derived directly from lipolysis, but also those already circulating in the blood. Some evidence that this type of co-ordinated control might occur in vivo is shown in Fig. 3. The injection of corticotropin into rats increased the concentrations of fatty acids in the blood by about 2-fold (21) and it decreased the activity of LPL by 25-40% (Fig. 3b). This decrease lasted for at least 360 min. The activity of the soluble PAP was decreased by 25-30% at 30 and 100 min after injection, but thereafter the PAP activity returned to control values. There was no increase in PAP activity in adipose tissue at 360 min after the injection of corticotropin, whereas in the livers of the same rats it was increased by 3-4-fold. These results, and the lack of a phosphatidate deacylase system in adipose tissue demonstrate a differential control of

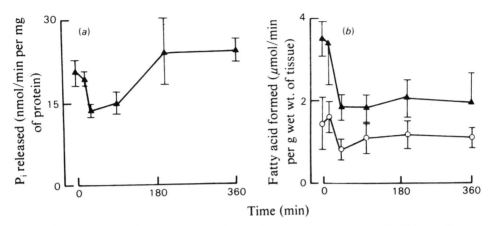

Time (min)

FIG. 3. <u>Effects of corticotropin injection on the activities of the soluble PAP (a), and on LPL (b) in rat adipose tissue</u>

Male rats were fed on starch (▲) and corn oil diets (O) for 3 weeks and they were injected with corticotropin at the time = 0 (20). Results are means ± S.D. for eight rats at time = 0, or for four rats at other times. This figure is reproduced with permission of Biochem. J. (21).

phosphatidate metabolism in the two organs (21).

The experiments described above do not establish whether the effects are produced solely by corticotropin, or whether other hormones such as catecholamines and glucagon are involved. It is known that these hormones, and other compounds that can increase cyclic-AMP concentrations and stimulate lipolysis in adipose tissue, can decrease LPL activity (8). Furthermore, nor-adrenalin can produce a rapid decrease in the PAP activity in adipocytes <u>in vitro</u>, and this effect can be blocked by propranolol and reversed by insulin (37). In other work <u>in vitro</u>, adrenalin, cyclic AMP-analogues and theophyline were reported to decrease the soluble PAP activity, but to increase PAP in the microsomal fraction. By contrast, corticotropin increased both microsomal and soluble PAP activities (28). Other work <u>in vitro</u> has demonstrated rapid changes in the activities of acyl-CoA synthetase, GPAT, DHAPAT and DGAT in adipocytes. In general catecholamines decrease these activities, whereas insulin opposes these changes (37).

At present it is not certain how important these changes are in terms of the physiological control of adipose tissue function. For instance, in starvation, the activity of LPL in adipose tissue was decreased by 62–72%, whereas the activities of acyl-CoA synthetase, the mitochondrial GPAT and the N-ethylmaleimide-insensitive DHAPAT fell by 25, 50 and 58% respectively (21). There were no changes in the activities of the microsomal GPAT and DGAT, or in the soluble PAP. Furthermore, changes in the composition of dietary fat and carbohydrate had little effect on the activities of the enzymes involved in glycerolipid synthesis, whereas high fat diets decrease LPL activities by about 50% (21). Increases in PAP activity have been reported in the adipose tissue of ob/ob mice (13) and in obese human beings (5), and these changes may be significant in producing accelerated triacylglycerol synthesis.

It seems clear that changes in the activity of LPL play an important part in controlling the uptake of fatty acids by adipose tissue. The enzymes of triacylglycerol synthesis can be regulated, particularly by rapid changes brought about by catecholamine, glucagon or corticotropin. However, there is very little information at present to show how important these changes are in vivo, when compared with those that occur in LPL activity.

CONCLUSION

This paper has reviewed some of the hormonal factors that control the synthesis and turnover of triacylglycerols in liver, muscle and adipose tissue. In particular, the importance of insulin action in relation to the effects of "stress" hormones such as glucocorticoids, corticotropin, catecholamines and glucagon has been emphasized. Glucocorticoids can either antagonise or complement the action of insulin. The antagonism is seen at the level of glycolysis, gluconeogenesis, protein synthesis and protein breakdown. It is also observed in hepatic triacylglycerol synthesis where insulin inhibits the effects of glucocorticoids in stimulating the activity of PAP. The glucocorticoid-induced increase in PAP activity has a number of metabolic consequences. First, it may enable the liver to maintain its synthesis of phosphatidylcholine and phosphatidylethanolamine when insulin concentrations are low. Secondly, it may help to protect the liver against the potentially toxic effects of high concentrations of fatty acids and acyl-CoA esters by facilitating the synthesis of triacylglycerols. Finally, it could enable the liver to secrete triacylglycerols in VLDL in times of metabolic stress.

In these conditions most of the VLDL can be metabolised in muscle tissue where the high glucocorticoid concentrations promote the activity of LPL. At the same time there is increased secretion of glucose and ketones from the liver. In this sense the secretion of triacylglycerol is part of a co-ordinated metabolic response that is analogous to that of gluconeogenesis. It enables the liver to provide extrahepatic tissue with a source of energy when insulin action is diminished. The hypertriglyceridaemia and hyperglycaemia that can result from this are both caused by increased secretion and by decreased peripheral uptake. The diminished effects of insulin would cause a decrease in the removal of VLDL by adipose tissue, and in the uptake of glucose by muscle and adipose tissue.

Obesity is accompanied by hyperglycaemia, insulin-resistance and an increased turnover and storage of triacylglycerol, even though hypertriglyceridaemia may not always occur. The increased storage of energy may also involve an interaction of insulin and glucocorticoids. In this case the actions of these two hormones are complimentary. They act together in stimulating the synthesis of glycogen, fatty acids and triacylglycerols, and the uptake of triacylglycerols by adipose tissue. Thus an improved understanding of how insulin interacts with "stress" hormones could provide a better insight into the changes in metabolism that accompany obesity.

ACKNOWLEDGEMENTS

We thank the Medical Research Council of Great Britain for financial support.

REFERENCES

1. Bates, E.J., and Saggerson, E.D. (1977): FEBS Lett., 84:229-232.
2. Bates, E.J., and Saggerson, E.D. (1979): Biochem. J., 182:751-762.
3. Bates, E.J., and Saggerson, E.D. (1981): FEBS Lett., 84:229-232.
4. Bates, E.J., Topping, D.L., Sooranna, S.R., Saggerson, E.D., and Mayes, P. (1977): FEBS Lett., 84:225-228.
5. Belfiore, F., Rabinazzo, A.M., Borzi, V., and Iannello, S. (1978): Diabetologia, 15:218.
6. Brindley, D.N. (1981): Clin. Sci., 61:129-133.
7. Cole, T.G., Wilcox, H.G., and Heimberg, M. (1982): J. Lipid Res., 23:81-91.
8. Cryer, A. (1981): Int. J. Biochem., 13:525-541.
9. Debeer, L.J., Declercq, P.E., and Mannaerts, G.P. (1981): FEBS Lett., 24:31-34.
10. Declercq, P.E., Debeer, L.J., and Mannaerts, G.P. (1982): Biochem. J., 202:803-806.
11. Diamant, S., and Shafrir, E. (1975): Eur. J. Biochem., 53:541-546.
12. Fallon, H.J., and Kemp, E.L. (1968): J. Clin. Invest., 47:712-719.
13. Fallon, H.J., Lamb, R.G., and Jamdar, S.C. (1977): Biochem. Soc. Trans., 5:37-40.
14. Haagsman, H.P., de Haas, L.G.M., Geelen, M.J.H., and van Golde, L.M.G. (1981): Biochim. Biophys. Acta, 664:74-81.
15. Herberg, L., and Coleman, D.L. (1977): Metabolism, 26:59-99.
16. Hülsmann, W.C., and Stam, H. (1979): In: Lipoprotein Metabolism and Endocrine Regulation, edited by L.W. Hessel and H.M.J. Krans, pp.289-297. Elsevier/North-Holland Biomedical Press, Amsterdam.
17. Ide, T., and Ontko, J.A. (1981): J. Biol. Chem., 256:10247-10255.
18. Jennings, R.J., Lawson, N., Fears, R., and Brindley, D.N. (1981): FEBS Lett., 133:119-122.
19. Kirk, C.J., Verrinder, T.R., and Hems, D.A. (1976): Biochem. J., 156:593-602.
20. Lawson, N., Jennings, R.J., Pollard, A.D., Sturton, R.G., Ralph, S.J., Marsden, C.A., Fears, R., and Brindley, D.N. (1981): Biochem. J., 200:265-275.
21. Lawson, N., Pollard, A.D., Jennings, R.J., Gurr, M.I., and Brindley, D.N. (1981): Biochem. J., 200:285-294.
22. Lawson, N., Jennings, R.J., Fears, R., and Brindley, D.N. (1982): FEBS Lett., 143:in the press.
23. Lehtonen, M.A., Savolainen, M.J., and Hassinen, I.E. (1979): FEBS Lett., 99:162-166.
24. Mangiapane, E.H., Lloyd-Davies, K.A., and Brindley, D.N. (1973): Biochem. J., 134:103-112.
25. Manning, R., and Brindley, D.N. (1972): Biochem. J., 130:1003-1012.
26. McGarry, J.D., and Foster, D.N. (1980): Ann. Rev. Biochem., 49:395-420.
27. Mitchell, M.P., Brindley, D.N., and Hübscher, G. (1971): Eur. J. Biochem.,18:214-220.
28. Moller, F., Wong, K.H., and Green, P. (1981): Can. J. Biochem., 59:9-15.
29. Murthy, V.K., and Shipp, J.C. (1977): Diabetes, 26:222-229.
30. Murthy, V.K., and Shipp, J.C. (1979): Diabetes, 28:472-478.
31. Murthy, V.K., and Shipp, J.C. (1980): J. Mol. Cell. Cardiol., 12:299-309.
32. Nimmo, H.G. (1979): Biochem. J., 177:283-288.

33. Nimmo, H.G., and Houston, D. (1978): Biochem. J., 176:607-610.
34. Pelech, S.L., Pritchard, P.H., and Vance, D.E. (1981):
    J. Biol. Chem., 256:8283-8286.
35. Pollard, A.D., and Brindley, D.N (1982): Biochem. Pharmacol.,
    30:1650-1652.
36. Roncari, D.A.K., and Mack, E.Y.W. (1981): Can. J. Biochem.,
    59:944-950.
37. Saggerson, E.D., Sooranna, S.R., and Cheng, C.H.K. (1979): In:
    Obesity - Cellular and Molecular Aspects, edited by G. Ailhaud,
    pp.223-238 Inserm, Paris.
38. Schlossman, D.M. and Bell, R.M. (1978): Arch. Biochem. Biophys.,
    182:732-742.
39. Soler-Argilaga, C., Russell, R.L., and Heimberg, M. (1977):
    Biochem. Biophys. Res. Commun., 78:1053-1059.
40. Soler-Argilaga, C., Russell, R.L., Werner, H.V., and Heimberg, M.
    (1978): Biochem. Biophys. Res. Commun., 85:249-256.
41. Sturton, R.G., and Brindley, D.N. (1980): Biochim. Biophys. Acta,
    619:494-505.
42. Van Tol, A. (1974): Biochim. Biophys. Acta, 357:14-23.
43. Whiting, P.H., Bowley, M., Sturton, R.G., Pritchard, P.H.,
    Brindley, D.N., and Hawthorne, J.N. (1977): Biochem. J.,
    168:147-153.
44. Wiegand, R.D., Rao, G.A., and Reiser, R. (1973): J. Nutri.,
    103:1414-1424.
45. Woods, J.A., Knauer, T.E., and Lamb, R.G. (1981): Biochim.
    Biophys. Acta, 666:482-492.
46. Yamada, K., and Okuyama, H. (1978): Arch. Biochem. Biophys.,
    190:409-420.
47. Young, D.L., and Lynen, F. (1969): J. Biol. Chem., 244:377-383.
48. Zammit, V.A. (1981): Biochem. J., 198:75-85.

The Adipocyte and Obesity: Cellular and Molecular Mechanisms, edited by A. Angel, C. H. Hollenberg, and D. A. K. Roncari. Raven Press, New York © 1983.

Lipid Transport in Tissue by Lateral Movement in Cell Membranes

*Robert O. Scow, *E. Joan Blanchette-Mackie, *Mary G. Wetzel, and **Alli Reinila

*Laboratory of Cellular and Developmental Biology, NIADDK, National Institutes of Health, Bethesda, Maryland 20205; and **Department of Pathology, University of Oulu, Oulu, Finland*

Triacylglycerol, cholesterol and phosphatidylcholine of chylomicrons are taken up directly by extrahepatic tissues (21,28). This process involves lipoprotein lipase (21,28), which hydrolyzes triacylglycerol to fatty acids and monoacylglycerol at the capillary luminal surface (20). There are two physical forms in which lipids might cross capillary endothelium, as components of lipoprotein particles and as individual molecules (20). There is no evidence that chylomicrons, intact or partially lipolyzed, cross capillary endothelium (20).

MOLECULAR TRANSPORT OF FATTY ACIDS

Three mechanisms have been proposed for transport of fatty acids in tissues: transport through aqueous phase and across cell membranes by molecular diffusion (7), transport by fatty acid-binding protein (14), and transport by lateral movement in a continuum of cell membranes (19). The concept of molecular diffusion of fatty acids requires concentration gradients across cell membranes, resulting from oxidation or esterification of fatty acids in cells, and presumes no difficulty in transfer of fatty acids across cell membranes or release of fatty acids from membranes to aqueous phase (7). However, transfer of fatty acids across membranes involves the flip-flop mechanism which is very slow (8), and desorption of long chain fatty acids from lipid-water interfaces to aqueous phase is negligible at pH 7.4 (14,22). Furthermore, long chain fatty acids are poorly soluble in aqueous medium at pH 7.4 (25), and their presence in cytosol as monomers has not been demonstrated. Transport of fatty acids by fatty acid-binding protein presumably occurs only in cytosol (14). Consequently, it too would require the slow flip-flop mechanism for transfer across cell membranes and molecular diffusion in aqueous phase for transfer through extracellular space.

Transport of fatty acids by lateral movement in cell membranes (19) is feasible because membranes are lipid bilayers (24), amphipathic lipids can move rapidly in the plane of membranes (8), and fatty acids are amphipathic (22,25). Studies with incubated chylomicrons (1) and lipid monolayers (22) showed that fatty acids and monoacylglycerol formed by action of lipoprotein lipase on triacylglycerol locate in the interface between lipid/gas and aqueous phase at pH 7.4, and spread in the interface toward zones of decreased surface pressure resulting from removal

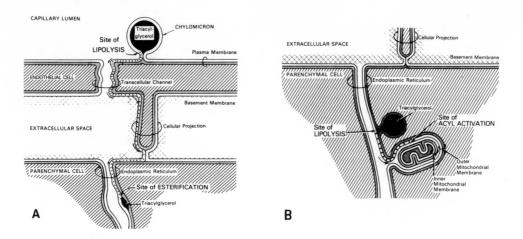

FIG. 1. Route for transport of fatty acids (A) from chylomicrons to
intracellular lipid droplets and (B) from lipid droplets to the interior
of mitochondria by lateral movement in an interfacial continuum of cell
membranes (5,20,26).

of lipolytic products from the interface or extension of the interface.

Transport between Capillary Lumen and Lipid Droplets in Cells

Transport of fatty acids from blood to tissue by lateral movement in
cell membranes presupposes an interfacial continuum between capillary
lumen and the interior of parenchymal cells (3,19). Capillary endothelium in adipose (3,19), muscle (23), and mammary tissue (19) have trans-
cellular channels which connect capillary lumen with extracellular
space (Fig. 1-A). Since the external (luminal) leaflet of the membrane
lining such channels connects the external leaflet of luminal plasma
membrane with that of basal plasma membrane, it provides an interfacial
continuum (broad white line in drawing) across capillary endothelium.
Recent studies in white adipose tissue (2), heart (26), muscular artery
(16), and brown adipose tissue (5) showed that cell processes of endothelial and parenchymal cells extend through basement membrane to make
contact with each other. Apparent continuity of the external leaflet
of plasma membrane of one cell with that of another cell was observed
in white adipose tissue (Fig. 2). Studies in white and brown adipose
tissues (2,4) showed that intracellular channels extend from extracellular space to the surface of lipid droplets in adipocytes. Thus,
the luminal leaflet of membranes lining these channels provides an interfacial continuum between the external leaflet of plasma membane and
the surface of lipid droplets (Fig. 1-A). The above constitute the
evidence for an interfacial continuum of membranes extending from the
luminal surface of capillaries to the surface of lipid droplets in
parenchymal cells.

Our model for transport of fatty acids by lateral movement in a continuum of cell membranes (19,20) proposes that fatty acids formed by action of lipoprotein lipase on chylomicron triacylglycerol enter the continuum at sites of lipolysis in capillaries, and move in the continuum

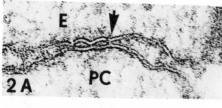

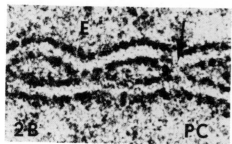

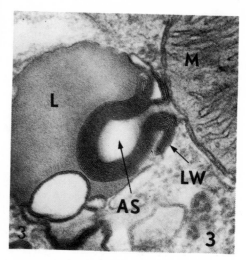

FIG. 2. A section of adipose tissue suggesting structural continuity between outer leaflet of plasma membrane of capillary endothelium (E) and that of parenchymal cell (PC). A. X160,000, B. X744,000. (Ref. 2). FIG. 3. A section of incubated-fixed heart showing in a myocyte a lamellar structure (LW) extending from periphery of aqueous space (AS) in lipid droplet (L) to outer chamber of mitochondrion (M). X84,000.

to endoplasmic reticulum of parenchymal cells where they can be reesterified to triacylglycerol and accumulate as lipid droplets between leaflets of the reticulum (Fig. 1-A). The model also proposes that fatty acids formed by action of tissue (hormone-sensitive) lipase (11,15) on intracellular triacylglycerol in adipose tissue reenter the continuum at sites of lipolysis in endoplasmic reticulum, and move in the continuum to capillary endothelium where they can bind to plasma albumin for transport to other tissues (3,20).

Lamellar structures with a periodicity of 40 A developed in glutaraldehyde-fixed white adipose tissue of young rats when incubated at 25°C (3). The lamellae were found in transendothelial channels, at sites of intercellular contact, and in channels that extended from extracellular space to intracellular lipid droplets in fat cells. They were found associated with chylomicrons in capillaries of tissue from fed rats, and near lipid droplets in fat cells of tissue from fasted rats. Similar findings were made in incubated-fixed heart (26), muscular (dorsalis pedis) artery (16), and brown adipose tissue (5) from fed rats. Lamellae developed under conditions causing lipolysis and accumulation of fatty acids in fixed tissues, and the amount and distribution of lamellae varied with incubation time and metabolic state of the tissue donor (3,5, 16,26). The lamellar structures in incubated-fixed tissues had the same periodicity, 40 A, as lamellae in sections of sodium oleate fixed with osmium (1). These findings indicate that the lamellar structures found in incubated-fixed tissues are probably fatty acids. We conclude from the above studies that fatty acids formed by lipolysis in fixed tissue locate and spread in an interfacial continuum of cell membranes extending from the capillary (arterial) lumen to intracellular lipid droplets. When fatty acids overcrowd the continuum, they form lamellar extensions into the aqueous phase at different sites marking the course of the continuum through the tissue.

Transport from Lipid Droplets to Mitochondria in Cells

Oxidation of fatty acids in mitochondria provides energy for muscular contraction in heart (10,13) and arteries (12), and heat production in brown adipose tissue (9). Fatty acids are delivered to these tissues by blood, as components of triacylglycerol in chylomcirons and VLDL, and as fatty acids bound to plasma albumin (10). Some of the fatty acids taken up are immediately oxidized (heart and artery), while others are esterified to triacylglycerol and stored temporarily as intracellular lipid droplets before being oxidized (brown fat, heart and artery). Movement of fatty acids from lipid droplets to mitochondria requires hydrolysis of triacylglycerol to fatty acids by tissue (hormone-sensitive) lipase (11,15). It is generally assumed that fatty acids are transported to mitochondria by molecular diffusion through cytosol (7,10). It has also been suggested that fatty acid-binding protein may be involved in transport of fatty acids to mitochondria (10,14). Limitations of these transport mechanisms were discussed above.

Our studies in incubated-fixed tissues showed that lamellar structures developed near and inside mitochondria in heart of fed and fasted rats (26), in smooth muscle cells of the muscular artery of rats infused intravenously with triacylglycerol (16), and in brown adipose tissue of young rats exposed to 4°C for 2 hr or unsuckled for 18 hr (5). In addition, intracellular lipid droplets decreased in size and aqueous spaces developed near lipid droplets during incubation (5,16,26). Lamellar whorls were also found in channels that extended from lipid droplets to the interior of mitochondria (Fig.3). This suggested that fatty acids could be transported from lipid droplets to mitochondria by lateral movement in an interfacial continuum comprised of the luminal leaflets of endoplasmic reticulum and outer mitochondrial membrane (Fig. 3). Evidence for membrane continuity between endoplasmic reticulum and outer mitochondrial membrane has been found in canine heart (6) and mouse oocytes (17). Therefore, we propose that when fatty acids are needed for oxidation, fatty acids formed by action of tissue lipase on intracellular triacylglycerol reenter the continuum at sites of lipolysis in the reticulum (Fig. 1-B), and move in the continuum to the outer mitochondral membrane where they are activated for transfer to the inner matrix for oxidation (10).

MOLECULAR TRANSPORT OF MONOACYLGLYCEROL, CHOLESTEROL AND PHOSPHOLIPID

Transport of monoacylglycerol, cholesterol and phosphatidylcholine from chylomicrons to parenchymal cells by molecular diffusion through aqueous phase is unlikely because these lipids are both strongly amphipathic and extremely insoluble in water (25). Exchange and carrier proteins have been proposed for transport of cholesterol (18) and phospholipid (27), but there is no evidence they are involved in lipid transport from capillary lumen to tissue cells.

We propose that these lipids are also transported by lateral movement in a continuum of cell membranes. Monoacylglycerol would enter the continuum at sites of lipolysis in capillaries, and leave the continuum in endoplasmic reticulum of parenchymal cells when reesterified to triacylglycerol (20). Cholesterol and phospholipid, in contrast, are present in the chylomicron surface film and would move in the continuum as the chylomicron core is reduced by lipolysis to contribute to membrane proliferation in cells during storage of triacylglycerol (19).

REFERENCES

1. Blanchette-Mackie, E.J., and Scow, R.O.(1976): J. Lipid Res., 17:57-67.

2. Blanchette-Mackie, E.J., and Scow, R.O.(1981): J. Ultrastruct. Res., 77:277-294.

3. Blanchette-Mackie, E.J., and Scow, R.O.(1981): J. Ultrastruct. Res., 77:295-318.

4. Blanchette-Mackie, E.J., and Scow, R.O.(1982): Anat. Rec., 203: No. 2.

5. Blanchette-Mackie, E.J., and Scow, R.O.: J. Lipid Res., (submitted).

6. Bowman, R.W.(1967): Tex. Rep. Biol. Med., 25:517-524.

7. Dietschy, J.M.(1978): In: Disturbances in Lipid and Lipoprotein Metabolism, edited by J.M.Dietschy, A.M.Gotto,Jr., and J.A.Ontko, pp.1-28. Am. Physiol. Soc., Bethesda, Maryland.

8. Edidin, M.(1974): Annu. Rev. Biophys. Bioeng., 3:179-201.

9. Hull, D.(1973): In: Comparative Physiology of Thermoregulation, edited by G.C.Whittow, pp. 167-200. Academic Press, New York.

10. Idell-Wenger, J.A., and Neely, J.R.(1978). In: Disturbances in Lipid and Lipoprotein Metabolism, edited by J.M.Dietschy, A.M.Gotto, Jr., and J.A.Ontko, pp. 269-284. Am. Physiol. Soc., Bethesda, Maryland.

11. Lech, J.J., Jesmok, G.J., and Calvert, D.N.(1977): Fed. Proc. 36:2000-2008.

12. Morrison, E.S., Scott, R.F., Kroms, M., and Frick, J.(1974): Biochem. Med. 11:153-164.

13. Neely, J.R., and Morgan, H.E.(1974): Ann. Rev. Physiol., 36:413-459.

14. Ockner, R.K., and Manning, J.A.(1974): J. Clin. Invest., 54:326-338.

15. Reed, N., and Fain, J.N.(1970): In: Brown Adipose Tissue, edited by O. Lindberg, pp. 207-224. Elsevier, New York.

16. Reinila, A., Blanchette-Mackie, E.J., and Scow, R.O.: Arteriosclerosis, (submitted).

17. Ruby, J.R., Dyer, R.F., and Skalko, R.G.(1969): Z. Zellforsch. Mikrosk. Anat., 97:30-37.

18. Scallen, T.J., Srikantaiah, M.V., Skrdlant, H.B., and Hansbury, E. (1972): FEBS Lett., 25:227-233.

19. Scow, R.O., Blanchette-Mackie, E.J., and Smith, L.C.(1976): Circ. Res., 39:149-162.

20. Scow, R.O., Blanchette-Mackie, E.J., and Smith, L.C.(1980): Federation Proc., 39:2610-2617.

21. Scow, R.O., Chernick, S.S., and Fleck, T.R.(1977): Biochim. Biophys Acta, 487:297-306.

22. Scow, R.O., Desnuelle, P., and Verger, R.(1979): J. Biol. Chem., 254:6456-6463.

23. Simionescu, N., Simionescu, M., and Palade, G.E.(1975): J. Cell Biol., 64:586-607.

24. Singer, S.J., and Nicolson, G.L.(1972): Science, 175:720-731.

25. Small, D.M.(1968): J. Am. Oil Chem. Soc., 45:108-117.

26. Wetzel, M.G., and Scow, R.O.: Am. J. Physiol., (submitted).

27. Wirtz, K.W.A.(1974): Biochim. Biophys. Acta, 334:95-117.

28. Zinder, O., Mendelson, C.R., Blanchette-Mackie, E.J., and Scow, R.O. (1976): Biochim. Biophys. Acta, 431:526-537.

The Adipocyte and Obesity: Cellular and Molecular Mechanisms, edited by A. Angel, C. H. Hollenberg, and D. A. K. Roncari. Raven Press, New York © 1983.

Cholesterol Turnover and Metabolism in Humans

DeWitt S. Goodman, Conrad B. Blum, Ralph B. Dell, Robert H. Palmer, and Rajasekhar Ramakrishnan

Arteriosclerosis Research Center and the Departments of Medicine and Pediatrics, Columbia University College of Physicians and Surgeons, New York, New York 10032

Two general experimental approaches have been used in recent years to investigate the in vivo parameters of body cholesterol metabolism in intact humans. In one of these, the sterol balance method, the daily turnover of cholesterol (in g/day) is determined directly by measurement of the fecal excretion products of cholesterol (fecal neutral sterols and bile acids) (7). The second, kinetic, approach has involved analysis of the turnover of plasma cholesterol following the injection of radioactively labeled cholesterol or a biosynthetic precursor of cholesterol (5). Estimates of the daily turnover of cholesterol obtained from kinetic studies agree well with estimates of this parameter determined by simultaneous sterol balance studies. Some investigators have also used combinations of kinetic and sterol balance experiments in particular studies (7,16).

Two mathematical approaches have been employed to analyze the results of kinetic studies: these are a model-free method (11,15), and a pool model or compartmental analysis method (5,4). Both methods (as well as the sterol balance methods) assume that the metabolism of cholesterol is constant from day to day (steady state) throughout the study. The principal difference between the model-free and the pool-model approaches is that the latter assumes that the turnover of cholesterol can be characterized by a small, finite number of pools, thereby obtaining more parameters.

Cholesterol Kinetics in Humans

A great deal has been learned from kinetic studies about cholesterol turnover and metabolism in intact humans. In 1968 it was reported from our laboratory (3) that the plasma cholesterol specific radio-activity-time curves obtained in experiments of about 10 weeks duration conformed to a simple two-pool model. Since then, this model has been used extensively in many laboratories to study cholesterol turnover in vivo. In 1970, however, Samuel and Perl reported (14) that in some patients, the slow slope of the plasma decay curve deviated from monoexponential behavior after approximately 20-25 weeks. This suggested that a multi-compartmental model of more than two pools was necessary to describe the long-term turnover of plasma cholesterol in man. Accordingly, the turnover of plasma cholesterol was studied by us for periods of 32-41 weeks in 6 subjects and, in each subject, the best description of the turnover curve was found to be a three-pool rather than a two-pool model (4).

We now report results obtained from long-term studies (32-49 weeks duration) of the turnover of plasma cholesterol carried out during the past decade in 82 subjects. Twenty-one subjects were normal, 22 had hypercholesterolemia alone, 25 had hypertriglyceridemia alone, and 14 had both hypercholesterolemia and hypertriglyceridemia. Many of the hyperlipidemic subjects had a familial form of hyperlipidemia. In every subject in this heterogeneous study population, the three-pool model provided the best fit to the long-term turnover data. Thus, this model seems to be generally valid for the study of cholesterol turnover in intact humans, and for comparison of hyperlipidemic patients with normals and with each other.

An extensive statistical analysis was conducted of the results obtained with the first 54 subjects studied (5). The objective of this analysis was to delineate any significant relationships that may exist between the model parameters of body cholesterol turnover and various physiological variables (body size, serum lipid levels, age, and sex). To this end, a search was conducted for correlations between many different forms of the model parameters as dependent variables and many different forms of the physiological variables as independent variables. A wide range of both linear and nonlinear relationships was explored, as well as possible relationships involving interactions between pairs of variables (cross-product terms). In all, 50 different forms of the model parameters and 53 forms of the physiological variables were examined.

In order to guard against declaring statistical significance when none was present, subjects were first randomly divided into two matched groups. In the first (hypothesis-generating) group of 36 subjects, more than 100,000 regression equations were considered for each form of the model parameters. After applying rigid statistical criteria and physiological considerations, 21 regression equations were found that were highly significant and that contained interesting physiological relationships for 4 model parameters and functions thereof. These equations were then tested for significance in the hypothesis-testing group of 18 subjects. Eighteen of the 21 equations were found to be significant in the testing group. From these, 6 equations were selected that accounted for a large part of the observed variation found between people in the 4 model parameters for which equations were found (production rate (PR), and the sizes of pool 1, pool 3, and total exchangeable body cholesterol).

The major determinant of cholesterol PR was body weight alone ($r = 0.80$). No function of serum lipid levels significantly influenced PR. Both body weight and the serum cholesterol level entered into the equations for cholesterol mass, i.e., for the sizes of pool 1, pool 3, and total exchangeable body cholesterol. Age influenced significantly the size of pool 3, suggesting that with time cholesterol deposition occurs in certain tissues and increases as cholesterol level increases. Serum triglyceride level only had an effect on the size of pool 1. Since these equations were generated in one subgroup of the study population and tested in another subgroup, it was felt that they could be considered as a confirmed set of predictive equations.

We have recently updated these equations by determining the coefficients that describe these relationships between model parameters and physiological variables for the larger study population of 82 subjects. The equations so obtained are given in Table 1. All of the multiple correlation coefficients shown are 0.72 or higher, so that the sets of physiological variables shown can account (as r^2) for 53 to 68% of the observed variation in the 4 model parameters listed.

Table 1. Equations for Major Model Parameters (82 subjects).

Dependent Variable[a]	Independent Variables and Regression Coefficients[b]			Intercept	Multiple r
PR	0.0213 Wt			− 0.386	0.77
M_1	0.291 Wt	+ 0.0397 Chol	− 1.63 TGGP	− 6.95	0.82
M_3min	0.659 Wt	+ 0.051 Chol	+ 0.536 Age	−52.1	0.73
M_3min	0.992 EWt	+ 0.375 Age		11.0	0.72
M_{tot}min	0.956 Wt	+ 0.091 Chol		−16.6	0.81
M_{tot}min	1.036 EWt	+ 0.00106 Chol·Wt		50.0	0.80

[a]PR = production rate (g/day): M_1 = size of pool 1 (g); M_3min = minimum estimate of the size of pool 3 (g); M_{tot}min = minimum estimate for total body exchangeable cholesterol (g).

[b]Wt = total body weight (kg); EWt = excess body weight (observed weight minus ideal weight, in kg); Chol = serum cholesterol concentration (mg/dl); TGGP = variable equal to 1, 2, or 3 depending on serum triglyceride concentration (<200, 200–300, or >300); Age (years); Chol·Wt = serum cholesterol concentration times body weight.

Body weight (or excess body weight) is the major determinant of the model parameter in each of the 6 equations shown in Table 1. The relationship between weight and total body exchangeable cholesterol (adjusting for the effects of serum cholesterol level) is shown in Figure 1; that between excess weight and the size of pool 3 (adjusting for effects of age) is shown in Figure 2.

Three-pool Model

Our mamillary three-pool model of cholesterol turnover consists of a central pool exchanging with two side pools (4,5). As discussed previously (4,5), it must be recognized that the three pools in the model represent mathematical constructs and do not have precise physical meaning. The finding that the long-term turnover of plasma cholesterol conforms to a three-pool model in humans means that the various tissue pools of exchangeable body cholesterol fall into three groups in terms of the rates at which they equilibrate with plasma cholesterol. Some information is available about the anatomic localization of the cholesterol molecules that comprise the three pools of the model. Pool 1, which consists of cholesterol in fairly rapid equilibrium with plasma cholesterol, mainly consists of cholesterol in plasma, blood cells, liver, and intestine. Pool 2 consists of cholesterol which equilibrates at an intermediate rate with plasma cholesterol, and probably includes some of the cholesterol in viscera, together with some of the cholesterol in peripheral tissues. Adipose

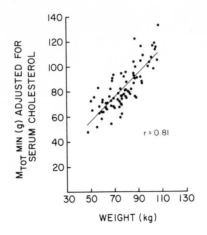

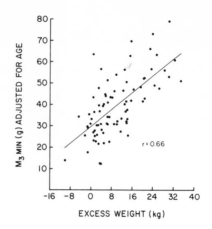

FIG.1. Relationship between M_{tot}min, adjusted for differences in serum cholesterol level, and body weight.

FIG.2. Relationship between M_3min, adjusted for differences in age, and excess body weight.

tissue cholesterol appears to be an important part of the most slowly turning over compartment, pool 3 (17). Cholesterol in other peripheral tissues, particularly connective tissue and skeletal muscle (1,19), and including arterial walls (8), also equilibrates slowly with plasma cholesterol; cholesterol in these tissue sites probably also constitutes a significant portion of pool 3.

In this three-pool model, the synthesis of cholesterol may take place in each of the three pools, while output is constrained to occur only through the rapidly miscible central pool, pool 1. The model has 8 unknown parameters. Since a sum of three exponentials has only 3 coefficients and 3 exponential constants, only 6 model parameters can be determined uniquely from an analysis of the plasma cholesterol turnover curve. The remaining ambiguity, in which the masses and synthesis rates of the side pools (pools 2 and 3) cannot be determined uniquely, may be termed nonuniqueness (12).

In our studies, this nonuniqueness has been recognized, and ranges of possible values have been calculated for the indeterminate parameters. In the three-pool model, minimum values for the side pool masses are obtained by setting side pool synthesis to zero: the maximum value for each side pool mass is obtained by setting the synthesis rate in that pool equal to the total endogenous synthesis rate. We have used this approach in our studies, and for each subject have computed minimum and maximum values for the sizes of pools 2 and 3, and intermediate values of these masses as well. The data analysis that was previously conducted (5) to search for relationships between model parameters and physiological variables included each of these mass estimates of pools 2 and 3 as dependent variables. Significant relationships were found for all of the estimates (minimum, intermediate, and maximum) of the size of pool 3, but for none of the estimates of the size of pool 2. As discussed (5,4), on physiological grounds it is highly probable that the true values for the sizes of pools 2 and 3 are closer to the minimum than to the maximum values.

Another approach would involve the injection of a biosynthetic precursor of cholesterol labeled with a different isotope, in addition to labeled cholesterol itself. Equations have been derived and reported (12) for calculating uniquely all of the parameters of a three-pool model following the injection of two such tracers. These equations could be used if a satisfactory precursor label were to be used along with a cholesterol label. There is a need to perform animal studies to establish that an injected precursor is incorporated at each synthetic site in an amount proportional to the rate of synthesis at that site. Until a validated precursor is available, the best approach is to calculate the ranges of the masses as discussed above.

Simplified Sampling Schedule

An extensive study has been conducted to assess the optimal sampling times and the minimal sampling frequency needed to estimate the parameters of the three-pool model. The approach used has been described in reference (2). In brief, for the three-pool model, only 6 accurate points, at critical times, are required to estimate the model parameters. Accuracy can be achieved by replicating the specific activity analyses at each critical sampling time. The first three critical times are 1, 7, and 24 days (for non-hypercholesterolemic subjects), or 1, 8, and 28 days (for hypercholesterolemic subjects). The last three times must be chosen for each subject individually, from the results of the first three samples and from prior information (derived from previously studied subjects).

This 6-point sampling schedule was compared with the usual schedule (36-points) in 26 normal and hyperlipidemic subjects. The results are shown in Table 2. We have compared the variation of the parameter estimates for the two schedules by expressing the standard deviation of the difference between the estimates from the two schedules as a percent of the mean estimate from the 36-point schedule (i.e., the coefficient of variation (C.V.) given in Table 2). The results for the 4 model parameters for which we have developed multiple regression equations (see (5) and Table 1) are shown. In Table 2, pool sizes (M values) are in g, and PR in g/day. The C.V.'s are quite small, and there is excellent agreement between the two sampling schedules for the mean parameter estimates for the 26 subjects. Thus, a convenient blood sampling schedule has been developed for determining the plasma cholesterol turnover curve, which has been tested on 26 subjects with good results. This simplified schedule is currently being used in all of our turnover studies.

Table 2. Model Parameters from Two Blood Sampling Schedules.

	PR	M_1	$M_3 min$	$M_{tot} min$
36-point mean	1.385	25.08	41.02	84.42
6-point mean	1.385	24.71	43.67	84.15
C.V. (%)	1.5	4.1	13.0	4.3

Lipoprotein Relationships

It is well established that plasma lipoproteins play an important role in the regulation of cholesterol metabolism and homeostasis in a variety of tissues. Currently, a great deal of interest exists about possible relationships between high density lipoprotein (HDL) metabolism and the metabolism of cholesterol in various cells and tissues. This interest has been stimulated in part by the now well established inverse relationship between HDL cholesterol levels and the prevalence of coronary heart disease (13,6).

The mechanism responsible for the protective role of HDL against coronary heart disease is not defined. A leading proposed mechanism is that HDL may reduce tissue stores of cholesterol, by transporting cholesterol from peripheral tissues,including the arterial wall,to the liver (9). Two sorts of evidence support this hypothesis. First, HDL or the apoproteins of HDL remove cholesterol from cells in culture (18). Secondly, a report published in 1976 (10) indicated that plasma HDL levels were found to be inversely related to the mass of slowly exchanging body cholesterol. A strong relationship, with a correlation coefficient of -0.88, was reported. However, this latter study suffered from two critical weaknesses: (i) the study was based on only 8 subjects; and (ii) only short-term cholesterol turnover studies were carried out (which do not give valid estimates of the mass of slowly exchanging pools of body cholesterol).

In order to evaluate this question definitively, we have conducted studies to determine whether HDL cholesterol or apoprotein levels are related to the mass of exchangeable pools of body cholesterol. The approach used was to carry out measurements of the plasma concentrations of HDL cholesterol, and of apoproteins A-I, A-II, and E, in the most recently studied 55 subjects among the group of 82 subjects discussed above. HDL cholesterol concentration was determined by standard precipitation techniques, and the levels of apoproteins were measured by specific radioimmunoassays. The subjects covered a very wide range of serum concentrations of cholesterol, triglyceride, HDL cholesterol, and the apoproteins. It was felt that the wide range of these variables would enhance our ability to detect any relationships which might exist between them and the parameters of body cholesterol metabolism.

For the present report, we have explored possible relationships between the levels of HDL cholesterol and the apoproteins (as independent variables), and 3 major model parameters (namely the minimum estimates of the mass of pool 3 (M_3min) and of total exchangeable body cholesterol ($M_{tot}min$), and cholesterol PR) as dependent variables. Similar results were obtained with other estimates of M_3 and M_{tot} than the minimum ones.

Simple univariate correlation analyses were first carried out to look for relationships between the HDL and apoprotein levels and the model parameters. The simple correlations with apoA-II and apoE were small and not significant. Statistically significant but rather weak correlations of HDL cholesterol and apoA-I with each of the three model parameters were found. The correlation coefficients for these relationships ranged from -0.36 to -0.42. Thus, in no case could more than 18% (r^2) of the variability of M_3min, $M_{tot}min$, or PR be described by variation in HDL cholesterol or apoA-I level. In contrast, the univariate relationships of the model parameters with body weight were much stronger, with correlation coefficients of 0.58, 0.78, and 0.76 for M_3min, $M_{tot}min$, and PR, respectively.

The results of univariate analyses may be misleading, since the HDL variables may be correlated with other physiological variables, notably with body size. A more definitive, multivariate regression analysis was therefore carried out to determine whether HDL cholesterol or the apoproteins could add to the description of model parameters given by the previously identified simple physiological variables (see (5) and Table 1). That is, we attempted to determine whether HDL cholesterol or apoproteins A-I, A-II, or E were independent determinants of PR, M_3min, or M_{tot}min, by using the regression equations previously identified.

For PR, adding HDL cholesterol or any of the apoprotein levels to the previously established independent variable, weight, did not explain any of the remaining variance. All of the partial correlation coefficients were very small and statistically insignificant. Similar results were found for the two previously established equations for M_3min (one with weight, cholesterol, and age, and the second with excess weight and age, as independent variables), and for the two previously established equations for M_{tot}min (see Table 1). With all four equations, adding HDL cholesterol or the apoprotein levels did not explain any of the remaining variance, and all of the partial correlation coefficients were very small and insignificant.

Thus, in summary, this study has shown that: (i) ApoA-II and apoE are not correlated with the cholesterol model parameters PR, M_3min, or M_{tot}min. (ii) There are weak univariate correlations of HDL cholesterol and apoA-I levels with the model parameters. (iii) In multivariate analyses, no relationship is apparent between HDL cholesterol or apoA-I levels and PR, M_3min, or M_{tot}min. (iv) Thus, the weak univariate correlations reflect relationships of HDL cholesterol and apoA-I with physiological variables such as body size which are primarily related to the model parameters. We conclude that the concentrations of HDL cholesterol and of these apoproteins are not significant determinants of cholesterol production rate, or of the mass of slowly exchanging or total exchangeable body cholesterol in humans.

Acknowledgement

This work was supported by Arteriosclerosis SCOR Grant HL 21006 from the National Heart, Lung, and Blood Institute.

References

1. Chobanian, A. V. and Hollander, W. (1962): J. Clin. Invest., 41:1732-1737.
2. Dell, R. B., and Ramakrishnan, R. (1982): In:Lipoprotein Kinetics and Modeling, edited by M. Berman and S. Grundy, pp. 313-330. Academic Press, New York.
3. Goodman, DeW. S., and Noble, R. P. (1968): J. Clin. Invest., 47:231-241.
4. Goodman, DeW. S., Noble, R. P., and Dell, R. B. (1973): J. Lipid Res., 14:178-188.
5. Goodman, DeW. S., Smith, F. R., Seplowitz, A. H., Ramakrishnan, R., and Dell, R. B. (1980): J. Lipid Res., 21:699-713.
6. Gordon, T., Castelli, W. P., Hjortland, M. C., Kannel, W. B., and Dawber, T. R. (1977): Amer. J. Med., 62:707-714.
7. Grundy, S. M. and Ahrens, E. H., Jr. (1969): J. Lipid Res., 10: 91-107.

8. Jagannathan, S. N., Connor, W. E., Baker, W. H., and Bhattacharyya, A. K. (1974): J. Clin. Invest., 54:366–377.
9. Miller, G. J., and Miller, N. E. (1975): Lancet, i:16–19.
10. Miller, N. E., Nestel, P. J., and Clifton-Bligh, P. (1976): Atherosclerosis, 23:535–547.
11. Perl, W., and Samuel, P. (1969): Circ. Res., 25:191–199.
12. Ramakrishnan, R., Dell, R. B., and Goodman, DeW. S. (1981): J. Lipid Res., 22:1174–1180.
13. Rhoads, G. G., Gulbrandsen, C. L., and Kagan, A. (1976): N. Eng. J. Med., 294:293–298.
14. Samuel, P., and Perl, W. (1970): J. Clin. Invest., 49:346–357.
15. Samuel, P., and Lieberman, S. (1973): J. Lipid Res., 14:189–196.
16. Samuel, P., Lieberman, S., and Ahrens, E. H.,Jr. (1978): J. Lipid Res., 19:94–102.
17. Schreibman, P. H., and Dell, R. B. (1975): J. Clin. Invest., 55:986–993.
18. Stein, O., Vanderhoek, J., Friedman, G., and Stein, Y. (1976): Biochim. Biophys. Acta, 450:367–378.
19. Wilson, J. D. (1970): J. Clin. Invest., 49:655–665.

The Adipocyte and Obesity: Cellular and Molecular Mechanisms, edited by A. Angel, C. H. Hollenberg, and D. A. K. Roncari. Raven Press, New York © 1983.

Lipoprotein Interactions and Cholesterol Metabolism in Human Fat Cells

A. Angel and B. Fong

Department of Medicine, Toronto General Hospital and University of Toronto, Toronto, Ontario, M5S 1A8 Canada

The ability of adipose tissue to accumulate, store and, under special circumstances, mobilize a large cholesterol pool is an important physiological property of this organ (4,10). In this paper the regulation of cholesterol accumulation in adipose tissue will be reviewed and its dynamic nature described. A concept of cholesterol flux in adipose tissue is presented in which lipoproteins play a critical role in both delivery and efflux of cholesterol. Evidence will also be presented showing that plasma membranes purified from homogenates of mature adipose cells contain multiple lipoprotein receptors that probably serve to regulate the amount of cholesterol delivered to the adipose storage pool.

REGULATION OF CHOLESTEROL ACCUMULATION IN ADIPOSE TISSUE

Human adipose tissue contains one of the largest pools of exchangeable cholesterol in the body. In normal man 25% of body cholesterol is found in fat tissue (Table 1). In the obese state, total body cholesterol increases progressively, and in massively obese patients well over half of total body cholesterol can be found in this tissue (2,22). There is a significant relationship between adipose cholesterol stores and plasma cholesterol levels, and plasma lipoprotein cholesterol equilibrates dynamically with this tissue pool (22). While adipose cholesterol turns

TABLE 1. Cholesterol content of human adipose tissue.

	Adipose mass	Adipose[a] cholesterol	Total body[b] cholesterol	% in adipose tissue
Normal man				
70 kg	12 kg	12x1.50=18g	70 g	26
Massive obesity				
140 kg	50 kg	50x1.85=92.5g	140 g	66

[a] Human adipose tissue contains approximately 1.5 mg cholesterol/gm and in massive obesity it is increased to 1.85 mg cholesterol/gm (2).

[b] Total body cholesterol is approximately 1 gm/kg (22).

over slowly in relation to other cholesterol pools such as plasma and liver, its flux in and out of adipose tissue occurs at a rate greater than that of stored triglyceride. The half-time of adipose cholesterol is approximately 40 days while that of triglyceride exceeds 100 days. Over the past decade a good deal has been learned about the regulation of adipose cholesterol stores, the size of which appears to be under nutritional control.

Adipose tissue cholesterol increases with age and dietary cholesterol load, and is specifically expanded in the obese state (4). Adipose cholesterol is reduced in chronic undernutrition and, in acute starvation, the adipose cholesterol pool is mobilized and excreted through the biliary system. Supersaturation of bile cholesterol has been noted during starvation and has been attributed to the mobilization of adipose cholesterol stores, thus explaining the increased risk of cholelithiasis and cholecystitis in these patients (8).

In man, unlike the rat or mouse, cholesterol synthesis in adipose tissue is negligible (2,22). Therefore, almost all the cholesterol in human fat cells is derived from circulating lipoproteins. While all major plasma lipoproteins are metabolized in adipose tissue, only HDL and LDL species distribute in the interstitial space where they are directly exposed to cell surfaces and interact with specific receptor sites (19). Approximately 30 to 40% of LDL and HDL distributes outside the plasma compartment in man; however, there are great variations in the concentration of lipoproteins in different interstitial compartments. In recent studies from our laboratory, Julien showed that the distribution and concentration of cholesterol-rich lipoproteins varies depending upon the lymph bed sampled. For example, cardiac lymph contained HDL and LDL at a concentration close to 50% that of plasma (12), whereas the concentration in peripheral lymph is only 10% that of plasma (19).

CHOLESTEROL FLUX IN ADIPOSE TISSUE: CELLULAR MECHANISMS, FIG. 1

The uptake, turnover and mobilization of cholesterol in adipose tissue can be conveniently divided into three phases. (I) The first involves cholesterol delivery through interactions of lipoproteins on the cell surface with specific recognition sites. (II) The second phase involves intracellular processing of lipoproteins with hydrolysis of cholesterol esters and liberation of free cholesterol. (III) The third phase is the mobilization of free cholesterol from the fat cell surface to available interstitial lipoprotein acceptors.

(I) Lipoprotein interactions have been demonstrated using mature adipose cells, cultured adipocyte precursors and purified plasma membranes. Human adipocytes prepared by collagenase digestion of surgical biopsy specimens of fat readily bind and internalize radio-iodinated human LDL (3). The reaction is time- and dose-dependent, saturable, and specific in that excess unlabelled LDL can competitively displace 80 to 90% of ^{125}I-LDL binding. Binding and internalization of LDL by fat cells is energy-dependent and a portion of it appears to be chloroquine-sensitive (Table 2). Degradation of LDL by mature fat cells incubated in vitro differs somewhat from that observed in cultured human skin fibroblasts and other mesenchymal cells, and appears to be a complex process involving more than one mechanism (3). Proteolytic degradation of LDL apoproteins by freshly-isolated intact fat cells occurs in the presence of a vast excess of medium albumin, thus excluding a simple nonspecific process. Degradation of ^{125}I-LDL is only partially inhibited by excess unlabelled LDL, indicating that at least a portion of the degradation is unrelated to high-affinity receptor binding. Proteolytic activity can be recovered in conditioned medium and this is only partially inhibited by trypsin inhibitors. Because degradation of LDL (as well as various HDL species) by mature adipocytes can occur without prior internalization of the particles, it is concluded that surface proteases exist which can de-grade lipoproteins or at least modify apoprotein structure to a signifi-cant extent.

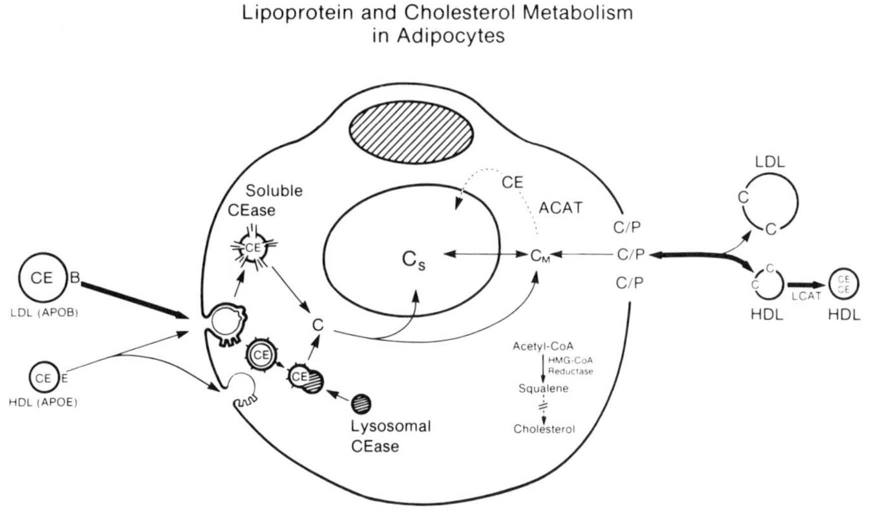

FIG. 1.   A schematic representation of lipoprotein interactions and chol-esterol flux in human fat cells.

Human low-density lipoproteins (LDL) and high-density lipoproteins (HDL) deliver cholesterol in ester form (CE) to fat cells. The particles bind to surface receptors and are internalized and degraded by lysosomal (pH5) and nonlysosomal (pH7) cholesterol ester hydrolases (CEase). Free cholesterol (C) is liberated and equilibrates with the large cholesterol storage pool (C_S) and membrane cholesterol (C_M). Cholesterol esterifica-tion by acyl cholesterol acyl transferase (ACAT) is shown as a broken line because the quantitative significance of this reaction is not estab-lished in human fat. Cholesterol efflux occurs by an exchange-transfer process and depends on the cholesterol/phospholipid (C/P) molar ratio gradient between the fat cell and the acceptor particles. Both HDL and LDL can act as cholesterol acceptors in vitro (7).

(11)   Entry of intact LDL particles occurs by adsorptive endocytosis in freshly-isolated adipocytes and is subject to hydrolytic degradation by a variety of acid hydrolases. Human fat cells contain both neutral and acid cholesterol ester hydrolase activity (Fig. 2) and it is these

activities which ensure conversion of all cholesterol esters to free
cholesterol which can equilibrate with the storage pool or with various
subcellular membrane fractions.

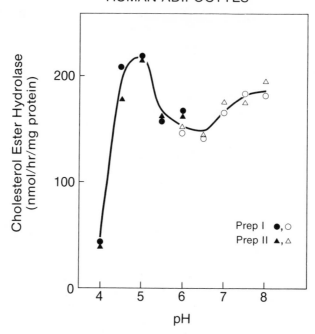

FIG. 2. Human adipocytes obtained from properitoneal (Prep I) or medi-
          astinal (Prep II) fat by collagenase digestion were washed 3
times in KRB buffer plus 2% BSA pH7.4, and 3 times with isotonic sucrose
pH7.5. The cells were homogenized by hand in isotonic sucrose 1 mM EDTA
and 10 mM HEPES buffer pH7.5, and spun at 5000 g for 20 min at 4°C, and
the aqueous supernatant was assayed at pH4-6 (acetate buffer) or pH6-8
(phosphate buffer) for cholesterol ester hydrolase activity. (Courtesy
Dr. D. Severson as described in Atherosclerosis 31:21-32, 1978.)

    While net entry of cholesterol into fat cells occurs as a result of
internalization of lipoproteins rich in cholesterol esters, almost all
the cholesterol found in human fat is in free form (10,22). This is un-
doubtedly a consequence of high levels of cholesterol ester hydrolase
activity in the tissue (13). It has been repeatedly noted that cholesterol ester hydrolase activity in adipose tissue is present in two forms,
that the neutral enzyme is indistinguishable from hormone-sensitive triglyceride lipase activity, and that the specific activity of this nonlysosomal (soluble fraction) enzyme is very high in fat tissue (14). This
ensures the complete hydrolysis of core neutral lipids of lipoprotein
particles entering the cell through adsorptive endocytosis. What has not
yet been established is the proportion of LDL uptake that is linked to
lysosomal processing. Because chloroquine only partially inhibits LDL
internalization, we conclude that both lysosomal and nonlysosomal processes are involved (Table 2).

TABLE 2.   Effect of chloroquine on ^{125}I-LDL binding and metabolism in
human adipocytes.

Additions	Binding	Internalization	Degradation
	μg LDL protein/gm cell lipid/4 hr		
^{125}I-LDL (10 μg/ml)	0.27±0.01	1.80±0.70	0.29±0.04
'' + unlabelled LDL (800 μg/ml)	0.04±0.02	0.05±0.01	0.10±0.04
'' + chloroquine (100 μM)	0.20±0.01	1.05±0.14	0.27±0.05

Adipose tissue was obtained from a 52-yr-old male patient at thora-
cotomy. Each flask contained 94 mg fat cells, 4% BSA in KRB buffer,
trypsin inhibitor 25 μg/ml. ^{125}I-LDL S.A. 6.35 x 10^4 cpm/μg protein. For
method details, see reference #3. Chloroquine partially inhibited LDL
binding and internalization but had no effect on degradation.

(III) Cholesterol mobilization from adipose tissue readily occurs and
one can calculate from published data what fraction of the adipose pool
is mobilized daily. In normal man approximately 250 to 500 mg of cholesterol are mobilized from adipose tissue stores per day. Exchange (uptake
and efflux) of free cholesterol between adipocytes and all serum lipoproteins has been demonstrated in vitro (15), but only LDL and HDL are present in significant amounts in the interstitial compartment in vivo, so
it is likely that only these species act as exchange acceptors. While HDL
is generally regarded as the preferred efflux acceptor for adipose cholesterol, LDL is also capable of exchange-transfer of cholesterol with fat
cells (7). Presumably net transfer of cholesterol from the fat cell surface to interstitial lipoproteins is determined by the relative choleste-
rol/phospholipid molar ratios of the interacting surfaces of the fat cell
and lipoprotein particles. Efflux of cholesterol to lipoproteins is not
dependent on binding of lipoproteins to receptor, which partially explains
the lack of specificity (7). The rate of cholesterol efflux from adipose
tissue is increased in starvation but little is known about the regulation of this process at the molecular level. It is known that mobilization of cholesterol from adipose tissue is slower than that of triglyceride stores, which explains the increased cholesterol/triglyceride ratio
in fat tissue from fasted patients despite an absolute decrease in cellular cholesterol content (2). As discussed below, large amounts of squalene are found in adipose tissue but little evidence exists to indicate
that it is released in significant amounts.

LIPOPROTEIN METABOLISM IN ADIPOCYTE PRECURSORS

Intact adipocytes studied in vitro present significant technical limitations: incubations are necessarily brief because the cells are so fragile. Thus time-dependent processes requiring prolonged incubation for
expression, e.g., up or down regulation of receptors, are difficult to
examine. Cultured adipocyte precursors provide a suitable model of adipocyte function because they express almost all the metabolic characteristics of mature fat cells, can be propagated, and can be maintained in
culture for many days. Adipocyte precursors store glycerolipids, assume a
signet ring appearance on maturation, elaborate lipoprotein lipase,

respond to lipolytic hormones and are insulin-sensitive (25). Cultured
adipocyte precursors also bind, internalize and degrade ^{125}I-LDL at significant rates and, like freshly-isolated mature fat cells, do not require
prior incubation in lipoprotein-deficient serum to express these properties (6). In further collaborative studies with Dr. Roncari, we have
demonstrated upregulation of LDL receptors following 18 hr incubation in
lipoprotein-deficient serum (Fig. 3). Additionally, adipocyte precursors
in culture degraded LDL in a manner similar to that of cultured fibroblasts, in that internalization of the particle by adsorptive endocytosis
was a prerequisite. This is evidenced by a long lag before the appearance
of TCA-soluble degradation products in the medium (Fig. 3, panel 3) and
contrasts with mature fat cells in which degradation begins immediately
on exposure of LDL to the incubation system (3). Furthermore, addition of
excess unlabelled LDL to adipocyte precursors in culture markedly inhibits
LDL binding and internalization, as well as degradation, which is consistent with the dependence of degradation on prior cellular internalization.

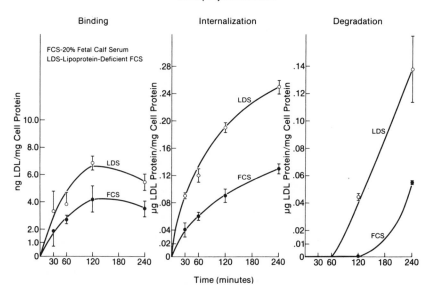

FIG. 3. The metabolism of ^{125}I-LDL in human adipocyte precursors. The
        cells were derived from omental fat taken from a 41-yr-old obese
male undergoing ileojejunal bypass surgery and were in their 4th subculture on day 15 of growth. 18 hr prior to the experiment the growth
medium was replaced with 20% fetal calf serum (FCS) or 20% lipoprotein-
deficient serum (LDS). Each flask contained 2.6 x 10^5 cells. The cells
were incubated with ^{125}I-LDL 10 µg/ml, S.A. 2.73 x 10^4 cpm/µg protein in
triplicate. Each value is mean±SEM. It is evident that prior exposure of
cells to LDS increased apparent binding, internalization and degradation
of ^{125}I-LDL. Thus exposure of the adipocyte precursors to lipoprotein-
deficient serum enhances binding, internalization and metabolism, presumably due to an increased number of surface recognition sites.

CHOLESTEROL SYNTHESIS IN ADIPOSE TISSUE

As noted earlier, almost all of the cholesterol in human fat tissue is derived from circulating lipoproteins as little is synthesized in situ. In studies on cholesterol synthesis in human adipose tissue from control and massively obese patients, in which ^3H_2O was used as the isotopic marker with glucose as substrate, formation of squalene and hydrocarbon precursors of cholesterol was evident but synthesis of sterol intermediates or cholesterol was negligible (2) (Fig. 4). The synthesis of squalene was readily apparent, indicating the presence of HMG-CoA reductase activity; however, a biosynthesis arrest beyond the squalene step was evident. In contrast, rat and mouse adipose tissue incubated in vitro synthesizes cholesterol at appreciable rates (21). There is as yet no explanation for the species difference. It is of interest that human adipose tissue is also a major storage site of squalene (24) and contains the highest concentration of this compound compared to all other tissues. It is tempting to speculate that the low rates of cholesterol biosynthesis in human fat reflect a feedback inhibitory reaction secondary to the large stores of cholesterol or squalene, but proof of this suggestion requires further experimentation. The synthesis of significant amounts of non sterol,

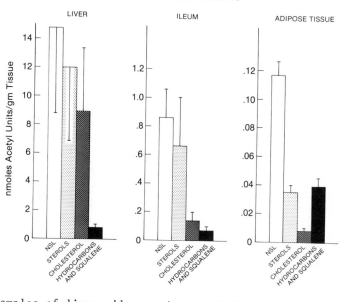

FIG. 4. Samples of liver, ileum and omental fat were obtained from 13 massively obese patients (wt 145-168 kg) during ileojejunal bypass surgery. The tissues were incubated in 5 ml KRB buffer, 5% BSA, 5.6 mM glucose and 10^{10} dpm/ml ^3H_2O, and incubated 4 hr in 95% O_2 at 37°C. The nonsaponifiable lipids (NSL) were obtained and fractionated by TLC. Absolute rates of lipid synthesis were calculated as described in reference #2. Cholesterol synthesis in adipose tissue was neglible compared to liver. Synthesis of nonsaponifiable lipids in adipose tissue in obesity may be important because of organ size.

hydrocarbons and other nonsaponifiable lipids suggests the presence of dolichol and ubiquinone biosynthetic pathways in human fat tissue. This will be a fruitful area for future research in adipose tissue mevalonate metabolism.

The free cholesterol in human adipose tissue is associated with cellular membrane elements but the majority is localized to the central lipid droplet. This contrasts again with rat adipose tissue which can esterify cholesterol (5) where 20 to 25% of the cholesterol is present as cholesterol ester (10). This may reflect a relative deficiency in ACAT activity (acyl cholesterol acyl transferase activity) in human adipose tissue so that little cholesterol re-esterification occurs following hydrolysis of internalized cholesterol esters (23). Cholesterol feeding to rats results in accumulation of cholesterol in adipose tissue and a significant portion of this cholesterol accumulates as cholesterol esters (16). It is not known whether cholesterol esters can accumulate in human fat. Thus, the ACAT reaction in Fig. 1 is shown as a broken line.

MULTIPLE LIPOPROTEIN RECEPTORS IN ADIPOSE TISSUE

Low-density lipoprotein binding and internalization readily occur in human adipocytes but this reaction lacks absolute specificity in that VLDL and HDL can inhibit these processes in vitro. This differs significantly from cultured human skin fibroblasts in which HDL has little or no effect on LDL binding, and where only HDL_c, the Apo E-rich lipoprotein isolated from plasma of cholesterol-fed dogs (17), has inhibitory effects. In isolated adipocytes, HDL and both its subfractions HDL_2 and HDL_3 are potent inhibitors of LDL binding and internalization and only partially inhibit LDL degradadation (1) (Table 3). These effects in fat cells of HDL and VLDL on LDL binding may be explained by the presence of the arginine-rich Apo E apoprotein in VLDL and HDL which interacts with the Apo B receptor site. The Apo B receptor is thus more appropriately designated as an Apo B-E recognition site (17).

To examine the characteristics of lipoprotein binding to fat cell surface membranes in more detail, studies were undertaken using a purified plasma membrane fraction. Purified plasma membrane has additional advantages of stability and eliminating the confounding effects of internalization and degradation which occur using intact cells. The purified plasma membranes were prepared from homogenates of freshly-isolated human adipocyte by the method of McKeel and Jarett (18) followed by purification on sucrose density gradients. The characteristics of LDL binding to adipocyte membranes differed markedly from that reported for cultured human skin fibroblasts, indicating the unique character of adipocyte lipoprotein recognition systems. Whereas LDL binding to fibroblasts is Ca^{++} dependent, EDTA sensitive, and completely inhibited by pronase treatment (9), LDL binding to human adipocyte membranes is not dependent on Ca^{++}, is sensitive to EDTA, and unaffected by pronase treatment (20). Initially, experiments were performed to optimize the binding assay, determine equilibrium times, and establish the specificity of the reaction. In Table 4 the maximum capacity of LDL binding to human adipocytes exceeds all other tissues previously reported and the Kd of LDL binding to adipocyte membranes was higher than fibroblasts. Thus human adipocytes possess high-capacity, low-affinity LDL binding sites (compared to fibroblasts) that appear to be active immediately upon removal from the body.

The LDL receptor on adipocyte membranes cross-reacted with both LDL and HDL_c. Apo E-rich HDL_c completely inhibited specific LDL binding to

TABLE 3. Effect of HDL_2 and HDL_3 on ^{125}I-LDL binding, internalization and degradation in human adipocytes.

Additions	Binding	Internalization	Degradation
	μg LDL protein/gm cell lipid/4 hr		
^{125}I-LDL (10.4 μg/ml)	0.24±0.010[a]	1.72±0.15	0.37±0.06
" + LDL 788 μg/ml	0.04±0.001	0.19±0.02	0.19±0.04
" + HDL_2 43.4 μg/ml	0.09±0.009	0.42±0.01	0.25±0.05
" + HDL_3 44.4 μg/ml	0.08±0.003	0.38±0.08	0.28±0.05

[a] Mean±SEM; n=3.

Adipose cells were prepared from tissue obtained from a male patient age 66 during elective cardiac surgery and incubated with ^{125}I-LDL S.A. 6.29 × 10^{4}cpm/μg LDL Prot. Each flask contained 80-100 mg fat cells and 2.5 μg/ml Trypsin inhibitor. For methodological details, see reference #3. Addition of HDL_2 (d 1.075-1.125) and HDL_3 (d 1.125-1.21) at concentrations similar to those found in peripheral lymph inhibited LDL binding and internalization. LDL degradation was partially inhibited by HDL_2 and HDL_3.

purified adipocyte membranes, which is consistent with the presence of an Apo B-E receptor site. An independent Apo E recognition site was also suggested in cross-competition studies using ^{125}I-HDL$_c$ as ligand and adding high concentrations of unlabelled LDL and HDL$_c$ as competitive inhibitors. Unlabelled LDL only partially (70%) inhibited ^{125}I-HDL$_c$ binding compared to unlabelled HDL$_c$ which displaced 95% of the ^{125}I-HDL$_c$ binding. That portion of ^{125}I-HDL$_c$ not inhibited by LDL is taken to represent the presence of a separate recognition site for Apo E-containing lipoproteins. Thus, human adipocytes contain at least two separate lipoprotein recognition sites, an Apo B-E and an Apo E receptor, that are fully expressed in freshly-isolated cell membranes (11). Whether these two sites are responsible for the unusual capacity of fat cells to bind and interact with VLDL, LDL, HDL_2, HDL_3, and HDL$_c$ remains to be established. Nevertheless, the relaxed specificity of the human fat cells promotes interactions with a wide variety of lipoprotein species and is consistent with its role as a cholesterol storage tissue, a function subserved by an extraordinary capacity to scavenge all manner of lipoprotein particles.

In summary, cholesterol turnover in adipose tissue is a regulated process and appears to be affected by a variety of nutritional and metabolic events. In obesity, cholesterol accumulates in fat tissue to a greater extent than that expected simply as a result of increased adipose mass. Entry of cholesterol into fat cells is achieved through selective binding and internalization of cholesterol-rich lipoprotein LDL and HDL found in the interstitial space. The lipoprotein particles are degraded and cholesterol esters hydrolyzed by neutral cholesterol ester hydrolase which is present in high amounts in human fat and indistinguishable from hormone-sensitive triglyceride lipase.

The free cholesterol equilibrates with a large pool of stored cholesterol in the central lipid droplet and with organelle membrane. Mobilization of cholesterol stored in adipose tissue seems to be a passive

TABLE 4. <u>LDL binding to membrane preparations from human tissues.</u>

Tissues	Kd	Vmax
Adipocytes	1.86×10^{-8} M	2870 ng/mg Prot.
Liver (adult)[a]	not detectable	< 1 ng/mg Prot.
Fibroblasts	$4-8 \times 10^{-9}$ M	300 ng/mg Prot.

[a] Data of Mahley et al. (1981): J. Clin. Invest., <u>68</u>:1197.

[b] Data of Basu et al. (1978): J. Biol. Chem., <u>253</u>:3852.

Adipose cells have the highest LDL binding capacity of tissues studied.

phenomenon involving exchange-transfer of cholesterol to acceptor lipoproteins in the environment. While relatively little is known about the
molecular regulation of cholesterol efflux from fat cells in vivo, both
LDL and HDL lipoprotein appear to be involved as efflux acceptors, and
this process does not depend on interactions with high-affinity lipoprotein receptors.

Freshly-isolated adipose cells, like most other mesenchymal cells, can
bind and metabolize Apo B- and Apo E-containing lipoprotein with high
capacity and somewhat relaxed specificity. Evidence has been presented
to indicate the presence of multiple lipoprotein receptors in human fat
cells that are active and functional immediately upon removal from the
body. The multiplicity of lipoprotein recognition activities may explain
the unique physiologic property of adipose tissue to take up and metabolize cholesterol-rich lipoprotein and act as a buffer storage pool of
cholesterol in vivo.

REFERENCES

1. Angel, A., and Asico, W. (1980): Effects of HDL subfractions on [125]I-
   LDL binding and metabolism in human adipocytes. Clin Res. <u>28</u>(2):
   #516A.
2. Angel, A., and Bray, G.A. (1979): Synthesis of fatty acids and cholesterol by liver, adipose tissue and intestinal mucosa from obese
   and control patients. Eur. J. Clin. Invest. <u>9</u>:355-362.
3. Angel, A., D'Costa, M.A., and Yuen, R. (1979): Low density lipoprotein in binding, internalization, and degradation in human adipose
   cells. Can. J. Biochem. <u>57</u>(6):578-587.
4. Angel, A., and Frakas, J. (1974): Regulation of cholesterol storage
   in adipose tissue. J. Lipid Res. <u>15</u>:491-499.
5. Angel, A., and Roncari, D.A.K. (1967): The control of fatty acid
   esterification in a subcellular preparation of rat adipose tissue.
   Biochim. Biophys. Acta <u>137</u>:464-474.
6. Angel, A., and Roncari, D.A.K. (1979): Low density lipoprotein binding, internalization and metabolism in human adipocytes and adipocyte precursors. Inserm <u>87</u>:103-122.
7. Angel, A., Yuen, R., and Nettleton, J.A. (1981): Exchange of free
   cholesterol between low density lipoproteins and human adipocytes.
   Can. J. Biochem. <u>59</u>(8):655-661.

8. Bennion, L.J., and Grundy, S.M.(1975): Effects of obesity and caloric intake on biliary lipid metabolism in man. J. Clin. Invest. 56: 996.

9. Brown, M.S., Kovanen, P.T., and Goldstein, J.L. (1981): Regulation of plasma cholesterol by lipoprotein receptors. Science 212:628-635.

10. Frakas, J., Angel, A., and Avigan, M.I. (1973): Studies on the compartmentation of lipid in adipose cells. II. Cholesterol accumulation and distribution in adipose tissue components. J. Lipid Res. 14:344-356.

11. Fong, B., Rodrigues, P., Julien, P., and Angel, A. (1982): Lipoprotein receptors in adult human adipocyte plasma membranes. Clin. Res. 30(2):#523A.

12. Julien, P., Downar, E., and Angel, A. (1981): Lipoprotein composition and transport in the pig and dog cardiac lymphatic system. Circ. Res. 49:248-254.

13. Khoo, J.C., Drevon, C.A., and Steinberg, D. (1979): The hydrolysis of cholesterol esters in plasma lipoproteins by hormone sensitive cholesterol esterase from adipose tissue. J. Biol. Chem. 254:1785-1787.

14. Khoo, J.C., Steinberg, D., Huang, J.J., and Vagelos, P.R. (1976): Triglyceride, diglyceride, monoglyceride, and cholesterol ester hydrolases in chicken adipose tissue activated by adenosine 3':5'-monophosphase-dependent protein kinase. J. Biol. Chem. 251:2882-2890.

15. Kovanen, P., and Nikkila, E.A. (1976): Cholesterol exchange between fat cells, chylomicrons and plasma lipoproteins. Biochim. Biophys. Acta 441:357-369.

16. Krause, B.R., Phares, F., Serbin, V., Krause, L., and Hartman, A.D. (1979): Adipocyte cholesterol storage: Effect of experimental hypercholesterolemia in the rat. J. Nutri. 109:2213-2225.

17. Mahley, R.W., Hui, D.Y., Innerarity, T.L., and Weisgraber, K.H. (1981): Two independent lipoprotein receptors on hepatic membranes of dog, swine and man. J. Clin. Invest. 68:1197-1206.

18. McKeel, D.W., and Jarett, L. (1970): Preparation and characterization of a plasma membrane fraction from isolated fat cells. J. Cell Biol. 44:417-432.

19. Reichl, D., Postiglione, A., Myant, N.B., Pflugg, J.J., and Press, M. (1975): Observations on the passage of apoproteins from plasma lipoproteins into peripheral lymph in two men. Clin. Sci. Mol. Med. 49:419-426.

20. Rodrigues, P., Fong, B., Roncari, D.A.K., and Angel, A. (June 1982): LDL receptors of adult human adipocytes differ from that of cultured skin fibroblasts (abstract). Proceedings of International Conference on the Adipocyte and Obesity (in press).

21. Rosenthal, J., Angel, A., and Frakas, J. (1974): Metabolic fate of leucine: A significant sterol precursor in adipose tissue and muscle. Am. J. Phys. 226(2):411-418.

22. Schreibman, P.H., and Dell, R.B. (1975): Human adipocyte cholesterol: Concentration, localization, synthesis and turnover. J. Clin. Invest. 55:986-993.

23. Steinberg, D., Pittman, R.C., Attie, A.D., Carew, T.E., and Joy, L. (1983): Uptake and degradation of low density lipoprotein by adipose tissue in vivo. In: The Adipocyte and Obesity: Cellular and Molecular Mechanisms, edited by A. Angel, C.H. Hollenberg, and D.A.K. Roncari, pp.   . Raven Press, New York.

24. Tilvis, R., Kovanen, P.T., and Miettinen, T.A. (1982): Metabolism of squalene in human fat cells. J. Biol. Chem. 257:10300-10305.
25. Van, R.L.R., Bayliss, C.E., and Roncari, D.A.K. (1976): Cytological and enzymological characterization of adult human adipocyte precursors in culture. J. Clin. Invest. 58:699-704.

ACKNOWLEDGEMENTS

The authors are grateful to Lily Lee and Laura Sheu for able technical assistance and Judy Botterill for manuscript preparation. Our thanks to Dr. B. Goldberg and H. Scully, Department of Cardiovascular Surgery, Toronto General Hospital, for their support in providing adipose tissue specimens, and to Dr. D. Roncari and D. Severson for helpful discussions. The research reported here was supported by grants from MRC and the Ontario Heart Foundation.

The Adipocyte and Obesity: Cellular and
Molecular Mechanisms, edited by A. Angel,
C. H. Hollenberg, and D. A. K. Roncari.
Raven Press, New York © 1983.

Cholesterol Ester Hydrolases in Adipose Tissue

David L. Severson

Faculty of Medicine, The University of Calgary, Calgary T2N IN4 Canada

Preincubation of hormone sensitive lipase (triacylglycerol ester hydrolase) preparations from adipose tissue with ATP and cyclic AMP resulted in a time-dependent increase in cholesterol ester hydrolase activity; activation ranged from 40% with preparations from rat adipocytes (16) to 235% with preparations from chicken adipose tissue (11). Since addition of a protein kinase inhibitor prevented this activation, presumably an endogenous protein kinase is responsible for the increase in cholesterol ester hydrolase activity; activation could be restored by the addition of excess exogenous protein kinase (11,16). Incubation of adipocytes or intact pieces of avian adipose tissue with either epinephrine (16) or glucagon (11) prior to homogenization result- ed in a decrease in the percentage activation of cholesterol ester hydrolase due to preincubation with ATP and cyclic AMP. This can be interpreted as evidence that the hormones have already converted the enzyme to an activated form by a mechanism that is the same as, or closely related to, the protein kinase-catalyzed activation. Reversible deactivation of cholesterol ester hydrolase in chicken adipose tissue by endogenous and exogenous phosphoprotein phosphatases has also been observed (23). Thus, the regulation of cholesterol ester hydrolase in adipose tissue by covalent modification (phosphorylation-dephosphoryla- tion) seems firmly established. Recently, the hormone sensitive lipase from rat adipose tissue has been purified 2000-fold to 50% protein pur- ity (7). The relative acyl hydrolase activity towards triacylglycerols and cholesterol esters remained relatively constant at various stages of the purification procedure. Also, various inhibitors did not discriminate between acyl hydrolase activity measured with triacyl- glycerols or cholesterol esters (7). Therefore, the same enzyme protein may hydrolyze both triacylglycerols and cholesterol esters. An activatable cholesterol ester hydrolase has also been observed in the adrenal cortex (4,12,13) and in macrophages (10).

PROPERTIES OF CHOLESTEROL ESTER HYDROLASES FROM PIGEON ADIPOSE TISSUE

Hydrolase activities in a lipase preparation from pigeon adipose tissue have recently been investigated (22). The effect of pH on chol- esterol ester hydrolase activity in this pigeon adipose tissue prep- aration is shown in Figure I. A glycerol-dispersed cholesterol oleate

substrate preparation was hydrolyzed with a distinct acid pH optimum
of 4.5 and a smaller neutral pH optimum of approximately 7. The
presence of both acid and neutral cholesterol ester hydrolases has
also been observed in enzyme preparations from rat fat pads (20) and
chicken adipose tissue (19). Previous investigations (11,16) on the
activatability of adipose tissue cholesterol ester hydrolase were
performed at pH values ranging from approximately 6 to 8.5. Riddle et
al (17) have reported that rat adipose tissue had some activity at acid

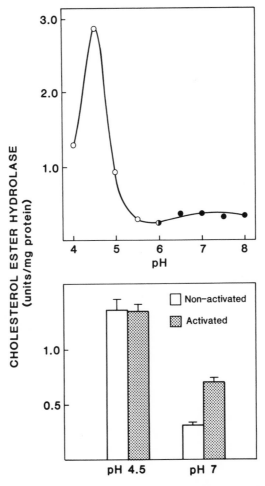

**CHOLESTEROL ESTER HYDROLASE ACTIVITY
IN PIGEON ADIPOSE TISSUE**

FIG. I. Top-panel: hydrolase activity was determined at the indicated
pH values with a glycerol-dispersed cholesterol oleate substrate
preparation (50 µM final concentration) containing lecithin
(350 µM). Lower panel: effect of preincubation with 5 mM $MgCl_2$
(non-activated) or with 5 mM $MgCl_2$, 0.5 mM ATP, 0.01 mM cyclic AMP
and 100 µg/ml protein kinase (Activated) on hydrolase activity measured
at pH 4.5 or 7 (mean ± SEM; n = 3). (Courtesty of NRC Canada).

pH values but much greater activity at neutral pH such that only a
single pH optimum of about 7 was observed. The absence of a distinct
acid pH optimum in the investigation by Riddle et al (17) may have been
due to their use of an acetone-dispersed cholesterol oleate substrate
preparation. Severson and Fletcher (19) have reported that an ethanol-
dispersed cholesterol oleate substrate was not hydrolyzed at acid pH
values and so a chicken adipose tissue preparation was characterized as
having a single pH optimum of approximately 7. However, when a glycerol
dispersed substrate was utilized as substrate, the cholesterol ester
hydrolase from chicken adipose tissue demonstrated two distinct pH
optima at 4.5 and 7 (19). Since the distribution of the acid cholesterol ester hydrolase in rat fat pad preparations was similar to that for
lysosomal marker enzymes, it was concluded that the acid hydrolase is
of lysosomal origin (20). Both acid and neutral cholesterol ester
hydrolases have been observed in the 3T3-LI preadipocytes (8).

Preincubation of the pigeon adipose tissue lipase preparation with
ATP, cyclic AMP, and protein kinase resulted in a 2 or 3-fold activation
of neutral cholesterol ester hydrolase activity (FIG. I); in contrast,
acid hydrolase activity was not increased by the preincubation with
nucleotides and protein kinase. A cyclic AMP-dependent protein kinase-
catalyzed activation of hydrolase activity measured at pH 7 could also
be determined with glycerol-dispersed substrate preparations of triolein
and methylumbelliferyl stearate (22). The kinetic characterization of
the protein kinase-catalyzed activation of pigeon adipose tissue cholesterol ester hydrolase has also been reported by Severson et al (22).
Activation resulted in an increase in V max from 0.8 to 2.5 units per
mg. protein with no change in the apparent Km of 70 µM (FIG. 2).

FUNCTIONAL SIGNIFICANCE OF ADIPOSE TISSUE CHOLESTEROL ESTER HYDROLASES

Cholesterol ester hydrolase activity has been implicated in the
uptake and degradation of internalized lipoprotein particles. Adipose
tissue is a major cholesterol storage organ, especially in human
obesity (6,18). In studies with sucrose-derivatized LDL (low density
lipoprotein), Pittman et al (14,15) have reported that adipose tissue
is an active extra-hepatic site for the degradation of LDL. Furthermore, Angel et al (3) have shown that human adipocytes will bind,
internalize and degrade LDL. Acid lysosomal cholesterol ester
hydrolases are usually implicated in the degradation of the cholesterol
ester component of the internalized lipoprotein particle (the LDL
receptor pathway described by Brown and Goldstein (5). However, Khoo
et al (9) have shown that the hormone sensitive cholesterol ester
hydrolase of adipose tissue will also hydrolyze the cholesterol esters
in plasma lipoproteins at neutral pH values. In addition, the hydrolysis of the lipoprotein cholesterol ester was increased following
preincubation of chicken adipose tissue lipase preparations with ATP,
cyclic AMP and protein kinase (9). This result is consistent with the
observations by Angel and Roncari (2) that hormones (catecholamines)
will enhance both the surface binding and internalization of LDL in
human adipocytes.

The majority (75-95%) of adipocyte cholesterol is free and
associated with the central oil (triacylglycerol) droplet (6,18).
Although some esterification of cholesterol was reported in rat
adipose tissue preparations (1), Severson and Fletcher were not able to
detect ACAT (acyl-CoA; cholesterol-acyl transferase) activity in rat

fat pad microsomes (21). The neutral cholesterol ester hydrolase in adipose tissue has been suggested to play a role in the mobilization of intracellular cholesterol esters as has been proposed for the

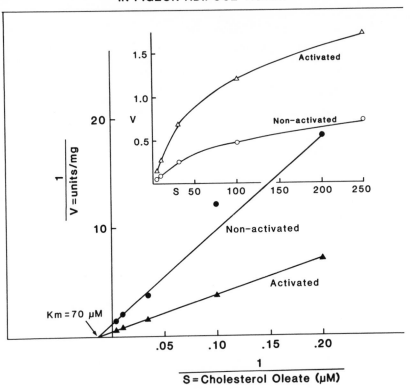

NEUTRAL CHOLESTEROL ESTER HYDROLASE IN PIGEON ADIPOSE TISSUE

FIG. 2. Double-reciprocal plot of the effects of substrate (glycerol-dispersed cholesterol oleate) on hydrolase activity determined with a non-activated and activated pigeon adipose tissue lipase preparation. (Courtesy of NRC Canada).

adrenal (4,12,13) and macrophages (10). The hydrolysis of these cholesterol esters may occur so that no relative accumulation of cholesterol esters occurs during the hydrolysis of the triacylglycerols. Since the enzymatic hydrolysis of a lipid is a heterogeneous reaction due to the fundamental insolubility of the lipid substrate in water, it follows that "physical state" of the lipid substrate will be an extremely important determinant of the expression of enzyme activity. It has also been suggested that the cholesterol ester hydrolase in adipose tissue could alter the surface of the neutral lipid droplet in order to augment the activity of the activated form of the hormone sensitive triacylglycerol ester hydrolase (16)

In summary, both acid and neutral cholesterol ester hydrolases are present in adipose tissue. The neutral ester hydrolase is activated by a cyclic AMP-dependent protein kinase-catalyzed phosphorylation. Both

the acid lysosomal cholesterol ester hydrolase and the protein kinase-
activated ester hydrolase may be involved in the degradation of
lipoprotein bound cholesterol esters. In addition, the neutral
cholesterol ester hydrolase may modify the lipolytic capability of the
hormone sensitive triacylglycerol ester hydrolase.

REFERENCES

1. Angel, A. and Roncari, D.A.K. (1967): Biochim. Biophys. Acta., 137: 464-474.
2. Angel, A., and Roncari, D.A.K. (1979) INSERM Colloq., 81: 103-122
3. Angel, A., D'Costa, M.A. and Yuen, R. (1979): Can. J. Biochem., 57: 578-587.
4. Beckett, G.J. and Boyd, G.S. (1977) Eur. J. Biochem., 72: 223-233
5. Brown, M.S., Kovanen, P.T. and Goldstein, J.L. (1981) Science 212: 628-635.
6. Farkas, J., Angel, A., and Avigan, M.I. (1973): J. Lipid. Res., 14: 344-356.
7. Frederikson, G., Stralfors, P., Nilsson, N.O. and Belfrage, P. (1981): J. Biol. Chem., 256: 6311-6320.
8. Kawamura, M., Jensen, D.F., Wancewicz, E.V., Joy, L.L., Khoo, J.C. and Steinberg, D. (1981) Proc. Natl. Acad. Sci. U.S.A. 78: 732-736.
9. Khoo, J.C., Drevon, C.A. and Steinberg, (1979): J. Biol. Chem., 254: 1785-1787.
10. Khoo, J.C., Mahoney, E.M. and Steinberg, D. (1981): J. Biol. Chem., 256: 12659-12661.
11. Khoo, J.C., Steinberg, D., Huang, J.J. and Vagelos, P.R. (1976): J. Biol. Chem., 251: 2882-2890.
12. Naghshineh, S., Treadwell, C.R., Gallo, L.L. and Vahouny, G.V., (1978) J. Lipid Res. 19: 561-569.
13. Pittman, R.C. and Steinberg, D. (1977): Biochim. Biophys. Acta. 487: 431-444.
14. Pittman, R.C., Attie, A.D., Carew, T.E. and Steinberg, D. (1979): Proc. Natl. Acad. Sci. U.S.A., 76: 5345-5349.
15. Pittman, R.C., Attie, A.D., Carew, T.E. and Steinberg, D. (1982): Biochim. Biophys. Acta., 710: 7-14.
16. Pittman, R.C., Khoo, J.C. and Steinberg, D.J. (1975): J. Biol. Chem. 250: 4505-4511.
17. Riddle, M.C., Fujimoto, W. and Ross, R. (1977): Biochim. Biophys. Acta., 488, 359-369.
18. Schreibman, P.H. and Dell, R.B. (1975): J. Clin. Invest. 55: 986-993.
19. Severson, D.L. and Fletcher, T., (1978): Atherosclerosis. 31: 21-32.
20. Severson, D.L. and Fletcher, T., (1981): Biochim. Biophys. Acta. 675: 256-264.
21. Severson, D.L. and Fletcher, T. (1981): Biochim. Biophys. Acta. 664: 475-486.
22. Severson, D.L., Fletcher, T., Groves, G., Hurley, B., and Sloan, S. (1981): Can. J. Biochem. 59: 418-429.
23. Severson, D.L., Khoo, J.C. and Steinberg, D. (1977): J. Biol. Chem., 252: 1484-1489.

The Adipocyte and Obesity: Cellular and Molecular Mechanisms, edited by A. Angel, C. H. Hollenberg, and D. A. K. Roncari. Raven Press, New York © 1983.

Uptake and Degradation of Low Density Lipoprotein by Adipose Tissue *In Vivo*

Daniel Steinberg, Ray C. Pittman, Alan D. Attie, Thomas E. Carew, and Lorna Joy

Division of Metabolic Disease, Department of Medicine, University of California at San Diego, La Jolla, California 92093

The unique specialized function of adipose tissue, of course, is the storage and subsequent mobilization of triglyceride fatty acids. These functions are discussed extensively in other contributions to this Symposium, including the role of lipoprotein lipase and of hormone-sensitive lipase. It is well-established that the triglycerides of chylomicrons and of very low density lipoproteins are mostly hydrolyzed before they are stored in the fat cells. Consequently, the delivery of chylomicron triglycerides or very low density lipoprotein triglycerides does not <u>necessarily</u> involve the uptake of any other components of the triglyceride-rich lipoproteins. From many studies on the fate of chylomicron remnants, we are quite sure that most of the cholesterol esters and of the apoprotein B return to the liver for ultimate uptake and degradation. The same may be true for very low density lipoproteins although we are less certain about that. Most studies have been carried out in the rat where remnant removal is clearly a predominantly hepatic function. More studies are needed in man and other mammals before the findings in the rat should be generalized.

Interest in the metabolism of lipoproteins by adipose tissue stems in part from the fact that a rather large fraction of the slowly turning over pool of body cholesterol is found in adipose tissue (1,2). A part of this is stored in the fat droplets and fluctuates with the mass of stored triglycerides in the adipose tissue (3,4). Another fraction represents cholesterol integral to the structure of the fat cell. Presumably the membrane cholesterol of the fat cell, like that in other cells, turns over at some rate and it may be that delivery of exogenous cholesterol in lipoproteins is needed under some circumstances, particularly during cell multiplication. Angel and co-workers have shown that there is a very significant rate of uptake and degradation of low density lipoproteins (LDL) by adipocytes <u>in vitro</u> (5). In this paper, we report observations on the rates of uptake and degradation of LDL by adipose tissue <u>in vivo</u> in three animal species. In addition, we present evidence for high-affinity, saturable uptake and degradation of LDL by 3T3-L1 cells (preadipocytes) and show that differentiation is accompanied by a marked increase in number of LDL receptors.

Assessing the absolute rate of degradation of a plasma protein by a given tissue <u>in vivo</u> presents difficult theoretical problems. If the arteriovenous difference is large enough to be measured, there is little difficulty. This is not the case for a plasma protein like LDL

because its half-life is long and the A-V difference too small. In any
case, the method would depend on finding a vascular bed bathing exclusively adipose tissue. Investigators have measured the initial rate of
tissue uptake of a plasma protein but this need not correlate with the
true steady-state rate of irreversible degradation in that tissue.
Basically, initial uptake measures the rate of penetration of the protein
from the plasma compartment into the intercellular spaces and into the
cells. Using conventional radioiodination, the degradation products
leave the tissue very quickly and thus measurement of the total radioactivity accumulating would underestimate true degradation. To deal
with these problems, we several years ago developed a new method that
should be applicable to the study of the sites of degradation of any
plasma protein (6-8). Advantage is taken of the fact that the sucrose
molecule cannot be degraded at any significant rate by lysosomal enzymes
and that it does not move readily across the lysosome membrane. These
properties have made free sucrose useful for measurements of fluid
endocytosis since sucrose taken up by endocytosis and delivered to the
lysosomal vesicle remains trapped there. What we did was to couple
^{14}C-sucrose covalently to LDL so that it would be carred with LDL into
the lysosome (see Figure 1).

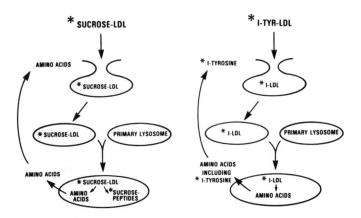

FIGURE 1.   PRINCIPLE UNDERLYING THE USE OF [^{14}C-SUCROSE]LDL TO DETERMINE
SITES OF IRREVERSIBLE DEGRADATION.

There the apoprotein undergoes degradation in the usual way, the free
amino acids escape rapidly but the labeled sucrose is trapped and
accumulates. Thus, the LDL degraded leaves behind as a "calling card"
its complement of [^{14}C]sucrose. The method for coupling [^{14}C]sucrose
covalently to the protein, and the validation that the labeling does not
alter the metabolic behavior of LDL has been previously presented in

detail (7,8). Briefly, it was shown that the uptake and degradation of ^{14}C sucrose LDL by fibroblasts in culture paralleled exactly that of iodinated LDL; it was shown that fractional catabolic rate of [^{14}C]-sucrose LDL in swine did not differ from that of coventionally iodinated LDL. The effectiveness of the trapping of the labeled sucrose was demonstrated using [^{14}C]sucrose asialofetuin as a model substance known to be taken up and degraded almost exclusively in the liver. One hour after intravenous injection into rats, almost 90% of the injected dose was found in the liver. After 24 hrs, the liver still contained about 70% of the injected dose and the bile accounted for an additional 20%. In other words, there was no evidence for loss of [^{14}C]sucrose back to the plasma compartment, but only secretion into the bile. The peripheral tissues examined showed no significant change in [^{14}C] sucrose content between 1 and 24 hrs. Additional data with regard to the rate of "leakage" are shown in Table 1.

FRACTIONAL RATE OF LOSS OF ^{14}C ACTIVITY OVER 5 DAYS
$$(D^{-1})$$

LIVER	-0.101 ± 0.015
KIDNEY	+0.106 ± 0.007
MUSCLE	-0.024 ± 0.013
ADRENAL	-0.046 ± 0.026
ADIPOSE TISSUE	-0.029 ± 0.017
SPLEEN	-0.083 ± 0.038

These data were obtained by injecting [^{14}C]sucrose LDL into a group of rats and sacrificing at daily intervals. Over 80% of the injected [^{14}C]sucrose LDL is taken up and irreversibly degraded in a day. As can be seen, the rate of loss is not more than 10% per day in any tissue examined and below that in several of them, including the adipose tissue.

The sites of degradation in rats (9) are shown in Tables 2 and 3. The predominant site of degradation of LDL was the liver and most of that occurred in the parenchymal cells. No other single tissue made a contribution to LDL degradation approaching that of the liver. The adipose tissue was one of the larger users accounting for about 3% of total body LDL degradation. When the data are expressed in terms of the degradation per unit weight of tissue (Table 3), the adrenal turns out to be the most active user of homologous LDL with the liver, ovary and spleen being comparably active.

TABLE 2.   Tissue sites of degradation of [^{14}C]sucrose labeled rat and human LDL.

Values for 'All tissues examined' represent recovery as % of calculated total catabolized; other values represent recovery as % of total ^{14}C recovered in all tissues.

Tissue	Rat LDL (n=5)	Human LDL (n=3)
All tissues examined	100±22	85±8
Liver	66.8±2.5	56.2±5.4
Small intestine	7.7±3.5	8.5±3.0
Kidney	3.8±1.1	3.1±0.8
Muscle	3.4±1.1	6.6±0.4
Skin	3.3±2.3	3.5±0.5
Adipose tissue	2.8±1.5	2.6±0.8
Spleen	1.8±0.7	6.7±5.3
Other tissues	3.2±0.6	4.7±2.7
Feces	4.9±2.9	6.7±7.2
Urine	3.1±2.5	2.8±2.0

TABLE 3.   Relative activities of rat tissues in degradation of [^{14}C]-sucrose-LDL.

Tissue	Relative content of ^{14}C/g wet wt. of tissue (liver = 100)	
	Rat LDL (n=5)	Human LDL (n=3)
Liver	(100)	(100)
Adrenal	119 ±55	78 ± 45
Ovary	91 ±30	41 ± 4
Spleen	76 ±28	228 ±114
Kidney	28 ± 5	28 ± 7
Small intestine	21 ± 9	21 ± 10
Large intestine	17 ± 4	15 ± 9
Adipose tissue	5 ± 5	3 ± 1
Skin	2.1± 1.1	1.8± 0.2
Muscle	0.6± 0.3	1.3± 0.2
Rest of tissues	<9	<20

The other tissues were much less active per unit weight. However, the data shown in Table 3 are expressed per gram of total wet weight. Because adipose tissue is about 90% inert stored triglyceride, the data if expressed per unit protein bring adipose tissue up to a ranking near the top, just behind adrenal, liver, ovary and spleen.

Data for degradation of LDL in three different species by adipose tissue compared to that in the liver are summarized in Table 4.

TABLE 4.   Percentage of total body LDL degradation attributable to liver and to adipose tissue.

	LIVER	ADIPOSE TISSUE
Pig	50%	6.8%
Rat		
Rat HDL	66%	2.8%
Human LDL	56%	2.6%
Rabbit	57%	1.6%

In pig, rat and rabbit, the liver is the dominant site of LDL degradation, much more active than the adipose tissue. If we express the data in terms of degradation rate per milligram tissue protein, the rankings are as shown in Table 5.

TABLE 5.   Tissues most active in LDL degradation per mg tissue protein

	RAT	PIG	RABBIT
1	ADRENAL	ADRENAL	ADRENAL
2	LIVER	LIVER	SPLEEN
3	OVARY	(N.G.)	LIVER
4	SPLEEN	SPLEEN	OVARY
5	ADIPOSE	ADIPOSE	ADIPOSE

In all three species studied, the adrenal was the most active tissue in LDL degradation. The liver, spleen and ovary were the next most active and the adipose tissue in each case took fifth place. (The "N.G." indicates that our pigs had "no gonads" left, a phenomenon apparently common in pig husbandry!)

From these findings it is evident that the adipose tissue, while relatively active in LDL degradation per milligram cell protein, does not make a major contribution to overall LDL degradation. Consequently, changes in uptake by the adipose tissue are unlikely to have much of an effect on ambient plasma LDL levels. On the other hand, the liver makes such a major contribution that changes in its activity, through regulation of receptors or by other mechanisms, will be determining with regard to plasma LDL concentrations. Evidence has been presented that the liver expresses a high-affinity LDL receptor and that it is indeed subject to regulation. On the other hand, the high activity of the adipose tissue relative to its mass of protoplasm is of interest with regard to the metabolism of the adipose tissue itself.

Is the uptake and degradation of LDL by adipose tissue receptor-mediated? Isolated adipocytes are relatively fragile and tend to lyse during prolonged incubation. To avoid this potential problem we have investigated the uptake and degradation of LDL by 3T3-L1 cells, the

model of preadipocytes first described by Green and Kehinde (10). Cells
were studied before and after differentiation induced by incubation in
the presence of dexamethasone and 1-methyl-3-isobutylxanthine (11).
Degradation was measured in terms of the generation of non-iodide radioactivity soluble in trichloroacetic acid. As shown in Figure 2 degradation was a linear function of time for at least 24 hrs, both in the
undifferentiated cells (Ll-) and in the differentiated cells (Ll+).
However, the rate of degradation was considerably greater in the
differentiated cells.

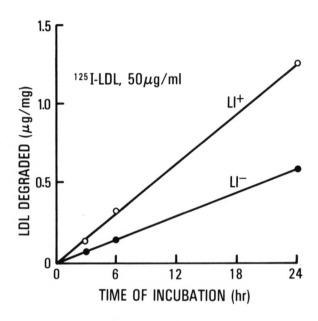

FIGURE 2. DEGRADATION OF ^{125}I-LDL, 50 ug/ml, AS A FUNCTION OF TIME IN
3T3-L1 CELLS BEFORE (●) AND AFTER (○)DIFFERENTIATION.

Degradation rate as a function of LDL concentration is shown in Figure 3.
Both the undifferentiated and differentiated cells yield a biphasic
curve indicating the participation of a saturable phase in the degradation, compatible with a receptor-dependent uptake mechanism. Again, the
rate of degradation in the differentiated cells was considerably greater
at all concentrations. Thus, it appears that differentiation of 3T3-L1
cells is accompanied by a significant induction of LDL receptors. It has
been shown previously that differentiation of these cells to the adipose-
like form is accompanied by a marked increase in hormone-sensitive lipase
as reviewed elsewhere in this symposium (12,13).

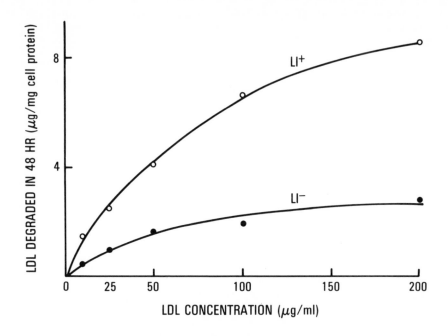

FIGURE 3. DEGRADATION OF ^{125}I-LDL AS A FUNCTION OF CONCENTRATION IN
3T3-L1 CELLS BEFORE (●) AND AFTER (○) DIFFERENTIATION (48 hr incubation).

   The LDL receptor of the 3T3 cells is subject to down regulation
analogous to that previously demonstrated for other cell types (14). As
shown in Table 6, prior incubation of differentiated cells in the presence of LDL for 24 hrs decreased the subsequent rate of LDL degradation
by approximately 50%; there was no such effect in the undifferentiated
cells, possibly reflecting the limited uptake by way of the LDL receptor.

TABLE 6.   DOWN-REGULATION OF 3T3-L1 LDL RECEPTOR

CELLS	^{125}I-LDL DEGRADATION* AFTER 24 H PREINCUBATION:	
	IN LDS	IN LDL + 200 µG/ML LDL
	(NG/MG PROTEIN)	
L+	438	269
L-	94	81

*5 H IN LDS PLUS 5 µG/ML ^{125}I-LDL

In fibroblasts, the uptake of LDL by way of the high-affinity pathway is accompanied by a marked stimulation of acylCoA:cholesterol acyltransferase (ACAT) (15). As shown in Table 7, we found no effect of LDL on this enzyme activity in 3T3, either before or after differentiation.

INCORPORATION OF [3H] OLEIC ACID INTO CHOLESTEROL ESTERS

CELLS	24-H PREINCUBATION IN:	(CPM/MG PROTEIN)
	LDS	6135
L+	LDL (100 μG/ML)	6079
	LDS	4146
L-	LDL (100 μG/ML)	3708

TABLE 7

The fraction of cholesterol stored in adipose tissue as cholesterol ester is very low. Most tissues when they accumulate cholesterol do so primarily in the ester form. In adipose tissue, 80% or more of the stored cholesterol is present in the free form. The failure of LDL to stimulate ACAT may account for this in part. In addition, it may be that cholesterol escaping from the lysosomes can be transported to the central fat droplet and thus avoid esterification by the ACAT of the microsomes.

In an attempt to estimate the fraction of uptake of LDL in vivo occurring by way of the receptor-mediated pathway, we have turned to the newly-described receptor-deficient rabbit (WHHL rabbit) (16). These animals have an almost complete deficiency of the high-affinity LDL receptors and their fractional catabolic rates for irreversible degradation of plasma LDL is only about one-third normal. By using [14C]sucrose LDL and comparing rates of degradation in the individual tissues of control rabbits versus WHHL rabbits, we were able to make an estimate of the receptor-dependent degradation in each tissue (17). The assumption is that receptor-independent pathways are unaffected in the mutant rabbit. As shown in Figure 4, a simple formula based on measurements of the fractional catabolic rate in each tissue can then be used to estimate the percentage of degradation occurring via the receptor. Calculations for the intact rabbit (based on fractional catabolic rate of plasma LDL) yield a figure of 62% receptor-mediated degradation. The calculated values for adrenal, liver and gut are all very high. Applying the same principle to the data for adipose tissue we obtain the values shown in Table 8. It should be stated at once that the variance among animals was very large and none of the data reached statistical significance. From the mean values for the four animals in each group, we would conclude that about 60% of LDL degradation in normal rabbit adipose tissue in vivo occurs by way of the LDL receptor. Additional studies will be needed before this value can be considered firm.

CALCULATED PERCENTAGE OF LDL DEGRADATION VIA THE LDL RECEPTOR-MEDIATED PATHWAY

$$\left[\frac{FCR_N - FCR_{WHHL}}{FCR_N} \times 100 \right]$$

TOTAL BODY	62%
ADRENAL	92%
LIVER	63%
GUT	83%

FIGURE 4. PERCENTAGE OF LDL DEGRADATION ATTRIBUTABLE TO CALCULATED LDL RECEPTOR-MEDIATED UPTAKE FROM DATA OBTAINED IN CONTROL AND RECEPTOR-DEFICIENT RABBITS.

TABLE 8. Adipose tissue degradation of LDL in control and in receptor-deficient rabbits

	Control rabbits (4)	Receptor-Deficient rabbits (4)
Percentage of total body LDL degradation occurring in adipose tissue	1.6	1.73
Clearance of plasma LDL pool (% $g^{-1}d^{-1}$)	0.010	0.004
Absolute rate of LDL delivery ($\mu g\ g^{-1}d^{-1}$)	1.94	5.7

REFERENCES

1. Nestel, P.J., Whyte, H.M. and Goodman, DeW. S. (1969):J. Clin. Invest. 48:982-991.
2. Farkas, J., Angel, A. and Avigan, M.I. (1973):J. Lipid. Res. 14: 344-356.
3. Bjorntorp, P. and Sjostrom, L. (1972):Eur. J. Clin. Invest. 2:78-84.
4. Angel, A. and Farkas, J. (1974): J. Lipid Res. 15:491-499.
5. Angel, A., D'Costa, M.A. and Yuen, R. (1979):Canad. J. Biochem. 57:578-587.

6. Pittman, R. and Steinberg, D. (1978):Biochem. Biophys. Res. Comm. 81:1254-1259.
7. Pittman, R.C., Green, S.R., Attie, A.D. and Steinberg, D. (1979): J. Biol. Chem. 254:6876-6879.
8. Pittman, R.C., Attie, A.D., Carew, T.E. and Steinberg, D. (1979): Proc. Natl. Acad. Sci. 76:5345-5349.
9. Pittman, R.C., Attie, A.D., Carew, T.E. and Steinberg, D. (1982): Biochim. Biophys. Acta 710:7-14.
10. Green, H. and Kehinde, O. (1974):Cell 1:113-116.
11. Rubin, C.S., Hirsch, A., Fung, C. and Rosen, O.M. (1978) J. Biol. Chem. 253:7570-7578.
12. Kawamura, M., Jensen, D.F., Wancewicz, E.V., Joy, L.L., Khoo, J.C. and Steinberg, D. (1981):Proc. Natl. Acad. Sci. USA 78:732-736.
13. Khoo, J.C., Yamamoto, M., Kawamura, M. and Steinberg, D. (1982) The Adipocyte and Obesity: Cellular and Molecular Mechanism, Raven Press, in press.
14. Goldstein, J.L. and Brown, M.S. (1977):Ann. Rev. Biochem. 46:897-930.
15. Brown, M.S., Dana, S.E. and Goldstein, J.L. (1975) J. Biol. Chem. 250:4025-4027.
16. Watanabe, Y. (1980) FEBS Lett. 118:81-84.
17. Pittman, R.C., Carew, T.E., Attie, A.D., Witztum, J.L., Watanabe, Y., and Steinberg, D. (1982) J. Biol. Chem., submitted for publication.

The Adipocyte and Obesity: Cellular and Molecular Mechanisms, edited by A. Angel, C. H. Hollenberg, and D. A. K. Roncari. Raven Press, New York © 1983.

Dietary and Pharmacologic Influences on Adipocyte Cholesterol Storage

*Arthur D. Hartman and **Brian R. Krause

*Department of Physiology, Louisiana State University Medical Center, New Orleans, Louisiana, 70119; and **Department of Pharmacology, Warner-Lambert/Parke-Davis, Pharmaceutical Research Division, Ann Arbor, Michigan 48105*

Although it is now well accepted that adipose tissue represents a major storage organ for cholesterol, the factors which regulate deposition and mobilization of cholesterol in adipocytes are still not well understood. These factors include adipocyte size (1-3), age (1-3), level of dietary cholesterol (4), de novo synthesis in situ (5,6), plasma cholesterol concentration (7) and the rate of turnover or mobilization of cellular triglyceride (1,4,8). Control of several of these variables under experimental conditions is difficult. For example, we have reported that both adipocyte size and plasma cholesterol in Sprague-Dawley rats vary as a function of age (2,3). As a result, in this strain of rat it is difficult, if not impossible, to determine independently the role of either of these two variables on adipocyte size. To circumvent the problems of changing cell size and plasma cholesterol with age we have utilized an animal model in which both of these variables remain constant for approximately one year after the rat achieves 9-12 months of age (7). This rat model is the Fisher 344 rat. We will report two experiments in which this model has been utilized to examine the regulation of adipocyte cholesterol.

In the first example the intent was to determine the relative contributions of dietary and plasma cholesterol levels on adipocyte cholesterol storage. One-year-old Fisher 344 rats were fed a cholesterol-free semi-purified diet to which was added either 0, 0.05, 0.5 or 5% cholesterol by weight (7). Since it has been reported that labeled adipocyte cholesterol disappears with a half-time of 27 days (9), we employed a feeding period of 90 days to assure ourselves of the ability to measure a change in mass if one should occur. Adipocyte free and esterified cholesterol were isolated prior to quantitation by a column procedure employing Sephadex LH-20 which efficiently separates these fractions in the face of large excesses of cellular triglyceride (10).

As expected, control rats fed a chow diet throughout the experimental period showed no significant alteration in total plasma cholesterol throughout the 90 day period. Plasma cholesterol in animals fed the experimental diets was not related to dietary level at the end of the experiment. In contrast to the plasma, both hepatic total cholesterol and cholesterol ester were directly related to the dietary load. Muscle cholesterol, on the other hand, was not affected by either dietary or plasma cholesterol with the exception of the group receiving 0.5% cholesterol which showed a significant increase. In contrast to liver and muscle, adipose tissue cholesterol storage was related to the plasma cholesterol concentration but not to that in the diet (Fig. 1). In all four depots when all data points were considered, total adipocyte cho-

lesterol was significantly correlated with the plasma cholesterol concentration. This observation was also true for adipocyte cholesterol
ester which was generally increased in cells with elevated cholesterol
storage. Similar results but with smaller changes were obtained in a
shorter feeding period limited to 70 days.

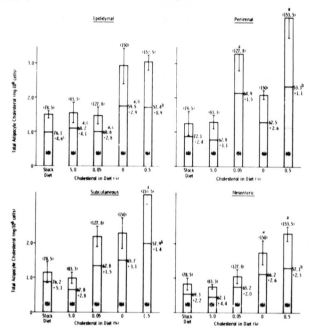

FIG. 1. Adipocyte cholesterol storage as a function of plasma cholesterol level in four adipose tissue depots of adult Fisher rats on day
90. Bars or numbers not sharing the same superscript are significantly
different at P < 0.05. Shaded area = free cholesterol fraction and
number of animals. Numbers above each bar = mean plasma total cholesterol value for each group in mg/dl. Numbers to the side of each bar =
percentage of cellular cholesterol in the free form (mean ± S.E.).
Ⓒ J. Nutr. American Institute of Nutrition.

These data allow several conclusions to be drawn:
1. Plasma cholesterol does not necessarily reflect the level of cholesterol in the diet.
2. Both hepatic total cholesterol and cholesterol ester, at least under
these experimental conditions, are directly related to dietary level.
3. Muscle cholesterol storage is generally not affected by either
dietary or plasma cholesterol level.
4. Adipose tissue cholesterol storage is related to plasma cholesterol
but not to dietary level under the conditions of this study.
5. Adipocyte cholesterol ester generally increases with increased cholesterol storage.
The second experiment was designed to study the converse of the first
study, i.e. to test the hypothesis that a decrease in plasma cholesterol
would mobilize adipocyte cholesterol independently of triglyceride.
This was accomplished by placing 9-12 month old Fisher 344 rats on a
semi-purified diet containing 0.5% cholesterol by weight for a period
of 90 days to preload the adipocytes with cholesterol as in the

preceding study. At the end of this time one group of rats was killed as a baseline control group while three other groups continued on the 0.5% cholesterol diet for an additional 90 days; a fifth group was fed a diet containing 1/10 the original amount of cholesterol. The three groups that continued on the "high" cholesterol diet were further subdivided into three subgroups, one which continued on the diet without further intervention, one which received 40 mg/day of oxandrolone while the third received a combination of clofibrate (0.25% w/w in the diet) and cholestyramine (2% w/w in the diet). The two drug regimens and the switch to the "low" cholesterol diet in the fifth group were designed to lower plasma cholesterol to test our hypothesis with regard to adipocyte cholesterol mobilization.

The two groups receiving the hypolipidemic drugs demonstrated prompt and significant 40% reductions in plasma cholesterol within two weeks while the "low" cholesterol diet produced no change in plasma cholesterol. At the end of the second 90 day period both drug-treated groups had significantly decreased plasma cholesterols whereas the "low" cholesterol group had plasma cholesterols equivalent to rats which continued on the "high" cholesterol diet throughout the study. Both the "low" cholesterol diet and the combination of clofibrate-cholestyramine significantly reduced hepatic total cholesterol and cholesterol-ester content whereas oxandrolone had no effect on either of these fractions. Adipocyte cholesterol in both drug-treated groups was significantly increased while subcutaneous adipocytes also contained more cholesterol especially in rats given oxandrolone (Fig. 2). These increases in adipocyte cholesterol were associated with decreases in the absolute amounts of apo AI and apo AIV both of which are associated primarily with HDL. The "low" cholesterol diet produced no change in either adipocyte cholesterol storage or apolipoprotein concentrations compared to the "high" cholesterol controls.

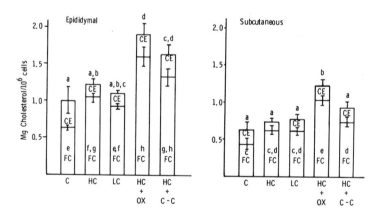

FIG. 2. Adipocyte total, free and esterified cholesterol in control (C) rats killed at Day 90 and in rats receiving the same high-cholesterol diet (HC), a low cholesterol diet (LC), the high cholesterol diet plus clofibrate-cholestyramine (HC+C-C) or the high-cholesterol diet plus oxandrolone (HC+OX) for an additional 90 days. Values are the mean ± S.E. of 6-8 rats/group. Groups with different letters (a,b,c, etc.) are significantly different at P < 0.05.

These data indicate that plasma cholesterol levels do not adequately reflect the cholesterol content of either liver or adipose tissue. Both drug treatments produced an increase in adipocyte cholesterol and decreased apo AI and AIV which is consistent with the reported effects of oxandrolone (11) and clofibrate (12) in decreasing rat HDL. These results are consistent with a possible imbalance between cholesterol delivery and reverse-cholesterol transport. Studies are currently underway to evaluate the effects of both exercise and alcohol consumption which both elevate HDL cholesterol to determine whether these interventions can decrease adipose tissue cholesterol storage.

Acknowledgement: These studies were supported by USPHS grant no. AM 19995.

REFERENCES

1. Kovanen, P.T., Nikkila, E.A. and Miettinen, T.A. (1975): J. Lipid Res. 16:211-223.
2. Krause, B.R. and Hartman, A.D. (1976): Biochim. Biophys. Acta 450: 197-205.
3. Hartman, A.D. and Krause, B.R. (1980): The Physiologist 23:34-43.
4. Angel, A. and Farkas, J. (1974): J. Lipid Res. 15:491-499.
5. Rosenthal, J., Angel, A. and Farkas, J. (1974): Am. J. Physiol. 226: 411-418.
6. Miettinen, T.A. and Tilvis, R.S. (1981): Int. J. Obesity 5:613-618.
7. Krause, B.R., Phares, F., Serbin, V., Krause, L. and Hartman, A.D. (1979): J. Nutr. 109:2213-2225.
8. Krause, B.R., Balzer, M. and Hartman, A.D. (1981): Proc. Soc. Exp. Biol. Med. 167:407-411.
9. Farkas, J., Angel, A. and Avigan, M.I. (1973): J. Lipid Res. 14:344-356.
10. Krause, B.R. and Hartman, A.D. (1978): J. Lipid Res. 19:774-777.
11. Freeman, M.W., Spring-Mills, E. and James, A.C. (1980):J. Gerontol. 35:31-38.
12. Day, C.E., Phillips, W.A. and Schurr, P.E. (1979): Artery 5:90-109.

The Adipocyte and Obesity: Cellular and
Molecular Mechanisms, edited by A. Angel,
C. H. Hollenberg, and D. A. K. Roncari.
Raven Press, New York © 1983.

Regulation of Estrogen Formation By Human Adipose Stromal Cells in Culture

Carole R. Mendelson, William H. Cleland, and Evan R. Simpson

*Departments of Biochemistry and Obstetrics-Gynecology and
The Cecil H. and Ida Green Center for Reproductive Biology Sciences,
The University of Texas Health Science Center at Dallas, Dallas, Texas 75235*

In the post-menopausal woman adipose tissue is the principal source of circulating estrogen (8). Unlike the ovary, in which the primary estrogen formed is estradiol, and its secretion is episodic, the principal estrogen produced by the adipose tissue is estrone and its secretion is continuous. The precursor utilized by adipose tissue for estrogen formation is circulating androstenedione produced primarily by the adrenal cortex. The fractional conversion of androstenedione to estrogen is increased with increased body weight (5,11) and with age (9). Increased estrogen formation in adipose tissue, as a function of aging and/or obesity, is believed to serve a role in the pathogenesis of endometrial cancer (4,10,11).

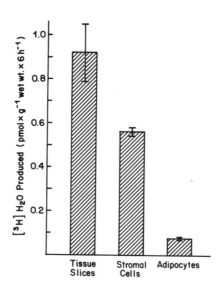

FIG. 1. Aromatase activity of tissue slices, stromal cells and adipocytes from human subcutaneous adipose tissue. (From Ackerman et al. (1) with permission).

In order to investigate the regulation of aromatase activity in human adipose tissue, it was our first objective to define the cellular localization of such activity. Human subcutaneous fat, obtained by informed consent from women undergoing elective surgery for a variety of benign gynecological disorders, was separated into adipocyte and stromal cell fractions by collagenase digestion as described previously (1). Adipose tissue slices, as well as aliquots of each cell fraction equivalent to 1 g wet weight of tissue, were incubated in suspension in the presence of [1-^{3}H]androstenedione (100 nM) for 6 h at 37°C and the incorporation of tritium into [^{3}H]water was assayed as an index of aromatase activity. The results of such a study are shown in Figure 1. Of the activity present in the adipose tissue slices some 67% was recovered in the isolated stromal cells and adipocytes. However, of the recovered activity, only 13% was present in the adipocytes, whereas the remaining 87% was present in the stromal cells. It is concluded, therefore, that most of the aromatase activity of human adipose tissue resides in the cells of the stroma, whereas the adipocytes manifest little of this activity.

These stromal cells are fibroblast-like, grow readily to confluence in monolayer culture and retain the capacity to aromatize androstenedione to estrone. Consequently, they provide an ideal model system for study of the regulation of aromatase activity. Addition of dexamethasone to the culture medium resulted in a 20-60 fold stimulation of conversion of androstenedione to estrone. The stimulatory effect of dexamethasone on aromatase activity was elicited only if fetal calf serum (FCS, 15%) was present in the culture medium (14). An

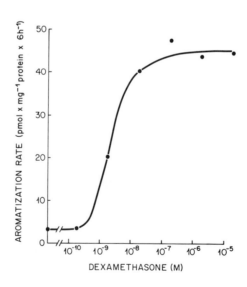

FIG. 2. Aromatase activity of adipose stromal cells in response to dexamethasone in various concentrations. (From Simpson et al. (14) with permission).

increase in aromatase activity was detectable within 4 hours of addition
of dexamethasone, and maximum stimulation of aromatase was observed
after 24 to 48 hours of addition of dexamethasone to the cultures.
When adipose tissue stromal cells were incubated in medium that contained FCS with dexamethasone in concentrations from 2.5×10^{-10} to
2.5×10^{-5} M for 48 h prior to aromatase assay, results such as those
presented in Figure 2 were obtained.   Dexamethasone stimulated the
conversion of androstenedione to estrone in a concentration-dependent
fashion; half-maximal stimulation was obtained at a concentration of
dexamethasone of about 2.5×10^{-9} M.   This proved to be similar to
the concentration of dexamethasone required to cause half-maximal
saturation of receptors in cytosolic fractions prepared from such
stromal cells (14).   These results are indicative that the action of
dexamethasone to stimulate aromatase activity in these cells is mediated
by its binding to a glucocorticosteroid receptor.   Further proof of this
contention was obtained by the finding that the order of potency of
various steroids to stimulate aromatase activity was dexamethasone >
cortisol > corticosterone.   Neither deoxycorticosterone nor progesterone
had the capacity to stimulate aromatase activity (14).   Furthermore,
the stimulatory effect of dexamethasone on aromatase activity was
blocked by cortisol-21-mesylate, an antagonist of glucocorticosteroid
receptor binding (14).   Both actinomycin D and cycloheximide blocked
the capacity of dexamethasone to stimulate aromatase activity (14),
suggestive that the stimulatory action of dexamethasone requires the
synthesis of new mRNA and protein.

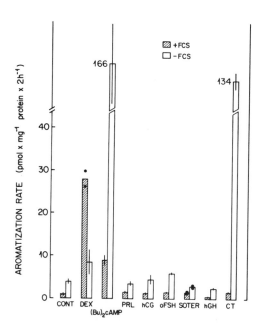

FIG. 3.   Effects of various agents on aromatase activity of cultured
adipose stromal cells after incubation for 5 days in the presence or
absence of FCS.   (From Mendelson et al. (12) with permission).

Aromatase activities of ovarian granulosa (3,6) and testicular Sertoli (2,7) and Leydig (15) cells are stimulated by gonadotropic hormones. The stimulatory effects of gonadotropins are thought to be mediated by an increase in cyclic AMP levels. Since the circulating levels of gonadotropins are increased with aging, as is the peripheral conversion of androstenedione to estrone, we investigated the capacity of gonadotropins and other hormones, as well as cyclic AMP, to stimulate aromatase activity in the cultured adipose stromal cells. In Fig. 3 are shown the effects of various agents on aromatase activity of adipose stromal cells incubated for 5 days in medium with or without fetal calf serum. Aromatase activity of control cells incubated in the absence of fetal calf serum was 4 pmol $\times$ mg^{-1} protein $\times$ 2 h^{-1}, and was 4-fold greater than the activity of cells maintained in serum-containing medium. Dexamethasone (10^{-7} M), in the presence of FCS caused a 30-fold increase in aromatase activity and its effect was diminished when FCS was absent from the culture medium. Neither bovine prolactin (bPRL, 2.5 µg $\times$ ml^{-1}), human chorionic gonadotropin (hCG, 50 ng $\times$ ml^{-1}), ovine follicle stimulating hormone (oFSH, 50 ng $\times$ ml^{-1}), soterenol (10^{-5} M), a β-adrenergic agonist, nor human growth hormone (hGH, 2.5 µg $\times$ ml^{-1}) significantly affected aromatase activity when added to cells maintained in the absence or presence of FCS. In contrast, a marked stimulation was observed when cells were incubated with either dibutyryl cyclic AMP ((Bu)$_2$cAMP, 10^{-3} M) or cholera toxin (CT, 10 µg $\times$ ml^{-1}) in medium that did not contain FCS. The stimulatory effect of these agents was markedly reduced when FCS was present in the culture medium (12). The stimulatory effect of (Bu)$_2$cAMP was also mimicked by 8-bromo cyclic AMP, and N-monobutyryl cyclic AMP but not by either sodium butyrate, cyclic AMP itself, or O-monobutyryl cyclic AMP. 1-Methyl-3-isobutylxanthine also caused a stimulation of aromatase activity. All of these agents were effective only when FCS was absent from the culture medium (12).

In addition to the differences in the serum requirement for aromatase induction by dexamethasone and (Bu)$_2$cAMP, the time courses of aromatase induction in response to these agents differed markedly. In response to dexamethasone in the presence of FCS, aromatase activity was increased about 30-fold by 18 h and this level was maintained through 72 h. In contrast, aromatase activity in response to (Bu)$_2$cAMP in the absence of FCS was increased only 4-fold by 18 h but continued to increase so that after 72 h of incubation, a 37-fold increase in enzyme activity was observed. Incubation of stromal cells for 8 days in the presence of (Bu)$_2$cAMP resulted in a 200-fold increase in aromatase activity (12). The difference in the time courses of aromatase activation by (Bu)$_2$cAMP and by dexamethasone, as well as the difference in the serum requirements are suggestive that these agents elicit their effects on aromatase induction by different mechanisms.

CONCLUSIONS

At present, the factors that regulate in vivo the extraglandular formation of estrogens are not known. It has been known for some time that cortisol production rates are elevated in obese subjects (13) as are the production rates of estrone from circulating androstenedione

(5,11). The fractional conversion of androstenedione to estrone is also increased in patients following the stress of surgery (P.C. MacDonald, personal communication). Thus, glucocorticosteroids may serve a role in the regulation of estrogen formation by human adipose tissue. Our findings are also indicative that cyclic AMP may mediate an increase in estrogen formation by human adipose tissue. The factors that increase adenylate cyclase activity in adipose stroma, however, are unknown. Our failure to find a stimulatory effect on aromatase activity of the β-adrenergic agonist, soterenol, or of the gonadotropins FSH and hCG, is indicative that either receptors for these hormones are absent from the stromal cells or, if present, that they are not coupled to adenylate cyclase. Studies are in progress to identify substances that elevate cyclic AMP levels in these cells and to define the molecular events that mediate aromatase induction by glucocorticosteroids and by cyclic AMP.

REFERENCES

1. Ackerman, G.E., Smith, M.E., Mendelson, C.R., MacDonald, P.C., and Simpson, E.R. (1981): J. Clin. Endocrinol. Metab., 53:412–417.
2. Dorrington, J.H., and Armstrong, D.T. (1975): Proc. Natl. Acad. Sci. USA, 72:2677–2681.
3. Dorrington, J.H., Moon, Y.S., and Armstrong, D.T. (1975): Endocrinology, 97:1328–1331.
4. Dunn, L.J., and Bradbury, J.T. (1967): Am. J. Obstet. Gynecol., 97:465–471.
5. Edman, C.D., and MacDonald, P.C. (1978): Am. J. Obstet. Gynecol., 130:456–461.
6. Erickson, G.F., and Hsueh, A.J.W. (1978): Endocrinology, 102:1275–1282.
7. Fritz, I.B., Griswold, M.D., Louis, B.G., and Dorrington, J.H. (1976): Mol. Cell. Endocrinol., 5:289–294.
8. Grodin, J.M., Siiteri, P.K., and MacDonald, P.C. (1973): J. Clin. Endocrinol. Metab., 36:207–214.
9. Hemsell, D.L, Grodin, J., Breuner, P.F., Siiteri, P.K., and MacDonald, P.C. (1974): J. Clin. Endocrinol. Metab., 38:476–479.
10. Knab, D.R. (1977): Obstet. Gynecol. Survey, 32:267–281.
11. MacDonald, P.C., Edman, C.D., Hemsell, D.L., Porter, J.C., and Siiteri, P.K. (1978): Am. J. Obstet. Gynecol., 130:448–455.
12. Mendelson, C.R., Cleland, W.H., Smith, M.E., and Simpson, E.R. (1982): Endocrinology, (in press).
13. Mlynaryk, P., Gillies, R.R., Murphy, B., and Pattee, C.J. (1962): J. Clin. Endocrinol. Metab., 22:587–591.
14. Simpson, E.R., Ackerman, G.E., Smith, M.E., and Mendelson, C.R. (1981): Proc. Natl. Acad. Sci. USA, 78:5690–5694.
15. Valladares, L.E., and Payne, A.H. (1979): Endocrinology, 105:431–436.

The Adipocyte and Obesity: Cellular and
Molecular Mechanisms, edited by A. Angel,
C. H. Hollenberg, and D. A. K. Roncari.
Raven Press, New York © 1983.

Control of Adipose Tissue Lipolysis by Phosphorylation/Dephosphorylation of Hormone-Sensitive Lipase

P. Belfrage, G. Fredrikson, H. Olsson, and P. Strålfors

Department of Physiological Chemistry 4, University of Lund, S-220 07 Lund, Sweden

Free fatty acids (FFA) are the quantitatively most important energy substrate in mammals. The flow of FFA is controlled by the hormonal and neural regulation of FFA mobilization from adipose tissue. The FFA mobilization rate mainly reflects the hydrolysis of the triacylglycerol stored in the adipose tissue, the process of adipose tissue lipolysis. Lipolytic hormones, *e.g.* catecholamines, glucagon and ACTH, stimulate, and insulin inhibits this process by regulating the activity of the rate-limiting enzyme, the hormone-sensitive lipase (HSL).

HORMONE-SENSITIVE LIPASE: FUNCTION AND PROPERTIES

The main reaction sequence of adipose tissue lipolysis is as follows: Triacylglycerol → 1,2-diacylglycerol + FFA → 2-monoacylglycerol + FFA → glycerol + FFA. Hormone-sensitive lipase catalyses the first two steps, the triacylglycerol hydrolysis being rate-limiting because of the lower enzyme activity towards this substrate (6). HSL is relatively specific for the primary ester-bonds of the acylglycerol substrates and has a relatively low activity against monoacylglycerols (6). The 2-monoacylglycerols are therefore probably hydrolysed by a separate enzyme, monoacylglycerol lipase, which has no positional specificity (12).

Rat adipose tissue HSL has recently been extensively purified and partially characterised (6). Microgram amounts of the enzyme at approximately 50% protein purity can be obtained from the epididymal adipose tissue of several hundred rats, after solubilization with non-ionic detergent and fractionation by modified ion-exchange and affinity chromatography (6). The enzyme has an apparent subunit molecular weight of 84,000 (SDS-polyacrylamide gel electrophoresis) and an apparent molecular size (gel chromatography) of 150,000, indicating that it is probably a dimer. Its relative enzyme activity against tri-, di-, monoacylglycerols and cholesterol esters is 1:10:4:1.5, respectively, and it has a molar specific activity against its favoured substrate, diacylglycerols, of 600 moles$\cdot$mol$^{-1}\cdot$s^{-1}. This high molar specific activity accounts for the high biological activity of the enzyme in spite of its low tissue concentration (1-2 μg/g adipose tissue). HSL is inhibited by micromolar concentration of DFP and Hg^{2+} and millimolar concentration of NaF. HSL with very similar properties has recently also been extensively purified from swine adipose tissue (F.T. Lee, S. Yeaman, G. Fredrikson, P. Strålfors and P. Belfrage, unpublished).

HSL catalyses the hydrolysis of cholesterol esters besides acylglyce-
rols, a substrate specificity which is notably different from pancreatic
lipase and lipoprotein lipase (4). This substrate specificity was
explained by recent collaborative work which demonstrated that the cytosolic neutral cholesterol ester hydrolase from bovine adrenal cortex was
very similar, or identical to HSL of adipose tissue (5). Moreover,
cholesterol ester hydrolase of corpus luteum has also been found to be
very similar, or identical, to HSL of rat adipose tissue (S. Yeaman,
personal communication). Thus, what has been thought of as a specific
adipose tissue enzyme may be a general hormonally controlled acylglyce-
rol/cholesterol ester lipase with different functions depending on its
tissue localisation: control of lipolysis in adipose tissue and control
of steroidogenesis in adrenal cortex.

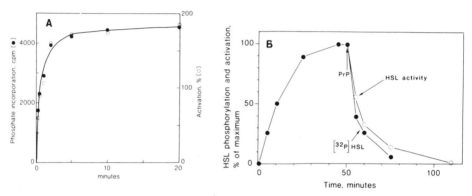

Fig. 1. Reversible phosphorylation and activation of HSL. A. The enzyme was
phosphorylated with the catalytic subunit of cAMP-PrK, 0.3 μM, in 5 mM
imidazole-HCl, pH 7.0, 1 mM DTE, 5 mM $MgCl_2$ and 0.1 mM $(\gamma-^{32}P)ATP$, 37°. At
the indicated time points incubations were interrupted by precipitation in
30% (v/v) acetone and 9% (w/v) trichloroacetic acid and subjected to
SDS-PAGE. Incorporation was determined after dissolution in H_2O_2 of gel-
slices containing HSL. Enzyme activation was determined against 1.5 mM
emulsified trioleoylglycerol after phosphorylation as above except that
unlabelled ATP was used and incubations were stopped by dilution in 5 vol.
of ice-cold 5 mM EDTA, in controls ATP was omitted. B. HSL was phosphorylated
and activated as in A. After 45 min the reaction was terminated by addition of
0.25 M glucose and 0.045 mg/ml hexokinase. The lipase was then incubated with
a protein phosphatase (indicated by PrP) isolated from adipose tissue in 1.25
mM Mn^{2+}, 1 mM DTE and 0.5 mg/ml BSA at 37°. At indicated time points aliquots
were withdrawn and assayed for HSL activity, or precipitated in 30% (v/v)
acetone and 9% (w/v) trichloroacetic acid and subjected to SDS-PAGE, and
autoradiography, for determination of ^{32}P-incorporation into HSL.

THE ACTIVITY OF ISOLATED HORMONE-SENSITIVE LIPASE IS CONTROLLED BY REVERSIBLE PHOSPHORYLATION

Extensive work by Steinberg and collaborators (10,11) during the
seventies had indicated that HSL activity was controlled by reversible
phosphorylation. However, no direct evidence for the phosphorylation/de-
phosphorylation of the enzyme was provided, since the enzyme protein had
not been identified. The identification (1) and subsequent extensive
purification of HSL (6) made this possible. Purified HSL is phosphorylated by cyclic AMP-dependent protein kinase (cAMP-PrK). The phosphorylation
is rapid (half-maximal within one minute) (Fig. 1A) and the rate of phos-

phorylation is comparable to that found in intact fat cells (see below). The phosphorylation of the enzyme is closely correlated with enhanced activity towards the triacylglycerol substrate (Fig. 1A). No intervening specific lipase kinase is necessary since the 50% pure enzyme is phosphorylated by the homogeneous catalytic subunit of cAMP-PrK and addition of the specific protein kinase inhibitor immediately arrests the phosphorylation of the lipase (6).

Purified, phosphorylated HSL is rapidly dephosphorylated in parallel with deactivation (Fig. 1B) by a protein phosphatase partially purified from rat adipose tissue (Olsson, H., Strålfors, P. and Belfrage, P., unpublished).

Phosphorylation by cAMP-PrK occurs exclusively on serine residues as demonstrated by high voltage electrophoresis after acid hydrolysis of the enzyme. After proteolytic fragmentation of HSL practically all phosphorylation can be shown to have taken place in a small (approximately 10 amino acids), acid (pI 2.5) peptide (Fig. 2). Manual Edman degradation indicates phosphorylation on the third residue from the amino terminal end of this peptide. From these findings and since the maximal

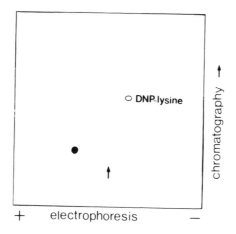

Fig. 2. Peptide mapping of proteolytic digests of phosphorylated HSL. Reduced and alkylated cAMP-PrK phosphorylated HSL obtained after SDS-PAGE was incubated in 0.5% (w/v) NH_4HCO_3 with 0.1 mg/ml of Staph. aur. V8 protease for 4 h at 37° and then with 10 μg/ml of trypsin for 15 h at 37°. After lyophilization the digest was redissolved in 33% (v/v) pyridine and subjected to peptide mapping on silicic acid TLC plates with electrophoresis at pH 3.4, 500 V, 60 min in the first dimension and ascending chromatography in butan-1-ol-pyridine-acetic acid-water (15:10:3:12) perpendicular to electrophoresis, and autoradiographed. Arrow indicates point of application.

phosphorylation seems to be 0.5-0.6 moles of phosphate per mole of enzyme subunit (6) it can be concluded that phosphorylation of the enzyme by cAMP-PrK occurs on a single serine residue.

HORMONE-SENSITIVE LIPASE IS PHOSPHORYLATED IN INTACT FAT CELLS

Phosphorylation of HSL in intact fat cells, stimulated with noradrenaline, has been demonstrated (2). HSL from fat cells preincubated with [^{32}P]orthophosphate and exposed to noradrenaline was extensively purified after detergent solubilization, through modified ion-exchange and affinity chromatography, to a protein purity of approximately 35%. The HSL thus isolated could be shown to have incorporated [^{32}P]orthophosphate (2). HSL is phosphorylated in intact fat cells also in the absence of any hormone stimulation, with no change of the biological activity of the enzyme. Recent experiments, employing proteolytic degradation of the phosphorylated enzyme from the cells, have indicated that two different sites are phosphorylated in HSL in the intact fat cells. Lipolytic hormones stimulate the phosphorylation of the same serine residue as that phosphorylated in the isolated enzyme with cAMP-PrK while a separate site is phosphorylated in the absence of hormones.

EFFECTS OF HORMONES ON THE PHOSPHORYLATION STATE AND ACTIVITY OF HORMONE-SENSITIVE LIPASE IN INTACT FAT CELLS

Determination of Activity and Phosphorylation State of the Hormone-Sensitive Lipase in Intact Fat Cells

A pH-stat titration technique has been developed which makes it possible to continuously monitor the biological activity of HSL in intact fat cells, as FFA-release into the medium (9). The phosphorylation state of HSL in intact fat cells is determined by measuring the ^{32}P content of the M_r 84,000 phosphopeptide band obtained by SDS-polyacrylamide gel electrophoresis of the total protein extract of fat cells preincubated with [^{32}P]orthophosphate (7). At least 70% of the ^{32}P-radioactivity in this 84,000 d band is due to HSL as verified by hydroxyapatite chromatography of the [^{32}P]phosphoprotein SDS-complexes eluted electrophoretically from the corresponding gel slice. Hormones effect mainly, possibly exclusively, the [^{32}P]HSL component (7). Moreover, the [^{32}P]phosphopeptide pattern of a proteolytic digest of the 84,000 d proteins was strikingly similar to the pattern obtained from [^{32}P]HSL purified extensively from intact fat cells. Thus, the ^{32}P-content of this band can be used as a valid measure of the HSL phosphorylation state in intact cells.

Lipolytic Hormones and Dibutyryl Cyclic AMP Stimulate the Lipolysis Rate in Intact Fat Cells by Increasing the Phosphorylation State of Hormone-Sensitive Lipase

In the absence of lipolytic hormones incubation of fat cells with [^{32}P]orthophosphate increased HSL ^{32}P-radioactivity to a steady state level after 40 min without any effect on the lipolysis rate, *i.e.* a basal phosphorylation of the enzyme occurred (Fig. 3). No significant effect on this basal HSL-phosphorylation was observed by exposure of the cells to 700 pM insulin during the entire preincubation with [^{32}P]orthophosphate, or by exposure of the cells to insulin immediately following this preincubation (8).

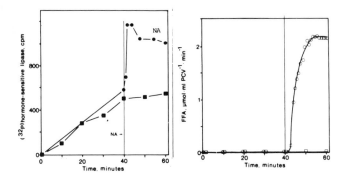

Fig. 3. Effects of noradrenaline on HSL phosphorylation and activity. Rat fat cells (5% v/v packed cell volume/ ml) were incubated in modified Krebs-Ringer medium with 3.5% bovine serum albumin and [^{32}P]orthophosphate (50 µM phosphate) for 40 min and hormone then added. The adipocyte proteins were defatted, subjected to SDS-PAGE and autoradiographed. HSL-activity was monitored continuously by pH-stat titration. NA, noradrenaline, 300 nM, added as indicated; squares, no hormone. Reproduced, by permission, from (7).

Noradrenaline addition rapidly increased the HSL phosphorylation state and, after a short time lag, the lipolysis rate, indicating an activation of HSL (Fig. 3) (7). The noradrenaline effect on HSL phosphorylation state and activity was related, in a dose dependent manner, to the peak of cyclic AMP concentration in the fat cells (Nilsson, N.Ö., Fain, J.N., and Belfrage, P., unpublished). The effect of noradrenaline was approximately half-maximal at a concentration of 25 nM (cell concentration 5%, v/v) (7). The effects of noradrenaline on the HSL phosphorylation and activity were rapidly reversed by exposure of the noradrenaline-stimulated cells to the β-adrenergic antagonist propranolol (8). The noradrenaline effects on the HSL phosphorylation state and activity could be mimicked by exposing the cells to millimolar concentration of dibutyryl cyclic AMP (13). As stated above data obtained from experiments with proteolytic degradation of ^{32}P-labelled HSL from intact fat cells indicated that noradrenaline induced phosphorylation of HSL at the same site as that phosphorylated on the isolated enzyme by cAMP-PrK.

Taken together the above results provide strong evidence that noradrenaline increases the activity of HSL in intact fat cells through increased phosphorylation of the enzyme with cyclic AMP-stimulated protein kinase.

Insulin Inhibits Hormone Stimulated Lipolysis in Intact Fat Cells through a Decrease of the Phosphorylation State of Hormone-Sensitive Lipase

Exposure of fat cells to insulin had no effect on the basal HSL phosphorylation state (see above). However, exposure of the fat cells to insulin after previous stimulation of the cells with noradrenaline rapidly decreased the HSL phosphorylation state followed by decreased HSL activity (Fig. 4A) (8). Insulin (700 pM) completely prevented the increase of HSL phosphorylation state and activity when added together with, or shortly before, noradrenaline (data not illustrated). Insulin inhibition of the lipolysis rate correlated closely with the effect of the hormone on the HSL phosphorylation state, when related to insulin concentration (Fig. 4B) (8). The half-maximal effect of insulin was found at 25 pM concentration (fat cell concentration 5%, v/v) (Fig. 4B).

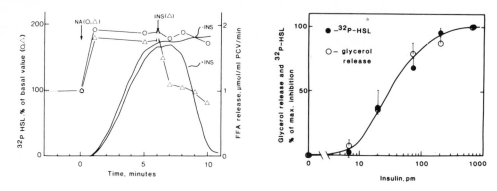

Fig. 4. <u>A</u>. Effect of insulin on HSL phosphorylation and activity in noradre-naline-stimulated adipocytes. Rat fat cells were incubated as in Fig. 3. Noradrenaline, 100 nM, and insulin, 700 pM, were added at the indicated times. Basal phosphorylation set to 100%. All experiments were performed with the same cell batch. <u>B</u>. Insulin inhibition of noradrenaline-stimulated HSL phosphorylation and activity. Rat fat cells were incubated as in Fig. 3 and 200 nM noradrenaline added after 40 min incubation followed 5 min later by varying concentrations of insulin. Glycerol release and HSL phosphoryla-tion was determined at the end of the incubation period. The values are based on duplicate samples obtained in each one of three separate experiments with different cell batches; S.E.M. is indicated by vertical bars. The data are expressed in relation to the maximal effect of insulin (700 pM), which was set to 100%.

Taken together the data above demonstrate that insulin inhibits the HSL activity, *i.e.* the lipolysis rate, in intact fat cells, by decreas-ing the HSL phosphorylation state, or by preventing the increase in the HSL phosphorylation state induced by lipolytic hormones. However, no information was obtained to indicate if this effect was due to a decrease of the phosphorylation rate or an increase of the dephosphorylation rate of HSL, or a combination of both.

Insulin did not affect maximally dibutyryl cyclic AMP-stimulated HSL phosphorylation and activity even when added in µM concentration (8). This might indicate that at least part of the insulin effect was mediat-ed by changes of the intracellular cyclic AMP level. Reduction of the peak cyclic AMP level obtained in noradrenaline-exposed cells was found when the cells had been previously exposed to insulin (Fig. 5) (Nilsson, N.Ö., Fain, J.N. and Belfrage, P., unpublished). However, the reduction of cyclic AMP peak level was only moderate and the effect on HSL phos-phorylation state and activity was much more pronounced than could be expected from this degree of reduction (Fig. 5). Moreover, the cAMP-PrK activity ratio (-cAMP/+cAMP) increased rapidly after noradrenaline, but was only partially reduced after exposure to insulin, while HSL phospho-rylation state was decreased to the basal level and the lipolysis rate was completely inhibited (Björgell, P. and Belfrage, P., unpublished).

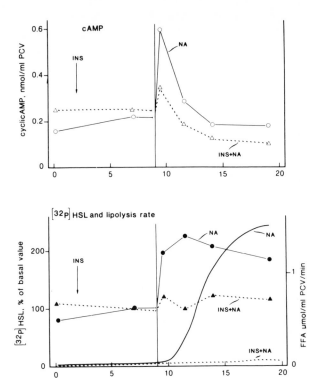

Fig. 5. Effects of insulin on cyclic AMP, HSL phosphorylation and activity in noradrenaline-stimulated
fat cells. Rat adipocytes were incubated as in Fig.
3. After 50 min preincubation noradrenaline (500 nM,
addition indicated by vertical line) was added to
cells, which had been incubated with or without insulin (700 pM), from the indicated time point. Each
value is the mean of duplicates and all experiments
have been performed with the same cell batch.

These data suggest that insulin decreased the extent of HSL phosphorylation state by some other mechanism in addition to its reduction of the
cellular cyclic AMP levels. This mechanism could be insulin-mediated
activation of the protein phosphatase(s) responsible for the dephosphorylation of HSL. This possibility is now under study in our laboratory.

ACKNOWLEDGEMENTS

Mrs Ingrid Nordh, Mrs Birgitta Danielsson and Miss Stina Fors gave
skilful technical assistance. The project was supported by grants from
the following foundations: Påhlssons, Malmö; Segerfalks, Helsingborg;
Nordic Insulin, Copenhagen; the Swedish Diabetes, Stockholm, and from
the Medical Faculty of the University of Lund and the Swedish Medical
Research Council (grant No. 3362).

REFERENCES

1. Belfrage, P., Jergil, B., Strålfors, P.,and Tornqvist, H. (1977): FEBS Lett.,75:259-264.
2. Belfrage, P., Fredrikson, G., Nilsson, N.Ö., and Strålfors, P. (1980): FEBS Lett.,111:120-124.
3. Belfrage, P., Fredrikson, G., Nilsson, N.Ö., and Strålfors, P. (1981): Int. J. Obesity,5:635-641.
4. Brockerhoff, H. and Jensen, R.G. (1974): Lipolytic enzymes. Acad. Press, New York.
5. Cook, K.G., Yeaman, J., Strålfors, P., Fredrikson, G., and Belfrage, P. (1982): Eur. J. Biochem. In press.
6. Fredrikson, G., Strålfors, P., Nilsson, N.Ö., and Belfrage, P. (1981): J. Biol. Chem.,256:6311-6320.
7. Nilsson, N.Ö., Strålfors, P., Fredrikson, G., and Belfrage, P. (1980): FEBS Lett.,111:125-130.
8. Nilsson, N.Ö. (1981): Studies on the short-term regulation of lipo-lysis in rat adipocytes, with special regard to the anti-lipolytic effect of insulin. Thesis. University of Lund, Lund, Sweden. ISBN 91-7222-402-9.
9. Nilsson, N.Ö. and Belfrage, P. (1981): Meth. Enzymol.,72:319-325.
10. Steinberg, D. and Huttunen, J.K. (1972): In: Advances in Cyclic Nucleotide Research,vol. 1, edited by P. Greengard, R. Paoletti and G.A. Robison, pp. 47-62, Raven Press, New York.
11. Steinberg, D. (1972): In: Advances in Cyclic Nucleotide Research, vol. 7, edited by P. Greengard and G.A. Robison, pp. 157-198, Raven Press, New York.
12. Tornqvist, H. and Belfrage, P. (1976): J. Biol. Chem.,251:813-819.

The Adipocyte and Obesity: Cellular and Molecular Mechanisms, edited by A. Angel, C. H. Hollenberg, and D. A. K. Roncari. Raven Press, New York © 1983.

Hormone-Sensitive Lipase System and Insulin Stimulation of Protein Phosphatase Activities in 3T3-L1 Adipocytes

J. C. Khoo, M. Yamamoto, M. Kawamura, and D. Steinberg

Division of Metabolic Disease, Department of Medicine, University of California at San Diego, La Jolla, California 92093

Because of the physiologic importance of fat mobilization, hormonal mechanisms regulating the process have been intensively studied. Figure 1 shows the lipolytic cascade summarized from our work on hormone-sensitive lipase in human, rat and chicken adipose tissue (5,7,8). Of particular value was the finding that the degree of activation demonstrable with the enzyme from chicken adipose tissue was much greater than that obtained with the enzyme from rat adipose tissue. Instead of the 50 to 100% increase seen with the rat enzyme, the chicken enzyme shows as much as a 50-fold activation by cAMP-dependent protein kinase. This huge activation allowed us to study the reversible deactivation by protein (lipase) phosphatase.

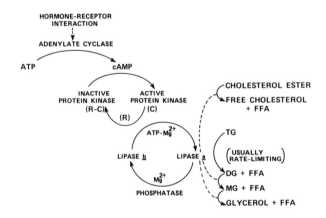

FIGURE 1. SCHEMATIC OUTLINE OF THE KEY STEPS REGULATING THE INTERCONVERSION OF HORMONE-SENSITIVE LIPASE a AND b. TG (triglyceride), DG (diglyceride), MG (monoglyceride), and FFA (free fatty acid).

Adipocytes isolated according to the method of Rodbell (15) from adipose tissue are fragile and difficult to use in experiments lasting for more than a few hours. For studies of longer term regulation it is necessary to have a stable cell system. We have found that 3T3-L1 cells express a hormone-sensitive lipase system similar in most respects to that of adipocytes and may be a useful cell line to which to study long-term regulation.

RESULTS AND DISCUSSION

Cell culture and glycerol release

Murine 3T3-L1 fibroblasts in monolayers (a gift of Dr. Howard Green) were grown in Dulbecco's modified Eagle's (DME) media containing 10% fetal calf serum. Cells reached confluency in 4 days (6). To initiate adipose conversion, the cells were treated with 0.25 μM dexamethasone (DEX) plus 0.5 mM 1-methyl-3-isobutylxanthine (MIX) for 2 days, as described by Rubin et al (16). After withdrawal of DEX and MIX, the cells were allowed to differentiate for an additional 4 to 6 days, during which time they accumulated multilocular fat droplets. To determine the rate of glycerol release, the culture media were replaced by Kreb's-Ringer bicarbonate buffer containing 2% bovine serum albumin and 10 mM glucose. As shown in Figure 1, the rate of glycerol release in control dishes was linear with time up to 2 hr; in the presence of 1×10^{-6} isoproterenol, the rate of glycerol release was stimulated six-fold. The data suggested the coordinated expression of a β-receptor-adenyl cyclase system and, possibly, the acquisition of a hormone-sensitive lipase.

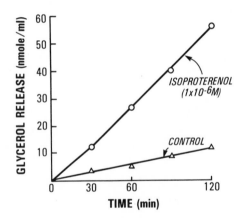

FIGURE 2. STIMULATION OF GLYCEROL RELEASE. Differentiated 3T3-L1 adipocytes in the absence and in the presence of isoproterenol.

Development of hormone-sensitive lipase system during adipose conversion.

Because differentiation is known to induce high levels of lipoprotein lipase (18) that might interfere with assays of neutral acyl-hydrolases, heparin (2U/ml) was added to the culture media for 1 hr at 37°C prior to harvesting to deplete the cells of lipoprotein lipase. The cells in monolayers were washed, harvested and homogenized in a buffer. The homogenates were centrifuged at 40,000 x g for 1 hr. The supernatant fraction was designated S_{40} and the pellet designated P_{40}.

The S_{40} fractions were assayed for tri-, di-, monoglyceride and cholesterol esterase activities at pH 7. As shown in Figure 3, the

activities prior to differentiation were very low. The activities increased markedly from day 2 to day 6 during differentiation. At day 6,
the tri-, diglyceride and cholesterol esterase increased 20- to 30-fold,
while the monoglyceride lipase increased somewhat less, but very significantly. In contrast, the activities in 3T3-C2 fibroblasts, a cell
line with a very low frequency of conversion to adipocyte-like form did
not increase when the cells were subjected to same treatment as 3T3-L1
cells.

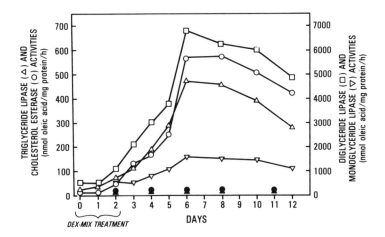

FIGURE 3. DEVELOPMENT OF TRIGLYCERIDE LIPASE ($\triangle$), DIGLYCERIDE LIPASE
($\square$), MONOGLYCERIDE LIPASE ($\triangledown$) AND CHOLESTEROL ESTERASE ($\bigcirc$) ACTIVITIES
IN THE S_{40} FRACTION OF DIFFERENTIATING 3T3-L1 CELLS AND OF TRIGLYCERIDE
LIPASE ($\blacktriangle$) AND CHOLESTEROL ESTERASE ($\bullet$) IN 3T3-C2 CELLS (from refer-
ence 6).

The pH activity profiles of triglyceride lipase before and after
differentiation at day 6 are shown in Figure 4. Prior to differentiation, the triglyceride lipase activity in the S_{40} fraction was extremely
low at all pH values. After differentiation, there was a huge increase
in triglyceride lipase activity with optimal activity at pH 7.4. The
P_{40} fractions were subjected to freezing and thawing 10 times to rupture
the lysosomes. In contrast to the striking increase in neutral triglyceride lipase, there was no significant change in the lysosomal lipase
activity which had optimal activity at pH 5.

Activation of neutral triglyceride lipase and neutral cholesterol esterase activity

Although hormonal stimulation of lipolysis has been shown in
adrenal, heart, muscle, and small intestines (1,3,4,17), it has not
been possible to demonstrate a protein kinase-activated triglyceride
lipase from any of these tissues, with the exception of the adrenal (14).
We examined the effect of protein kinase on the neutral triglyceride
lipase in the S_{40} fraction prepared from differentiated 3T3-L1 cells.
As shown in Figure 5, incubation of the S_{40} fraction with cAMP, ATP and
Mg^{2+} increased the triglyceride lipase by about 2-fold. The addition of
a specific inhibitor of cAMP-dependent protein kinase at progressively

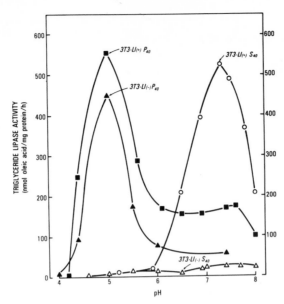

FIGURE 4. pH-ACTIVITY PROFILES FOR TRIGLYCERIDE LIPASE OF THE S40 AND P40 FRACTIONS OF 3T3-L1 CELLS. △,○, S40 before and after differentiation; ▲,■, P40 before and after differentiation (4 days after exposure to DEX/MIX. Between pH 4 and pH 6, assays were carried out with substrate mixtures containing 50 mM acetate buffer, between pH 6.5 and 8, assays were carried out with substrate mixtures containing 50 mM phosphate buffer (from reference 6).

increasing concentrations blocked activation which then could be restored by adding back increasing concentrations of purified cAMP-dependent protein kinase, thus demonstrating the dependency of the reaction on protein kinase. The neutral triglyceride lipase activity in the S40 fraction prepared from undifferentiated 3T3-L1 and 3T3-C2 fibroblasts was not activated by protein kinase, suggesting the acquisition of the protein kinase activatable neutral triglyceride lipase on adipose conversion. Protein kinase also had no effect on the acid triglyceride lipase (data not shown).

To further characterize the enzyme, we applied the methods used to purify the enzyme from chicken adipose tissue to the S40 fraction of differentiated 3T3-L1 cells. As shown in Figure 6 (panel A), after isoelectrofocusing in 1% agarose tube gel, the enzyme has a major component with a pI of 6.7 and a minor component with pI of 6.1. When the same enzyme fraction was first phosphorylated with protein kinase system in the presence of (γ-^{32}P)ATP and then subjected to isoelectrofocusing, the pI of the major peak shifted from 6.7 to 6.1 (Figure 6, panel B). The enzyme activity in the first dimensional isoelectrofocusing gel was found to be associated with ^{32}P-labeled protein of $Mr = 84,000$.

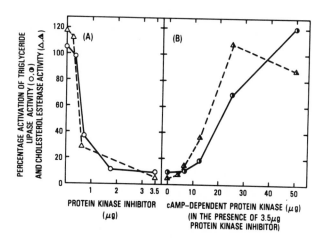

FIGURE 5. EFFECTS OF PROTEIN KINASE INHIBITOR AND PROTEIN KINASE ON TRIGLYCERIDE LIPASE AND CHOLESTEROL ESTERASE ACTVITIES. Aliquots of S_{40} fraction prepared from differentiated 3T3-L1 cells were incubated with MgATP and cAMP or with Mg^{2+} only in 25 mM Tris-HCl (pH 8) for 5 min at 30°C. Triglyceride lipase activity was assayed with a substrate mixture containing 50 mM Tris-HCl at pH 7.4. Cholesterol esterase activity was assayed with a substrate mixture containing 50 mM Tris-HCl at pH 8. (A) Percentage activation of triglyceride lipase activity (O) and cholesterol esterase activity (△) with increasing concentrations of protein kinase inhibitor. (B) Percentage activation of triglyceride lipase activity (●) and cholesterol esterase activity (▲) with increasing concentrations of purified protein kinase in the presence of a constant amount of protein kinase inhibitor (3.5 ug) (from reference 6).

Neutral cholesterol esterase of differentiated 3T3-L1 cells and adipose tissue

As mentioned earlier, neutral cholesterol esterase activity increased markedly during differentiation. The level of activity was about 5 times higher than that of mouse adipose tissue. It was activated 2.2-fold by protein kinase (Figure 5). The neutral cholesterol esterase activity in the S_{40} fraction of undifferentiated 3T3-L1 cells and 3T3-C2 cells was not activated by protein kinase, again implying the synthesis of this unique enzyme during adipose conversion. We have demonstrated that the protein kinase-activated cholesterol esterase of adipose tissue (9) was able to hydrolyze the cholesterol esters in intact plasma lipoproteins (11). The role of this neutral cholesterol esterase has not been established but two possibilities have been suggested. First, it may play a role in the mobilization of stored cholesterol esters. The second possibility is that this enzyme might play a role in the hydrolysis of cholesterol esters of lipoproteins as they are taken into the cell. Studies in cultured rat hepatocytes have revealed a low-affinity pathway (2) that may deliver lipoproteins into the cytoplasmic compartment.

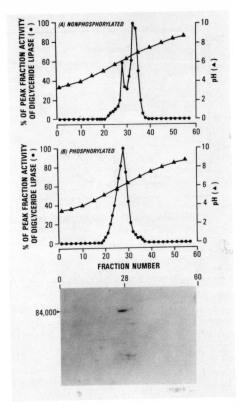

FIGURE 6. ISOELECTROFOCUSING AND TWO-DIMENSIONAL GEL ELECTROPHORESIS OF
A PARTIALLY PURIFIED ENZYME PREPARATION. The S40 fraction was treated
with Triton X-100 (0.6 mM) and NaCl (50 mM) for 12 hr. The solubilized
enzyme preparation was chromatographed on a hydroxyapatite column. The
peak fraction was subjected to isoelectrofocusing in 1% agarose tube gel
(A). The activity profile of a protein kinase phosphorylated enzyme
fraction (B). Autoradiography to demonstrate ^{32}P-labeled band in the
second-dimensional SDS-polyacrylamide gel (C). (from reference 12).

Mechanism of action of insulin

        A number of hypotheses have been presented with regard to the
mechanism by which insulin regulates the enzymes of glycogen and lipid
metabolism. The proposal that it acts through regulation of cAMP levels
is supported by some studies, but this does not adequately explain all
of the observations. The studies of Larner and co-workers were the
first to demonstrate insulin regulation of skeletal muscle glycogen
synthase in the absence of measurable change in cAMP (13). This, of
course, suggested the possibility that control might be exercised on
the activating enzyme, glycogen synthase phosphatase. We have considered the lipase phosphatase a good possibility based on our work with
chicken adipose tissue. As shown in Figure 7, the activated lipase
showed a progressive fall in activity during incubation with a highly
purified protein phosphatase. At 20 min, an aliquot was removed and
again incubated (10 min) with protein kinase. This restored lipase
activity to that of the fully activated preparation. Unfortunately,

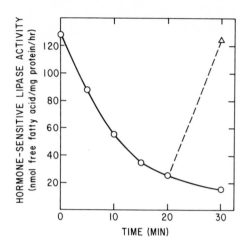

FIGURE 7. REVERSIBLE DEACTIVATION OF HORMONE-SENSITIVE LIPASE. Chicken adipose tissue 5.2 P was fully activated with cGMP-dependent protein kinase. The activated enzyme preparation was immediately passed through a Sephadex G-50 column to remove ATP, cGMP, and Mg^{2+}. The enzyme eluted in the void volume was supplemented with 5 mM Mg^{2+} and purified bovine heart protein phosphatase, and incubation was carried out at 30°C (O). Reactivation of the deactivated lipase was effected at 20 min by ATP, 10 μM cGMP, and cGMP-dependent protein kinase and incubating for 10 min at 30°C(10).

chicken adipose tissue shows very little response to insulin. Because of the small degree of activation of hormone-sensitive lipase in 3T3-L1 cells (about 2-fold) we have difficulty in demonstrating the process of reversible deactivation. Thus, it is still not possible to study the effects of insulin on lipase phosphatase activity directly.

However, our preliminary data show that in differentiated 3T3-L1 cells, insulin stimulates some protein phosphatase activities. Fully differentiated 3T3-L1 cells were incubated in DME media without glucose and fetal celf serum for 12 hr prior to study. At that time insulin (50,100 or 200 uU/ml) and 5 mM glucose were added to the media in 10 dishes of cells for each insulin concentration. Glucose only (5 mM) was added to another 10 dishes. Incubation was carried out for 15 min at 37°C at which time the cells were harvested for assay of phosphatase activities. As shown in Table 1, a small but statistically significant effect was obtained at all concentrations. A maximum effect was seen at 100 uU/ml for glycogen synthase phosphatase activity (82.4% stimulation). The degree of stimulation of histone phosphatase activity was less (maximum stimulation 25%, but the difference was statistically highly significant ($p<0.001$).

To test whether the differences observed might reflect the presence of glucose-6-phosphate (or other allosteric activators) or some other change in the composition of the homogenate, the 1,000 x g supernatant fractions were subjected to chromatography on Sephadex G-25 and the void volume fractions were taken for enzyme assays. The stimulating

TABLE 1. Effects of insulin on glycogen synthase phosphatase and histone phosphatase activities in 3T3-L1 adipocyte-like cells.*

Insulin (uU/ml)	Glycogen synthase phosphatase activity	Histone phosphatase activity
	Δ units synthase **I**/mg protein/hr	pmol/mg protein/ min
0	2.78±0.17	18.26±0.54
50	3.23±0.12[a] (16.2%)[e]	19.75±0.66 (8.2%)
100	5.07±0.15[b] (82.4%)	22.82±1.01[d] (25.0%)
200	4.21±0.08[c] (51.4%)	21.42±0.85 (17.3%)

*Values reported are mean ± SEM
[a,b,c,d]Statistically significant from control values (p<0.001)
   [e]Percentage increased above control value.

effects of insulin on glycogen synthase and histone phosphatase activities were still readily demonstrated. The results suggest but do not
prove that the effect of insulin was due to some relatively stable
modification of the protein phosphatase(s) or some factor binding
tightly to the enzyme(s). Insulin had no such effect on 3T3-L1 cells
prior to their differentiation nor on a related cell line (3T3-C2)
that does not share the property of differentiating into adipocyte-like
cells. The results are compatible with the possibility that some of the
regulatory effects of insulin in adipose tissue occur via regulation of
protein phosphatase.

SUMMARY

(1) During differentiation to adipocyte-like form, 3T3-L1 cells develop
a hormone-sensitive lipase system similar in all respects to the components of hormone-sensitive lipase in adipose tissue.
(2) Hormone-sensitive lipase in 3T3-L1 cells was identified as a [32]P-
labeled protein with a minimum molecular weight of approx. 84,000 (similar to that of rat adipose tissue).
(3) Preliminary data show that insulin stimulates protein phosphatase
activities in 3T3-L1 cells.
(4) This stable cultured cell line of adipocyte may be useful in
further elucidating regulatory mechanism, particularly those that
require longer incubation time.

REFERENCES

1. Abumrad, N.A., Tepperman, H.M., and Tepperman, J.(1980): J. Lipid
    Res., 21:156-161.
2. Attie, A.D., Pittman, R.C., and Steinberg, D.(1980): Proc. Natl.
    Acad. Sci., 77:5923-5927.
3. Grass, M.F., III(1977): Fed. Proc., 36:1995-1999.
4. Hulsman, W.C., Stam, H., and Geelhold-Mieras, M.M.(1979): In:
    Obesity-Cellular and Molecular Aspects, edited by G. Ailhaud,
    pp. 179-191. Insern, Paris.

5. Huttunen, J.K., and Steinberg, D.(1971): Biochim. Biophys. Acta, 239:411-427.
6. Kawamura, M., Jensen, D.F., Wancewicz, E.V., Joy, L.L., Khoo, J.C. and Steinberg, D.(1981): Proc. Natl. Acad. Sci., 78:732-736.
7. Khoo, J.C., and Steinberg, D.(1974): J. Lipid Res., 15:602-610.
8. Khoo, J.C., Aquino, A.A., and Steinberg, D.(1974): J. Clin. Invest., 53:1124-1131.
9. Khoo, J.C., Steinberg, D., Huang, J.J., and Vagelos, P.R.(1976): J. Biol. Chem., 251:2880-2890.
10. Khoo, J.C., Sperry, P.J., Gill, G.N., and Steinberg, D.(1977): Proc. Natl. Acad. Sci., 74:4843-4847.
11. Khoo, J.C., Drevon, C.A., and Steinberg, D.(1979): J. Biol. Chem., 254:1785-1787.
12. Khoo, J.C., Kawamura, M., Jensen, D.F., Wancewicz, E.V., Joy, L.L., and Steinberg, D.(1981): In: Cold Spring Harbor Conference on Cell Proliferation Vol. 8: Protein Phosphorylation, edited by E.G. Krebs and Rosen, O.M., pp. 675-685. Cold Spring Harbor Laboratory, New York.
13. Larner, J., and Villar-Palasi, C.(1971): In Curr. Top. Cell. Regul., 3:195-236.
14. Pittman, R.C., and Steinberg, D.(1977): Biochim. Biophys. Acta, 487:431-444.
15. Rodbell, M.(1964): J. Biol. Chem., 239:375-380.
16. Rubin, C.S., Hirsch, A., Fung, C., and Rosen, O.M.(1978): J. Biol. Chem., 253:7570-7578.
17. Rudman, D., and Garcia, L.A.(1960): Endocrinology, 78:1087-1088.
18. Spooner, P.M., Chernick, S.S., Garrison, M.M., and Scow, R.O.(1979): J. Biol. Chem., 254:1305-1311.

ACKNOWLEDGMENT

We are indebted to Mr. Edward Wancewicz, Mr. Dennis Jensen, and Ms Lorna Joy for excellent technical assistance. This work was supported by National Institutes of Health Research Grant HL 22053, and a grant from the Kroc Foundation.

The Adipocyte and Obesity: Cellular and
Molecular Mechanisms, edited by A. Angel,
C. H. Hollenberg, and D. A. K. Roncari.
Raven Press, New York © 1983.

Pharmacological Characterization and Regulation of Adrenergic Receptors in Human Adipocytes

Thomas W. Burns, Paul E. Langley, Boyd E. Terry, and
David B. Bylund

*Departments of Medicine, Surgery and Pharmacology,
University of Missouri School of Medicine, Columbia, Missouri 65212*

Fifteen years ago, Robison et al. (23) postulated that metabolically active cells may contain dual adrenergic receptors mediating divergent effects on cyclic AMP and hormone expression. Subsequently, we and others produced evidence indicating that the human fat cell is endowed with both beta and alpha adrenergic receptors (6,21). Activation of beta sites increases adenylate cyclase activity, the concentration of cyclic AMP and the rate of lipolysis while stimulation of alpha receptors has opposite effects. When human adipocytes are exposed to epinephrine, an agonist at both alpha and beta receptors, the beta activity predominates and lipolysis is increased. To determine if both alpha and beta sites are operative *in vivo*, volunteers were infused with epinephrine alone, and with epinephrine in combination with phentolamine or propranolol (8). The changes noted in the plasma concentration of free fatty acids were consistent with the earlier *in vitro* results. Infusion of epinephrine alone prompts a modest rise in plasma FFA and glycerol. When phentolamine is added to the infusion, FFA and glycerol increase substantially while the addition of propranolol is associated with a decline in FFA and glycerol concentrations to levels below preinfusion baselines.

Beta receptors have been divided into beta-1 and beta-2 subgroups (17) as have the alpha receptors (18). Both beta-1 and beta-2 receptors appear to activate the adenylate cyclase system. The effects of alpha-2 stimulation are generally believed to be mediated by adenylate cyclase while the action of alpha-1 receptors is associated with an increase in phosphatidylinositol turnover and calcium mobilization (10). To further characterize the adrenergic receptors of human adipocytes, studies were conducted using appropriate radioligands and selective agonists and antagonists.

PHARMACOLOGICAL CHARACTERIZATION OF THE ADRENERGIC RECEPTORS OF HUMAN ADIPOCYTES

Radioligand Binding Studies. Three distinct adrenergic receptor binding sites were identified by radioligand binding studies (7): beta ([^{3}H]dihydroalprenolol, DHA); alpha-1 ([^{3}H]WB 4101); and alpha-2 ([^{3}H]p-aminoclonidine, PAC and [^{3}H]yohimbine). Saturation experiments, conducted using conventional methods and membranes prepared from properitoneal adipose tissue, indicated that each ligand binds to a single class of high affinity sites. The K_D (affinity) and B_{max} (receptor density) values are given in Table 1. The densities of the three receptors differ only about two-fold. The difference in the B_{max} values for [^{3}H]PAC and [^{3}H]yohimbine may result from the agonist (PAC) labeling only part of the receptors (those in the high affinity state) while the antagonist (yohimbine) labels the total receptor population (19).

TABLE 1. Adrenergic Receptor Binding in

Human Adipocyte Membranes[a]

Adrenergic Receptor	Radioligand	n	B_{max} (pmol/g prot)	K_D (nM)
Beta	[^{3}H]Dihydroalprenolol	13	296 ± 25	0.56 ± 0.07
Alpha-1	[^{3}H]WB4101	7	298 ± 34	0.91 ± 0.06
Alpha-2	[^{3}H]p-Aminoclonidine	13	197 ± 33	0.90 ± 0.13
Alpha-2	[^{3}H]Yohimbine	9	585 ± 62	0.41 ± 0.01

[a]Membranes were prepared from isolated adipocytes. B_{max} (density of receptor binding sites) and K_D (equilibrium dissociation constant) were derived from saturation experiments.

Pharmacological Characterization of Beta and Alpha-2 Receptors. Beta and alpha-2 receptors were further characterized by examining the effects of adrenergic drugs on adenylate cyclase activity, cyclic AMP content and glycerol release (an index of lipolysis) (7). Isoproterenol (beta agonist) is very potent in stimulating lipolysis, while epinephrine (alpha and beta agonist) is less active, and methoxamine (alpha-1 agonist) has no effect. By contrast, clonidine (alpha-2 agonist) depresses lipolysis. When cells are incubated in the presence of epinephrine and with increasing concentrations of the antagonists, both yohimbine (alpha-2) and phentolamine (alpha-1 and alpha-2) substantially increase the effect of epinephrine on lipolysis while prazosin (alpha-1) has no effect.

These adrenergic drugs have similar effects on cellular cyclic AMP concentration. Isoproterenol markedly increases the cylic AMP concentration, while methoxamine is without effect and clonidine depresses the nucleotide content below the basal levels. When cells are incubated in the presence of epinephrine, both yohimbine and phentolamine markedly enhance the stimulatory effect of epinephrine on cyclic AMP, while prazosin is without effect. We also studied the effects of these drugs on the enzyme, adenylate cyclase, using adipocyte ghosts. Both yohimbine and phentolamine enhance the effect of epinephrine on adenylate cyclase, while prazosin has no effect. Clonidine reduced adenylate cyclase activity below basal, while methoxamine did not affect the enzyme.

Characterization of Alpha-1 Receptors. To evaluate human adipocytes for the presence of alpha-1 adrenergic receptors, the effects of epinephrine alone and in combination with antagonists were studied (7). The phospholipid composition and the incorporation of radioactive phosphate into the major phospholipids in human cells are similar to those observed in rat and hamster fat cells (7,11,12). Epinephrine produces a dose-dependent increase in the incorporation of labeled phosphate into phosphatidylinositol and phosphatidic acid. Isoproterenol is without effect on the labelling of phosphatidylinositol and phosphatidic acid, indicating that this action of epinephrine must be mediated by alpha receptors. Selective antagonists block the stimulation by epinephrine of ^{32}P incorporation into the phosphatidylinositol and phosphatidic acid. The potency order is prazosin > phentolamine > yohimbine. Prazosin is about 1000-fold more potent than yohimbine indicating that this action of epinephrine is mediated by alpha-1 receptors. None of the antagonists, when studied alone, affected the labeling of the phospholipids.

The major conclusion of the foregoing studies is that the human adipocyte has three distinct types of adrenergic receptors, each coupled to its own biochemical response: beta, activation of adenylate cyclase, alpha-2, inhibition of adenylate cyclase and alpha-1, stimulation of phosphatidylinositol turnover.

DESENSITIZATION OF THE ADRENERGIC RECEPTORS OF HUMAN ADIPOCYTES

Desensitization (i.e., a substantial reduction in cellular response to a second exposure to a hormone or agonist) of adrenergic receptors has been studied extensively. Desensitization of beta receptors has been assessed in a number of tissues including frog erythrocytes (11) and alpha desensitization has been studied with rat parotid aciner cells (15). We sought to determine if the beta and alpha-2 receptors of human adipocytes undergo desensitization and, if so, whether associated changes in radioligand binding occur.

Beta Receptor Desensitization. To evaluate the possibility of desensitization of beta receptors, cells were preincubated for three hours with or without 10 µM isoproterenol, washed for one-half hour and then assayed for isoproterenol-stimulated adenylate cyclase activity (Fig. 1). In these studies, cyclic AMP concentration was used as the end-point rather than glycerol release since we have established that only modest increases in cyclic AMP (e.g. 5-fold) result in maximal increases in glycerol release. Cyclic AMP concentration, on the other hand, can increase markedly (50-fold or more) with increasing stimulation. Cells preincubated in the absence of isoproterenol are just as responsive as cells which were not preincubated. However, preincubation in the presence of isoproterenol reduces the response to a second exposure of catecholamine by 60%. We interpret this reduction to represent desensitization of the beta receptors.

Alpha-2 Receptor Desensitization. To evaluate alpha receptor desensitization the same experimental design described for beta receptors was used with the exceptions that epinephrine was used rather than isoproterenol and all incubations contained 30 µM propranolol (to block beta receptors) and 1 mM theophylline during both preincubation and incubation. The results obtained are shown in Fig. 2. The basal level of cyclic AMP is reduced by alpha-2 stimulation. The difference in the magnitude of cyclic AMP concentration between these two groups reflects the unopposed alpha-2 activity of epinephrine. Preincubation of cells for 3 hours with epinephrine does not diminish their response to subsequent exposure of epinephrine. Thus, desensitization of alpha-2 receptors was not demonstrated under these experimental conditions.

Requirement for Beta Desensitization. The next experiments were done to test the hypothesis that desensitization requires, or is associated with, a large production of cyclic AMP rather than beta receptor occupancy

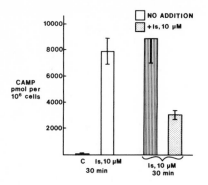

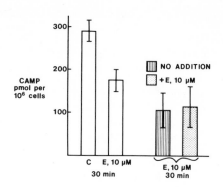

Fig. 1. The effect of preincubation with isoproterenol on the
subsequent   beta   adrenergic
response. Flasks represented by
the first two bars were not preincubated. Bars 3 and 4 represent
3 hr preincubations without and
with 10 µM isoproternol, respectively. Preincubation with isoproterenol was associated with a
diminished response to subsequent
exposure to the catecholamine. The
heights of the bars denote the mean
values of 3 experiments.

Fig. 2. The effect of preincubation with epinephrine on the alpha
adrenergic response. The conditions were the same as in Figure 1
except that epinephrine was used as
the   agonist   and   all   flasks
contained 30 µM propranolol and 1
mM theophylline. Preincubation
with epinephrine for 3 hours did
not   diminish   the   effect   of
epinephrine noted in the subsequent incubation. The heights of
the bars denote the mean values of
3 experiments.

with little or no increase in cyclic AMP formation. Cells were incubated
for three hours with either no addition, with epinephrine, or with
isoproterenol. Following preincubation, all cells were washed and then
assayed for isoproterenol activity. We have shown that epinephrine alone
causes a modest increase in cyclic AMP, usually less than two-fold, while
exposure to isoproterenol results in a marked increase in cyclic AMP. In
the present experiments the level of cyclic AMP during the preincubation
in the cells preincubated with isoproterenol was presumably about 50 times
higher than in cells preincubated with epinephrine. However, both sets of
cells responded similarly to the subsequent exposure to isoproterenol.
This finding suggests that desensitization is not dependent on the
production of large quantities of cyclic AMP.

Radioligand Binding Studies. In other systems, desensitization of the
beta adrenergic receptor-adenylate cyclase complex is accompanied by the
loss of receptor sites as determined by the ^{3}H-antagonist binding. To
determine if this down regulation occurs with human adipocytes, cells were
preincubated for three hours with and without 10 µM isoproterenol, just as
in the experiments described above for the evaluation of beta
desensitization by measuring cyclic AMP levels. Membranes were then
prepared from the washed cells and saturation analysis performed using
[3]H]DHA. There was a significant 20-25% decrease in the B_{max} of ^{3}H]DHA
binding in the cells which had been preincubated with isoproterenol, as

compared to the control cells. The affinity (K_D) of the radioligand for the receptor was not altered by incubation with the beta agonist. These results indicate that conditions which result in a decreased responsiveness of beta adrenergic-stimulated cyclic AMP levels also result in a down regulation or loss of beta adrenergic receptor binding sites.

In similar experiments membranes were prepared and alpha-2 adrenergic receptors assayed following a three-hour preincubation of cells with and without 10 μM epinephrine. Incubation with epinephrine does not alter the binding of [^{3}H]yohimbine but does result in a 43% decrease in the B_{max} for [^{3}H]PAC binding. These data suggest that there may be an excess number ("spare receptors") of alpha-2 receptors, and the loss of 40% of them is not sufficient to decrease the extent of inhibition of adenylate cyclase. Furthermore, if the adipocyte is similar to other cells in that [^{3}H]PAC only labels those receptors in the high affinity agonist conformation, then the preincubation with epinephrine may simply decrease the percent of the receptors in high affinity state thus decreasing [^{3}H]PAC binding without altering the total number of receptors ([^{3}H]yohimbine binding). In any case, a preincubation time of greater than three hours may be necessary in order to observe desensitization and down regulation.

THE EFFECT OF FORSKOLIN ON HUMAN ADIPOCYTES

The diterpine, forskolin, has been shown to activate adenylate cyclase in membrane preparations and to increase cyclic AMP in intact cells from a variety of tissues (26). In rat adipocytes, forskolin increases cyclic AMP and lipolysis and markedly potentiates the cyclic AMP response to isoproterenol. The manner in which forskolin activates cyclase is unclear. Of considerable interest is the observation that forskolin is active with the cyclase in the cyc mutant of the S49 mouse lymphoma cell line which appears to lack the guanine nucleotide regulatory protein (25). We evaluated the activity of forskolin with human adipocytes.

<u>Effects of Forskolin on Cyclic AMP Concentration</u>. Incubation of isolated human adipocytes with 10 μM forskolin for 30 minutes causes a 100-fold increase in the level of cyclic AMP (Fig. 3). The beta adrenergic antagonist, propranolol, 30 μM, has no effect on either the basal or on the forskolin-stimulated cyclic AMP concentration. Isoproterenol also causes a 100-fold increase in the cyclic AMP level, but consistent with previous studies this increase is completely blocked by the addition of propranolol. When adipocytes are incubated with both isoproterenol and forskolin the effect is more than additive resulting in a 300-fold increase in cyclic AMP concentration. The addition of propranolol to this combination reduces the nucleotide accumulation to that seen with forskolin alone. Epinephrine increases cyclic AMP levels by 4.5-fold while epinephrine plus propranolol decreases the cyclic AMP levels due to the unopposed inhibitory effect of epinephrine mediated by alpha-2 adrenergic receptors. The combination of epinephrine and forskolin, similar to the combination of isoproterenol and forskolin, gives a much greater than additive effect, increasing cyclic AMP levels nearly 250-fold over basal. The effect of alpha-2 adrenergic activation on forskolin-stimulated cyclic AMP accumulation was studied using epinephrine and propranolol with forskolin. The accumulation of cyclic AMP observed with this combination of agents is only 10% of that seen with forskolin alone. Furthermore, the alpha-2 antagonist yohimbine completely reversed the epinephrine inhibition (Fig. 4). The quantities

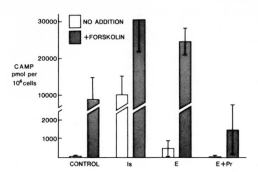

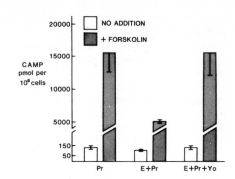

Fig. 3. The effect of forskolin on the cyclic AMP content of human fat cells. Forskolin (10 µM) was included for 30 minutes with adipocytes alone and with 10 µM isoproterenol, 10 µM epinephrine and with the combination of 10 µM epinephrine plus 30 µM propranolol. Due to the large range of cyclic AMP concentrations, the scale on the ordinate is discontinuous. The heights of the bars denote the mean values of 3 experiments.

Fig. 4. Reversal of alpha-2 adrenergic inhibition of cyclic AMP by yohimbine. The combination of epinephrine plus propranolol substantially reduced forskolin-stimulated cyclic AMP levels (bar 4) as compared to propranolol alone (bar 2). Yohimbine completely reversed this alpha adrenergic inhibition (bar 6). The concentrations of drugs were the same as in Figure 3. The heights of the bars denote the mean values of 3 experiments.

of glycerol released when human adipocytes were incubated with forskolin alone, or in combination with propranolol, epinephrine and isoproterenol, are those expected from the changes observed in cyclic AMP levels just described.

The effect of alpha-2 adrenergic receptor activation on forskolin stimulated adipocytes was investigated further in a series of dose response studies. Cells were incubated with varying concentrations of forskolin either alone or with 10 µM epinephrine and 30 µM propranolol. Each 10-fold increase in concentration of forskolin is associated with an increase in cyclic AMP content. Alpha-2 adrenergic activation, achieved by epinephrine plus propranolol, substantially reduces the response to forskolin at each concentration point, shifting the dose-response curve to the right approximately 8-fold (Fig. 5). The changes in glycerol release are those one would expect from the cylic AMP values.

<u>Effects of Forskolin on Adenylate Cyclase Activity.</u> We also studied the effects of forskolin on adenylate cyclase by measuring the enzyme activity in membrane preparations (Fig. 6). Forskolin at 0.1 mM causes a 4- to 5-fold activation of adenylate cyclase over basal activity, while propranolol has no effect on either basal or forskolin-stimulated enzyme activity. Isoproterenol at 100 µM causes a 3-fold increase in enzyme activity. This is completely blocked by the addition of propranolol. The combination of isoproterenol and forskolin activates the enzyme nearly 10-fold over basal, which is a greater effect than one would have expected

if the effects of isoproterenol and forskolin are simply additive. The combination of isoproterenol, propranolol and forskolin give the same value of adenylate cyclase activity as is obtained with forskolin alone. Epinephrine at 0.1 mM increases adenylate cyclase activity 3-fold and again the effect of epinephrine plus forskolin is more than additive. Epinephrine plus propranolol inhibits both the basal and the forskolin stimulated adenylate cyclase activity. Sodium fluoride, 10 mM, increased adenylate cyclase activity about 8-fold. The combination of forskolin and sodium fluoride results in a level of enzyme activity which is approximately additive. These results show that forskolin readily activates adenylate cyclase and acts synergistically with a beta adrenergic agonist. Furthermore, alpha-2 receptor activation inhibits forskolin-stimulated cyclase activity.

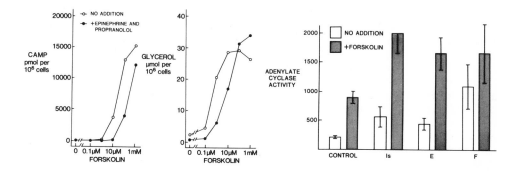

Fig. 5. Forskolin dose-response curves. Forskolin-stimulated increases in cyclic AMP (left panel) and glycerol release (right panel) in a dose dependent fashion. Alpha adrenergic stimulation, achieved with 10 μM epinephrine and 30 μM propranolol shifted the dose-response curves about 8-fold to the right. The data shown are from a representative experiment.

Fig. 6. The effect of forskolin on adenylate cyclase activity. Forskolin (10 μM) stimulated basal adenylate cyclase activity 5-fold and enhanced the effect of 10 μM isoproterenol (bar 4), 10 μM epinephrine (bar 6) and 10 mM fluoride (bar 8). The units of adenylate cyclase activity are pmol of cyclic AMP per min per mg protein. The heights of the bars denote the mean values of 3 experiments.

THE EFFECT OF FASTING ON THE ADRENERGIC RECEPTORS OF HUMAN ADIPOCYTES

Modulation of Epinephrine Effect by Fasting. The discovery that human adipocytes are endowed with both alpha and beta adrenergic receptors that mediate opposite effects on lipolysis raises the question of the physiological significance and regulation of this dual system. As mentioned above, early in vitro and in vivo studies indicated that beta effects predominate. Thus, exposure to the mixed agonist, epinephrine, leads to an increase in lipolysis. In 1971, Kjellborg and Ostman (16) reported on the effects of fasting on the adrenergic activity of adipose tissue.   Tissue obtained from normal subjects before fasting responded positively to epinephrine, while samples taken during fast reacted negatively, i.e., the catecholamine caused a reduction in cyclic AMP and lipolysis. We have done experiments to determine if a similar reversal could be demonstrated with isolated fat cells (5). Tissue was obtained before and following three to eight days of fasting. Consistent with past observations epinephrine prompted an increase in both cyclic AMP and lipolysis when incubated with cells from fed subjects. In contrast, the catecholamine was associated with a decrease in the nucleotide and in lipolysis when incubated with adipocytes from fasted individuals.

To determine whether this altered pattern of response was due to a heightened alpha activity or to a diminished beta effect, studies were done with the beta blocker, propranolol, and the alpha agonist, phentolamine. When propranolol was included in the incubation flasks, thus blocking beta sites and leaving alpha receptors to act unopposed, there was little or no difference in the level of cyclic AMP and lipolysis between cells from fed and fasted subjects. Thus, there did not appear to be an enhanced alpha effect during fasting. On the other hand, fasting greatly dimished the level of cyclic AMP and lipolysis caused by the combination of phentolamine and epinephrine. The magnitude of the beta effect can be estimated by subtracting basal cyclic AMP and lipolysis values from those obtained in the presence of phentolamine and epinephrine. When this was done, the beta effect noted in terms of cyclic AMP and lipolysis with cells from fasted subjects was considerably less than the values found with adipocytes from fed subjects. Our findings are at variance with those of Ostman's group (2,16). They found enhanced alpha effect and no change in beta activity using tissue fragments (rather than isolated cells) obtained from subjects fasted for one week. Subsequently, they presented data suggesting that during fasting there is a correlation between fat cell size and receptor responsiveness and that catecholamines may be involved in regulating cell volume (1).

Recently Berlan et al. (4) assessed the influence of hypocaloric diets on the alpha adrenergic responsiveness of subcutaneous adipocyte sites from obese subjects. Cells were prepared from abdominal wall subcutaneous tissue obtained from two groups of obese subjects; Group 1 was fed a normal hospital diet of 1900 calories and Group 2 was fed a hypocaloric diet of 800-1000 calories per day. Biopsies were done on the 13th to 15th day of diets. Basal lipolysis was substantially increased with cells from the hypocaloric group, and the lipolytic response to epinephrine was reversed with these cells. In agreement with Kjellberg and Ostman (16) this change appeared to be explicable by enhanced alpha activity rather than by diminished beta effect. In contrast to the findings of Arner et al. (1), Berlan et al. (4) found no apparent influence of cell size on alpha receptor activity; there was no difference in cell size in adipose tissue samples taken from the isocaloric and hypocaloric groups. Studies designed to assess the binding characterisitcs of the adrenergic receptors of human adipocytes obtained from calorie-deprived human subjects will be important in the resolution of the conflicting data.

THE EFFECT OF THYROID HORMONE ON THE ADRENERGIC RECEPTORS OF HUMAN ADIPOSE TISSUE

The considerable body of literature relative to the influence of thyroid hormone on adipose tissue, recently reviewed by Fain (24), indicates that tissue from hypothyroid animals is less responsive to lipolytic hormones while the converse is true relative to tissue from hyperthyroid animals. There is evidence suggesting that these changes may be in part explicable in terms of alterations in the adrenergic receptors of the fat cell. Rosenquist (24) found that adipose tissue samples from hypothyroid patients had dimished lipolytic responses to catecholamines. Studies with blockers suggested that this change was due to enhanced alpha activity rather than to diminished beta effect. Reckless et al. (22), however, found no such effects in adipocytes from their hypothyroid subjects. Arner et al. (3) reported finding an increased lipolytic responsiveness to catecholamines with adipose tissue from hyperthyroid patients; they attributed this change to augmented beta receptor activity. As with the case with the effects of fasting on the adrenergic receptors of human adipocytes, there is no information concerning the influence of thyroid hormone on the binding characteristics of the adrenergic receptors of human cells. There are, however, some data available from animal studies. Guidicelli (13) for example, found a marked reduction in [^{3}H]DHA binding to fat cell membranes obtained from hypothyroid rats. Subsequently, Guidicelli et al. (14) used [^{3}H]-dihydroergocryptine to identify alpha adrenergic receptors in crude adipocyte membrane fractions obtained from hyper-, hypo-, and euthyroid hamsters. These workers concluded that hyperthyroidism was associated with a 40% decrease in the number of these binding sites while binding affinity was unaffected. In parallel experiments, a 50% reduction in alpha adrenergic responsiveness, as reflected by the increment in epinephrine-stimulated cyclic AMP synthesis induced by phentolamine, was found with adipocytes from hyperthyroid animals. Adipocytes from hypothyroid hamsters responded in a manner similar to that of cells from euthyroid animals. Sorely needed, however, are in vitro studies relative to the binding characteristics of adrenergic receptors of cells from hypo- and hyperthyroid subjects.

REFERENCES

1. Arner, P., Engfeldt, P., and Ostman, J. (1979): Metabolism 28:198-209.
2. Arner, P., and Ostman, J. (1976): Acta Med. Scand. 200:273-279.
3. Arner, P., Wennlund, A., and Ostman, J. (1979): J. Clin. Endocrinol. Metab. 48:416-419.
4. Berlan, M., Dang-Tran, L., Lafontan, M., and Donald, Y. (1981): Int. J. Obes. 5:145-153.
5. Burns, T.W., Boyer, P.A., Terry, B.E., Langley, P.E., and Robison, G.A. (1979): J. Lab. Clin. Med. 94:387-394.
6. Burns, T.W., and Langley, P.E. (1970): J. Lab. Clin. Med. 75:983-997.
7. Burns, T.W., Langley, P.E., Terry, B.E., Bylund, D.B., Hoffman, B.B., Tharp, M.D., Lefkowitz, R.J., Garcia-Sainz, A., and Fain, J.N. (1981): J. Clin. Invest. 67:467-475.
8. Burns, T.W., Mohs, J.M., Langley, P.E., Yawn, R., and Chase, G.R. (1974): J. Clin. Invest. 53:338-341.
9. Fain, J.H. (1980): In: Biochemical Actions of Hormones, Vol. 7, edited by G. Litwack, pp. 119-204. Academic Press, New York.
10. Fain, J.N., and Garcia-Sainz, J.A. (1980): Life Sci. 26:1183-1194.

11. Garcia-Sainz, J.A., and Fain, J.N. (1980): Biochem. J. 186:781-789.
12. Garcia-Sainz, J.A., Hoffman, B.B., Li, S.Y., Lefkowitz, R.J., and Fain, J.N. (1980): Life Sci. 27:953-961.
13. Giudicelli, Y. (1978): Biochem. J. 176:1007-1010.
14. Giudicelli, Y., Lacasa, D., and Acli, B. (1980): Biochem. Biophys. Res. Comm. 94:1113-1122.
15. Harper, J.R., and Brooker, G. (1978): Mol. Pharmacol. 14:1031-1045.
16. Kjellberg, J., and Ostman, J. (1971): Acta Med. Scand. 19:191.
17. Lands, A.M., Arnold, A., McAuliff, J.P., Ludueno, F.P., and Brown, T.G. (1967): Nature 214:597-598.
18. Langer, S.Z. (1974): Biochem. Pharmacol. 23:1793-1800.
19. Lefkowitz, R.J., DeLean, A., Hoffman, B.B., Stadel, J.M., Kent, R., Michel, T., and Lumbird, L. (1981): In: Advances in Cyclic Nucleotide Research, Vol. 14, edited by J.E. Dumont, Greengard, D., and Robison, G.A., pp. 145-161. Raven Press, New York.
20. Lefkowitz, R.J., and Williams, L.T. (1978): In: Advances in Cyclic Nucleotide Research, Vol. 9, edited by W.J. George, and Ignarro, L.J., pp. 1-17. Raven Press, New York.
21. Ostman, J., and Efendic, S. (1970): Acta Med. Scand. 187:471-476.
22. Reckless, J.P., Gilbert, C.H., and Galton, D.J. (1976): J. Endocrinol. 68:419-430.
23. Robison, G.A., Butcher, R.W., and Sutherland, E.W. (1967): Ann. N.Y. Acad. Sci. 139:703-723.
24. Rosenqvist, U. (1972): Acta Med. Scand. (Suppl.). 532:1-28.
25. Seamon, K.B., and Daly, J.W. (1981): J. Biol. Chem. 256:9799-9801.
26. Seamon, K.B., Padgett, S.J., and Daly, J.W. (1981): Proc. Natl. Acad. Sci. USA 78:3363-3367.

The Adipocyte and Obesity: Cellular and
Molecular Mechanisms, edited by A. Angel,
C. H. Hollenberg, and D. A. K. Roncari.
Raven Press, New York © 1983.

Regional Differences and Effect of Cell Size on Lipolysis in Human Adipocytes

Ulf Smith

Department of Medicine II, Sahlgren's Hospital, Gothenburg, Sweden

I. Effect of cell size on lipolysis

The fat cell is uniquely adapted for its function to store energy as triglyceride in the cell and to release the stored lipids as fatty acids (FA) when needed by the body. The cell is capable of changing its diameter at least 10-fold to accomodate the stored triglyceride. The degradation of the stored lipid (lipolysis) is under precise neural and humoral control. Catecholamines are the most important lipolytic agents in man while insulin exerts a potent antilipolytic action (c.f. 15).

The enlargement in fat cell size occurring during periods of affluence associated with expanding adipose tissue mass leads to perturbations in cell metabolism (review in ref 3). Concurrent with the expanding cell size metabolic processes involved in both lipid accumulation and lipid degradation increase. Thus, an increased turn-over of the stored triglyceride occurs. At the cellular level the increased lipolysis seen in the large fat cells is associated with higher cAMP levels (1) in spite of higher phosphodiesterase activity (5).

These findings with human fat cells are partly at variance with those reported in experimental animals such as the rat. Here, however, increasing obesity is seen in old rats and, thus, the effect of age is superimposed on the effect of obesity.

One important reason for the increased enzyme activities reported in large fat cells of obese humans is the associated hyperinsulinemia. Even though insulin clearly is an antilipolytic hormone it also influences protein turn-over and the activity of various enzymes. This adaptation is probably mostly dependent on the ambients, basal insulin levels. It has been shown in culture, for instance, that chronically elevated insulin levels increase both basal and catecholamine-stimulated lipolysis (13).

In accordance with this we have recently shown that both glucose metabolism and basal lipolysis of human fat cells in vitro are correlated with the fasting plasma insulin levels (14). Furthermore, following weight reduction and diminished cell size the metabolic rates of the adipocytes in vitro are reduced. The degree of reduction in metabolism is correlated with the concurrent fall in plasma insulin levels (14).

Not only is an increase in lipolytic responsiveness to

245

catecholamines seen in large fat cells but also the antilipolytic effect of insulin is enhanced (6). However, the
cellular sensitivity to either of these hormones remains
unchanged (6). This finding is in clear contrast to the
insulin resistance in large fat cells from obese subjects
on the side of glucose metabolism (6,11). This discrepancy
for two main insulin actions is not consonant with the concept that the insulin resistance on glucose uptake is largely due to alterations in insulin binding (11). In fact, in
our hands the number of insulin receptors is normal in large
fat cells (to be published). The reason for this discrepancy
between different investigations is unclear but may be due
to technical differences.

In summary, adipocyte enlargement is associated with increased rates of lipid accumulation and lipid degradation.
These perturbations in metabolism reflect, at least in part,
the associated hyperinsulinemia. It may also be concluded
that the development of obesity is not due to diminished
mobilization of fat from the adipocytes. There is no evidence of resistance to the antilipolytic effect of insulin in
large fat cells from obese subjects.

II. Regional differences in fat cell metabolism
and possible consequences in vivo

Metabolism in vitro of fat cells from different regions

Several findings suggest that the adipose tissue of different regions respond differently to various hormones as well
as to changes in the nutritional state. Experimental studies
in the rat have shown, for instance, that insulin administration leads to expansion of the subcutaneous fat cells in
particular while estrogen seems to exert a predominant effect
on the parametrial fat (9). Furthermore, the redistribution
of the fat following corticosteroid administration is well-
known. The abdominal fat cells are more susceptible to body
fat changes than those in peripheral regions (4).

There may be various reasons for these findings such as
differences in blood flow, innervation and/or cellular metabolism. Although virtually nothing is known about the first
two possibilities several recent studies have shown differences in the activity and hormonal responsiveness of various
metabolic pathways between fat cells from different regions.
As far as lipid mobilization is concerned it is quite clear
that the responsiveness to catecholamines is several fold
higher in the abdominal than in the femoral fat cells (7,8,
10,14,18). The omental fat cells seem to be the most responsive of the abdominal cells to catecholamines. Although the
femoral fat cells also seem to be less sensitive to the hormones (14) the most pronounced differences are found for the
responsiveness.

Thus, under lipolytic conditions the abdominal region
contributes more to the energy supply of the body than the
mere proportion of the abdominal fat to the total body fat
would suggest. The omental fat cells may be particularly
important in this respect in two ways; not only are the

cells the most responsive to catecholamines but the venous
blood is drained through the portal vein to the liver.

The concept that the abdominal fat cells are of greater
quantitative importance for the FA supply than more dis-
tally located adipocytes is supported by our observation
that arterial FA levels are correlated with the lipolysis
in vitro of the abdominal but not the femoral fat cells (14).

Mobilized fatty acids (FA) may, under appropriate conditions, be converted to VLDL-triglycerides in the liver. The
association between obesity and hypertriglyceridemia is well-
recognized. Whether excessive supply of FA to the liver and
other organs may also be involved in the production of other
metabolic aberrations of the obese state, such as hyperinsulinemia and propensity for diabetes, is presently unknown.

Metabolic differences between fat cells of various regions have also been shown to involve the action of insulin.
Thus, the antilipolytic effect of the hormone is drastically
reduced in femoral as compared to abdominal cells (14). This
insensitivity to insulin is entirely due to post-receptor
events since the number of insulin binding sites is at least
as high in femoral as in abdominal cells (to be published).

The reason for these differences in metabolic rates and
hormonal effects in fat cells from different regions is presently unknown but does suggest the possibility that the
adipose tissue is a polyclonal tissue derived from different
stemcells.

Possible importance of the abdominal fat for the metabolic aberrations in obesity

As discussed above, the abdominal fat cells are metabolically more responsive and mobilize fat at a considerably
higher rate than peripheral adipocytes. What is the available evidence that the abdominal region is particularly important for the development of the metabolic aberrations of
obesity? Such a question implies a direct association between
these metabolic perturbations and the adipose tissue which
seems reasonable. The elevated triglyceride levels in obesity are in all likelihood an effect of the increased FA
mobilization discussed above.

Definite proof for the concept that increased FA levels
lead to reduced glucose uptake and, thus, propensity for
diabetes as suggested by Randle and collegues (12) is lacking. Still, however, recent studies suggest a closer association between the abdominal type of obesity and the metabolic changes associated with the obese state than with a
peripheral type of obesity. Furthermore, various characteristics of the obese state have been reported in patients
with a "regional abdominal adiposity" even in the absence
of an increased total body fat mass (16).

The idea that the distribution of the body fat is of importance for the associated metabolic changes was suggested
long time ago by Vague (c.f. review in ref. 17). His classi-
fication, however, based on measurements of the various skin-
folds did not provide any pathophysiological understanding

of these differences. Consequently, it may not be the best
way to classify types of obesity and their association to
metabolic aberrations.

We recently studied a patient with the rare condition of
Werner's syndrome (16). This syndrome is, among other things,
associated with partial lipodystrophy and a high prevalence
of diabetes. Ultrasound measurements showed a "regional abdominal adiposity" in this patient and a reduced total body
fat mass. The abdominal fat cells were extremely large,
probably in an attempt to accomodate as much lipid as possible to compensate for the reduced peripheral depots. This
cell enlargement was associated with an elevated rate of
lipolysis of the fat cells in vitro (16). A number of metabolic aberrations were found in the patient which are characteristic of the obese state such as elevated glucose
levels, hyperinsulinemia, insulin resistance, elevated FA
levels and low growth hormone levels. These findings, together with our in vitro data discussed above, made us
suggest that abdominal obesity is particularly associated
with the metabolic aberrations of the obese state (16).
This concept was further strengthened by the work of Björntorp and collaborators (see review in ref. 2) showing that
the blood insulin and triglyceride levels correlated with
the size of the abdominal but not the femoral fat cells.

This hypothesis has recently been tested in two situations. It is well-recognized that abdominal obesity is typical for men while females have a more peripheral distribution of the body fat. This observation was verified by
ultrasound measurements of different regions in a large
sample of obese men and women (n=930). Men were also found
to be more susceptible to the effect of obesity on metabolism (to be published). Thus, for the same amount of body
fat men were found to have higher triglyceride-, insulin-
and glucose levels. The blood pressure was also higher in
the men. Only in the most extremely obese individuals was
an equality between the sexes found. Thus, from this investigation it may be concluded that males have an abdominal
type of obesity and also show greater susceptability to the
metabolic aberrations associated with obesity.

Since it may be argued that these differences between
males and females are due to the sex rather than the distribution of the fat further analyses were carried in obese
females only (to be published). Thus, women with a large
waist: hip ratio (abdominal type) were compared to those
with a smaller ratio (peripheral female type). Again, clear
evidence (Table 1) was found that women with the abdominal
type of obesity showed greater metabolic changes than those
with the peripheral type. The prevalence of diabetes was
also higher in these women. Similar results have recently
been reported by Kissebah and collaborators (8).

To conclude, the evidence so far obtained supports the
hypothesis that abdominal obesity is more clearly associated
with the metabolic complications of the obese state. Apart
from the cardiovascular riskfactors of elevated lipid levels
and propensity for diabetes the blood pressure is also

higher in this group. It may, thus, become feasible not only to diagnose obesity in patients but also to classify the type of obesity in order to obtain an estimate of its impact on the risk profile of the patient.

Table 1. Influence of type of obesity on metabolic variables in women with the same amount of body fat. A comparison is made of changes seen in abdominal obesity (A.O.) in comparison with peripheral obesity (P.O.).

Metabolic variable	Change in A.O. compared to P.O.
Body fat	→
Epigastric fat cell size	↑
Fasting insulin	↑
Fasting glucose	↑
Triglyceride	↑
Cholesterol	→
Blood pressure	↑
Prevalence of diabetes	↑

↑ = increase

→ = no change

References

1. Arner, P., Engfeldt, P., and Östman, J. (1979): Metabolism 28:198-209.

2. Björntorp, P. (1974): Metabolism 11:1091-1102.

3. Björntorp, P., and Smith, U. (1976): Front. Matrix Biol. 2:37-61.

4. Björntorp, P., Carlgren, G., Isaksson, B., Krotkiewski, M., Larsson, B., and Sjöström, L. (1975): Am. J. Clin. Nutr. 28:445-452.

5. Engfeldt, P., Arner, P., and Östman, J. (1980): J. Lipid Res. 21:443-448.

6. Jacobsson, B., Holm, G., Björntorp, P., and Smith, U. (1976): Diabetologia 12:69-73.

7. Kather, H., Zöllig, K., Simon, B., and Schlierf, G. (1977): Eur. J. Clin. Invest. 7:595-597.

8. Kissebah, A., Vydelingum, N., Murray, R., Evans, D., Hartz, A., Kalkhoff, R., and Adams, P. (1982): J. Clin. Endocrinol. Metab. 54:254-260.

9. Krotkiewski, M. (1976): Academic Dissertation, University of Gothenburg, Sweden.

10. Lafontan, M., Dang-Tran, L., and Berlan, M. (1979): Eur. J. Clin Invest. 9:261-266.

11. Olefsky, J., and Kolterman, O. (1981): Am. J. Med. 70: 151-168.

12. Randle, P., Garland, P., Hales, C., and Newsholme, E. (1963): Lancet 1:785-789.

13. Smith, U., Boström, S., Johansson, R., and Nyberg, G. (1976): Diabetologia 12:137-143.

14. Smith, U., Hammarsten, J., Björntorp, P., and Kral, J. (1979): Eur. J. Clin. Invest. 9:327-332.

15. Smith, U. (1980): Eur. J. Clin. Invest. 10:343-344.

16. Smith, U., DiGirolamo, M., Blohme, G., Kral, J., and Tisell, L.-E. (1980): Int. J. Obesity 4:153-163.

17. Vague, J., Rubin, P., Jubelin, J., Lan-Van, G., Aubert, F., Wassermann, A., and Fondarai, J. (1974): In: Regulation of the Adipose Tissue Mass, edited by J. Vague, and J. Boyer, pp. 296-310.

18. Östman, J., Arner, P., Engfeldt, P., and Kager, L. (1979): Metabolism 28:1198-1205.

Acknowledgement

The studies referred to in this article were supported by the Swedish Medical Research Council (project 03X-3506).

The Adipocyte and Obesity: Cellular and
Molecular Mechanisms, edited by A. Angel,
C. H. Hollenberg, and D. A. K. Roncari.
Raven Press, New York © 1983.

Effect of Obesity on Human Energy Expenditure

J. S. Garrow

Nutrition Research Group, Clinical Research Centre, Harrow, Middlesex, HA1 3UJ England

Thirty years ago experienced clinicians stood no nonsense from their obese patients: they knew how much weight an obese patient should lose on a prescribed reducing diet and "we categorically accuse each subject of dietary errors whenever they fail to equal at least 85% of prediction" (6). However we now know that two people of similar age, sex, body composition and pattern of activity may differ in energy expenditure by 40% (12) so we cannot predict weight loss in an individual patient without a great deal of tedious investigation (5). Since the range of total daily energy expenditure, or of resting metabolic rate, is so wide within groups of lean or obese subjects it is always possible to find an individual in either group with a strikingly high, or low, value. Many obese patients give dietary histories which imply astonishingly low energy requirements, but we know that dietary histories may be misleading, even in intelligent well-motivated subjects (1). Furthermore evidence has accumulated that in certain circumstances the thermogenic response of obese subjects is reduced compared with lean controls.

The pendulum of opinion has now swung so that the obese patient is no longer automatically accused of gluttony. In the last ten years research has focussed on metabolic tricks by which some obese people might remain obese despite a modest energy intake, while some lean people remain lean because they can in some way avoid depositing excess dietary energy as fat.

However, the laws of thermodynamics inexorably apply to man, as to the remainder of the natural world. Whatever the intermediate metabolic steps if energy intake exceeds energy output by all routes the excess energy must be stored in some form. If the cumulated excess over several months exceeds 20 MJ (say 5000 kcal) the only available storage space is as fat in the adipocyte. It is therefore relevant to the topic of this conference to examine the evidence that, in general or in particular circumstances, groups of obese people have lower energy requirements than groups of lean people studied under similar conditions, and hence that the obese group would have a greater tendency to store fat if the dietary intake of the two groups was similar.

UNITS OF MEASUREMENT

Obesity and energy expenditure can be expressed in many units. It is convenient for this review to compare degrees of obesity between subject groups using the Quetelet Index, or Body Mass Index, obtained by dividing the subjects' weight in kg by height in m (W/H^2). This is because there are many methods for estimating body fat which are not strictly interchangeable, but data on height and weight are usually given. In fact W/H^2 correlates well with other measures of fatness if the subjects do not include athletes or old people (3).

When the rate of energy expenditure is measured by direct calorimetry the observed heat loss is expressed in watts. This is the most accurate method available, so other estimates of energy expenditure have been converted to watts to permit comparison. The conversion factors are given in the table below.

TABLE 1. Conversion factors for rates of energy expenditure

1 watt = 1 J/sec
1 kcal = 4.18 kJ
1 litre oxygen = 21 kJ
100 watts = 8.64 MJ/day
100 watts = 2067 kcal/day
100 watts = 286 ml oxygen/minute

DAILY ENERGY EXPENDITURE AND RESTING METABOLISM

Daily energy expenditure obviously varies with the pattern of physical activity. Whenever the heat loss of a subject is measured in a calorimeter chamber it cannot be assumed that this is typical of the heat loss of the subject during ordinary life, since any chamber enclosing the subject may well affect the normal pattern of activity. This is even more true if the measurement is made by indirect calorimetry using a close-fitting face mask. However the workers at the University of Lausanne have recently published an excellent study of the energy expenditure of lean and obese men and women measured in a large comfortably furnished respiration chamber, with an internal volume of 31 m^3 (10). The movement of subjects inside the chamber was monitored by a radar device. At the end of a 24-hour period of observation a resting metabolic rate was measured on each subject. The results for daily energy expenditure and resting metabolism for 14 men and 16 women are shown in Fig 1.

It is evident from this study that with increasing obesity (indicated by the increasing value of W/H^2) both resting metabolism and total energy expenditure tend to increase in both men and women. This trend cannot be explained by any difference between the lean and obese group in their pattern of physical activity. The authors calculate that 92% of the increased metabolism in the obese group, compared with the lean controls, was accounted for by the higher resting metabolic rate in the obese group, and only 8% by other factors, such as the extra energy cost of moving the extra weight of adipose tissue.

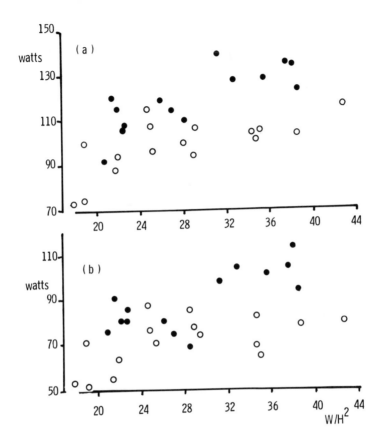

FIG. 1. Total daily energy expenditure (a) and resting metabolic rate
(b) among 14 men (●) and 16 women (o) studied by Ravussin et al (1982)
in a large respiration chamber. Resting metabolism accounted for
about 73% of total energy expenditure under these experimental
conditions (10).

METABOLISM IN FAMILIAL OR EARLY-ONSET OBESITY

It could be argued that the failure of the Lausanne group to find any
evidence of depressed metabolism among their obese subjects might be
explained by the fact that their obese subjects were not very obese, and
perhaps did not include individuals with a genetic predisposition to
obesity. To check this hypothesis we have reviewed our own data on
the relation of W/H^2 to resting metabolism among 65 women in whom we
had data concerning the age of onset of obesity and history of obesity
among first-degree relatives. These data are set out in Fig 2 (4).
The series includes some very obese individuals, and the upward trend
of resting metabolism with increasing W/H^2 is seen even more clearly
than in the results of Ravussin et al (10). However there is no suggestion that early-onset obesity, or a family history of obesity, is
associated with a lower resting metabolism than is found in similarly-
obese individuals without a history suggesting genetic predisposition
to obesity.

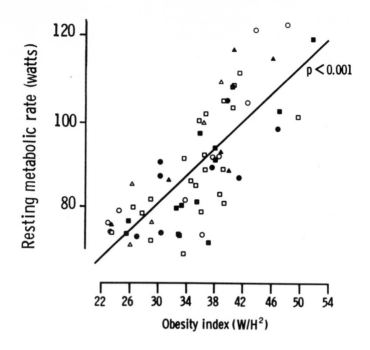

FIG 2. Relation of resting metabolism to W/H² among 65 women whose onset of obesity was in childhood (circles), or adolescence (triangles) or adult life (squares). Those individuals who gave a history of obesity in a majority of first degree relatives are shown in filled symbols, and those without a family history of obesity in open symbols (4).

METABOLISM OF LEAN AND OBESE SUBJECTS BEFORE AND AFTER A MEAL

Pittet et al (9) were the first group of workers to report that obese subjects showed a smaller thermogenic response to a meal than lean controls. Since that publication several studies have shown this effect with various types of meal. Studies in which lean and obese subjects were compared are tabulated in Table 2.

Although the absolute metabolic rate ascribed to lean and obese subjects varies between studies there is no exception to the rule that each study has found a higher fasting metabolic rate among obese subjects compared with lean, as the previous review suggests. Furthermore, although some studies report a smaller thermic response to food in obese subjects, there is still no exception to the rule that the absolute energy expenditure of each obese group after the meal was still greater than that of the lean controls. Indeed the average value for heat loss in fed lean subjects (87.1 watts) is still slightly below the average baseline value for obese subjects (88.4 watts). Thus it is difficult to sustain the argument that a decreased thermic response to food can be an important factor in maintaining obesity.

TABLE 2. Metabolic rate (watts) in lean and obese subjects before and
after a meal of various composition

Meal Nutrient	Energy MJ	Obese subjects		Lean subjects		Reference
		Before	After	Before	After	
Glucose	0.84	86.7	91.2	80.6	91.1	(9)
Protein	0.82	127.1	131.0	86.8	101.3	(7)
Protein	4.18	78.8	94.6	72.7	93.5	(13)
Protein	2.09	78.0	84.4	65.1	79.2	(13)
Mixed	2.33	74.8	79.6	61.7	71.7	(11)
Glucose	1.25	88.2	97.8	75.8	83.8	(8)
Protein	1.25	86.7	102.1	76.9	93.7	(8)
Fat	1.25	87.1	98.7	76.0	82.3	(8)
Mean		88.4	97.4	74.5	87.1	
Increase		9.0		12.6		

THERMIC RESPONSE TO HEAT, COLD, FOOD AND EXERCISE

A rather thorough investigation of the effect of moderate warmth, cool, food and exercise on the total daily energy expenditure of obese and lean women has been undertaken by Blaza (3). The total heat loss of five obese and five lean women was studied by 24-hour direct calorimetry under five experimental conditions, using a Latin square design. Each subject spent one day in the calorimeter at the upper end of the thermal comfort zone for that subject, another at the lower end of the comfort zone, another with the addition of an extra 800 kcal (3.4 MJ) of food to the basal diet, another with the equivalent of 5 miles cycling on a bicycle ergometer, and a fifth control day at the middle of the thermal comfort zone and with no extra food. The thermal comfort zones were similar for lean and obese groups of subjects (23.2 to 26.4°C). The effect of these stimuli on the heat loss of the lean and obese group is shown in Fig 3.

Under control conditions the obese group had a mean energy expenditure of 96.1 watts, while that of the lean group was 61.7 watts. This difference of 34.4 watts in baseline energy production was far larger than the thermogenic response to any of the stimuli. After food and exercise there was an increase above baseline of 3.4 and 10.1 watts in the obese group, and of 3.0 and 10.3 watts in the lean group. In each case the magnitude of the increase was similar to that which is observed by indirect calorimetry after similar stimuli. However there was a difference in the pattern of response to warm and cool conditions between the two groups. In cool conditions the obese group showed no thermogenic response: their mean energy expenditure actually fell 2.0 watts below baseline. The lean group however showed an increase of 4.8 watts over baseline values. In warm conditions the lean group showed no change from baseline, while the obese group showed an increase of 3.8 watts. It is obvious from Fig 3 that there is no situation in which any difference in thermogenic response between obese and lean subjects results in the former having a lower energy expenditure than the latter.

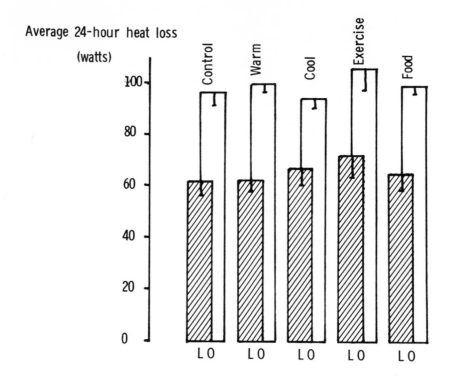

FIG 3. The average 24-hour heat loss of a group of five lean women "L" shaded columns (W/H^2 = 20.4 ± 1.0) and five obese women "O" open columns (W/H^2 = 36.0 ± 2.7) who were maintained on a uniform diet supplying 3.4 MJ/day throughout the study (data of Blaza 1980).

CHANGE IN METABOLIC RATE WITH WEIGHT LOSS IN OBESE PATIENTS

It is a common observation that severely obese patients who have lost a substantial amount of weight tend inexorably to regain this weight despite trying to keep to a low energy diet. This suggests that the process of weight loss may lead to a hypometabolic state in which energy requirements are extraordinarily low. To test this hypothesis Doré et al (2) performed a regression analysis of resting metabolic rate on body weight and composition among 140 obese women, and found that the best fit equation was

RMR = 99.8 + (1.155 x W) + (0.02227 x TBK) - (0.4563 x A) where RMR is resting metabolic rate (ml O$_2$/min) W is weight (kg), TBK is total body potassium (mmol) and A is age in years.

This regression was applied to 19 severely obese women before weight loss: their weight was 104.5 ± 9.05 kg, their total body potassium was 3245 ± 363 mmol, their age 31 ± 9 years and their predicted metabolic rate was 290 ± 33 ml O$_2$/min. At that stage their observed metabolic rate was 278 ml O$_2$/min, which is 4% higher than prediction. After weight loss their weight was 73.7 kg, total body potassium 2761 ± 290 mmol, and age 32 ± 9 years. Using the same regression equation their predicted resting metabolic rate after weight loss was 232 ± 26 ml O_2/min, and their observed resting metabolic rate was 234 ml O_2/min, which is 1% higher than predicted.

Since the observed metabolic rate agrees well with the prediction both before and after weight loss we conclude that, although obese patients will have lower energy requirements after weight loss, their new level of metabolism is similar to that found in people of similar body composition who have not experienced massive weight loss. However this will not necessarily be true of obese patients who lose weight very rapidly, for example by total starvation, since this involves excessive loss of lean tissue, and hence excessive decrease in resting metabolic rate and energy expenditure (3,10).

SUMMARY

The most striking difference between the energy expenditure of lean and obese groups of individuals is that the obese group has a higher resting metabolic rate. To some extent this is explained by the higher lean body mass in obese subjects. Although some, but not all, studies of thermogenesis in obese human subjects have shown a decreased response to food, cold, and the infusion of noradrenalin, the higher energy expenditure of the obese group, relative to the lean, persists even after these thermogenic stimuli. After massive weight loss the energy expenditure of obese patients is reduced, but not to an extent which is unusually low for their new body composition.

All the foregoing statements apply to groups of subjects, but not necessarily to individuals, since the variation of metabolic rate within groups of obese and lean individuals is often greater than the difference in the average value of the two groups.

We must conclude that a low basal energy expenditure, or decreased thermogenesis to a variety of stimuli, cannot be a major factor in causing or maintaining obesity in man, although in certain rodents decreased thermogenesis is certainly important in the aetiology of genetically determined obesity. This conclusion will be greeted with disbelief by many obese patients, who will remain convinced that their energy requirements are abnormally low, and that their adipocytes enlarge on a very modest diet. However from the viewpoint of the clinician the conclusion is encouraging, since it implies that obesity can be effectively treated if only the energy intake of the obese patient can be restricted for a sufficiently long time.

REFERENCES

1. Acheson, K.J., Campbell, I.T., Edholm, O.G., Miller, D.S. and Stock, M.J. (1980): Am. J. Clin. Nutr., 33:1147-1154.
2. Doré, C., Hesp, R., Wilkins, D. and Garrow, J.S. (1982): Hum. Nutr: Clin. Nutr., 36C:41-48.
3. Garrow, J.S. (1981): Treat Obesity Seriously: A Clinical Manual. Churchill Livingstone, Edinburgh.
4. Garrow, J.S., Blaza, S.E., Warwick, P.M. and Ashwell, M.A. (1980): Lancet, i: 1103-1104.
5. Garrow, J.S., Durrant, M.L., Mann, S., Stalley, S.F. and Warwick, P. (1978): Int. J. Obesity, 2: 441-447.

6. Jolliffe, N. and Alpert, E. (1951): <u>Postgraduate Medicine</u>, 9: 106-115.

7. Kaplan, M.L. and Leveille, G.A. (1976): <u>Am. J. Clin. Nutr.</u>, 29: 1108-1113.

8. Nair, K.S., Garrow, J.S. and Halliday, D. (1982): <u>Clin. Science</u>, 62: 43-44P.

9. Pittet, Ph., Chappuis, Ph., Acheson, K., de Techtermann, F. and Jéquier, E. (1976): Br. J. Nutr., 35: 281-292.

10. Ravussin, E., Burnand, B., Schutz, Y. and Jéquier, E. (1982): <u>Am. J. Clin. Nutr.</u>, 35: 566-573.

11. Shetty, P.S., Jung, R.T., James, W.P.T., Barrand, M.A. and Callingham, B.A. (1981): <u>Clin. Sci.</u>, 60: 519-525.

12. Warwick, P.M., Toft, R. and Garrow, J.S. (1978): <u>Int. J. Obesity</u>, 2: 396.

13. York, D.A., Morgan, J.B. and Taylor, T.G. (1980): <u>Proc. Nutr. Soc.</u>, 39: 57A.

The Adipocyte and Obesity: Cellular and Molecular Mechanisms, edited by A. Angel,
C. H. Hollenberg, and D. A. K. Roncari.
Raven Press, New York © 1983.

Role of Thermogenesis in Brown Adipose Tissue in the Regulation of Energy Balance

Jean Himms-Hagen

Department of Biochemistry, University of Ottawa, Ottawa, Ontario, K1H 8M5 Canada

Thermogenesis in brown adipose tissue [BAT] has only recently been recognized as playing an important role in overall energy expenditure and thus in energy balance. For over twenty years this tissue has been known to have the specific function of heat production (60). However, only in the last four years has a major role in two forms of facultative thermogenesis, *cold-induced nonshivering thermogenesis* [CINST] and *diet-induced thermogenesis* [DIT] been established (19-21,29,56,58,59,61). The recognition of this major role has led to the study of the importance of defective thermogenesis in BAT in certain forms of obesity characterized by low energy expenditure and high metabolic efficiency and to the concept that thermogenesis in BAT is regulated to buffer energy intake over a fairly wide range so as to minimize changes in body fat content. A corollary of this concept is that defective caloric buffering by BAT may contribute to the development of obesity.

CINST is an increase in metabolic rate that occurs at temperatures below thermoneutrality. It is switched on by the increased sympathetic activity brought about by the exposure to cold and is due primarily to a metabolic effect of noradrenaline [NA] on BAT (20,21). It must be distinguished from shivering thermogenesis, an increase in metabolic rate that may also occur at temperatures below thermoneutrality due to muscle activity. DIT is an increase in metabolic rate that occurs in response to ingestion of food. It is mediated by the increased sympathetic activity engendered by the diet (39,40) and, like CINST, is due primarily to a metabolic effect of NA on BAT (56,58,59,81). DIT is not to be confused with the thermic effect of food (formerly referred to as specific dynamic action) which is the immediate energy expenditure obligatorily involved in ingestion, digestion, absorption and the initial processing of the food components themselves. The increase in metabolic rate after a meal thus has two distinguishable components, the thermic effect of the food itself, and the sympathetic-mediated DIT (55). DIT may, however, persist long after the ingested food has been initially processed, depending on the amount and composition of the food ingested (55,58,61).

BAT is an organ distinct from white adipose tissue and may be characterized by its smaller multilocular cells, its numerous and large mitochondria with many cristae and its rich sympathetic innervation. It is scattered in many fairly small deposits throughout the body, primarily in the interscapular, subscapular, cervical, axillary and perirenal regions, along the great vessels in the thorax and between the ribs.

CONTROL OF BAT THERMOGENESIS

Thermogenesis in BAT

BAT thermogenesis is switched on by NA liberated from the sympathetic nerve endings on the BAT cells. NA reacts with the BAT β-adrenergic receptors to activate adenylate cyclase and thus to initiate a cyclic AMP-mediated activation of lipolysis. The exact nature of the link between acceleration of lipolysis and activation of the unique thermogenic process in BAT mitochondria is uncertain but the lipolytic products, either the fatty acids themselves (6,44) or acyl CoA derived from them (8), may be directly involved.

BAT mitochondria differ from mitochondria of other tissues in that they possess a proton conductance pathway. When activated this pathway provides a means for short-circuiting the usual proton cycling (which occurs through the pumping out associated with electron transport and reentry via the mechanism associated with oxidative phosphorylation, see FIG.1). When this short-circuiting occurs (FIG.1), the rate of electron transport, no longer restrained by the proton gradient, rises to a maximum, and available substrates are oxidized much more rapidly so that there is a large increase in heat production (7,50). In the resting BAT cell the pathway is inhibited by the binding of purine nucleotides to a specific polypeptide component of the mitochondrial inner membrane (of molecular weight 32,000 daltons) (7,50).

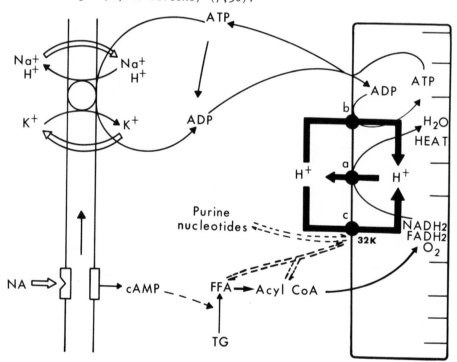

FIG.1. Control of BAT mitochondrial thermogenesis by noradrenaline [NA]. The inner mitochondrial membrane contains [a] the electron transport system, [b] oxidative phosphorylation, and [c] the proton conductance pathway. See text for explanation. (Based on references 6-8, 44, 50).

BAT Thermogenesis: Acute Changes

Acute stimulation of BAT by administration of NA or by exposure of the animal to cold for a few hours produces certain changes in the mitochondria which can be observed by electron microscopy of the intact cells (62,63,72) and by electron microscopy and biochemical studies of mitochondria isolated from the tissue (13-15). At this early stage no changes can be detected in the polypeptide composition of such isolated mitochondria (13,15). However, a consistent finding is an increase in the capacity of the isolated mitochondria to bind purine nucleotides (13, 15). The effect is mediated by NA (13) and is rapidly reversible (FIG.2).

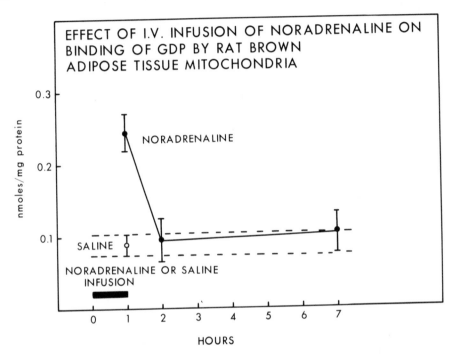

FIG.2. Effect of intravenous infusion of NA on binding of GDP by isolated BAT mitochondria of the rat. Conscious rats with an indwelling venous cannula were infused with NA or saline for 1 h (see 13 for technical details). Rats were killed at the end of the infusion or 1 or 6 h later. Note that the unmasking response to NA (increase in GDP binding) has reversed within 1 hour.

The increase in binding does not require protein synthesis (31), is not associated with any detectable change in mitochondrial polypeptide composition (15) and appears to be due to a structural reorganization of mitochondrial membranes and unmasking of binding sites already present (14). The functional significance of this "unmasking response" is not understood. The response does, however, serve as a very sensitive and readily measurable index of the thermogenic state of BAT mitochondria. It is seen, for example, in cafeteria-fed rats, in which an increase in BAT mitochondrial GDP binding occurs (4,32) in the absence of any change in polypeptide composition (32). It fails to occur in thyroidectomized rats and requires permissive amounts of thyroid hormones (47,70).

Acute stimulation of BAT thermogenesis is also associated with a very large increase in blood flow (20,21). The increase is not mediated directly by the noradrenergic innervation of BAT blood vessels (which appears to have a vasoconstrictor function) but is secondary to the BAT hypermetabolism and brought about by an as yet unknown mediator (18).

BAT Thermogenesis: Long-term Adaptive Changes

BAT enlarges when there is an increased need for its thermogenic function, as in animals living at low temperatures or in animals that are overeating. This is a true growth, accompanied by cell proliferation (5). The increase in metabolic size of BAT can be readily measured from the increases in total DNA, protein and cytochrome oxidase content (as measures of cellularity, active tissue mass and mitochondrial mass). The measurement of wet weight alone is not a useful assessment of the amount of metabolically active BAT present, since changes in wet weight may result from changes in triglyceride stored in the tissue. A rough estimate of the total amount of functional BAT present in an animal can be obtained from the size of the maximum thermogenic response of the animal to NA, as determined from measurements of oxygen consumption.

Not only does the mitochondrial mass increase during the growth of BAT but the composition of the mitochondria may also change. In cold-acclimated rats the mitochondria of the enlarged BAT have a relative increase in the amount of the 32,000 dalton polypeptide associated with the thermogenic proton conductance pathway (15,52,54) and a marked change in composition of phospholipid fatty acids, which become more saturated (53,54). The change in polypeptide composition occurs only in response to some growth-promoting stimuli (acclimation to cold)(15,52,54) and not to others (cafeteria feeding) (32) and is associated with a selective change in the synthesis of mitochondrial proteins (31).

The stimulation of the growth of BAT is mediated, at least in part, by increased sympathetic activity. Chronic treatment of rats with catechol-amines can mimic this effect (13,28). Cold-induced growth requires only permissive amounts of thyroid and adrenal cortical hormones and does not require the direct participation of any of the pituitary hormones (17,70); it does not occur in denervated BAT (Park, Himms-Hagen, unpublished results). In contrast, the nature of the presumed hormonal mediator that brings about the change in mitochondrial polypeptide composition is at present unknown. It does not appear to be any of catecholamines, thyroid hormones, adrenal cortical hormones or pituitary hormones (13,17, 70). The change in mitochondrial fatty acid composition is also not observed in BAT of animals treated chronically with catecholamines (46).

BAT THERMOGENESIS AND ENERGY BALANCE IN NORMAL ANIMALS

A major role for BAT thermogenesis in energy balance has been quantitatively established for two types of normal animal, the cold-acclimated rat and the cafeteria-fed rat.

The cold-acclimated rat (one that has lived at a low temperature, usually 4°C, for 2-3 weeks) is hypermetabolic and hyperphagic, eating twice as much as a rat kept at thermoneutrality (28°C for the rat) (26). Most of the extra heat is produced in BAT (21). Despite its hyperphagia the cold-acclimated rat is very lean; sympathetic-mediated thermogenesis in BAT plays a major role in the maintenance of energy balance and lean-ness in these animals. BAT grows rapidly during the initial phase of cold-acclimation so that the cold-acclimated rat has a greatly increased capacity for CINST (up to 3-4 times its resting metabolic rate).

The cafeteria-fed rat (one that has eaten, in addition to the regular chow, a variety of highly palatable foods) is also hyperphagic and hyper-metabolic (56) and becomes less obese than would be expected from its excess energy intake. Most of the extra heat is produced in BAT and is sympathetic-mediated (56,58,59,81). BAT grows in response to cafeteria feeding so that the capacity of the cafeteria-fed rat for CINST (as well as for DIT) is greatly increased (32,56,57).

In both these two types of hypermetabolic animal the increased thermo-genesis (CINST or DIT) is sympathetic-mediated and occurs primarily in BAT. The efferent pathway (NA-stimulated thermogenesis in BAT) is identical but the afferent pathways and central integrative mechanisms must differ.

BAT THERMOGENESIS IN ANIMALS WITH GENETIC OBESITY

BAT has been studied extensively in three strains of laboratory animals in which obesity is inherited (autosomal recessive). These are the genetically obese mouse [ob/ob], the genetically diabetic-obese mouse [db/db] and the Zucker "fatty" rat [fa/fa].

The ob/ob mouse is hyperphagic but hypometabolic at all temperatures below thermoneutrality (30-33°C for the mouse) (67). It is extremely cold-sensitive, becoming hypothermic and dying in a few hours at 4°C (67). The major thermogenic defect in the ob/ob mouse can be attributed to a failure of NA-mediated CINST and DIT in BAT. Thus the cold-exposed ob/ob mouse fails to activate thermogenesis in its BAT (as indicated by the lack of increase in mitochondrial GDP binding (30,34)). Cold-exposure does accentuate sympathetic activity in BAT of the ob/ob mouse (38,82). The defect appears to lie in a refractoriness of BAT to the thermogenic action of NA, a conclusion in keeping with the low capacity of the ob/ob mouse to respond thermogenically to injected NA (35,67). The defective thermogenic responsiveness of BAT (present in normal amounts) can quantitatively account for the reduced capacity of the ob/ob mouse to respond thermogenically to NA (64). In the ob/ob mouse, despite the defective acute thermogenic responsiveness of BAT to cold-exposure, the growth response of BAT to prolonged acclimation to mild cold (14°C) is normal (34), indicating an independence of these two responses.

The low metabolic rate of the ob/ob mouse has suggested that it might be hypothyroid. However, the ob/ob mouse appears to have no major hypo-thalamic-pituitary-thyroid abnormality (3) and the T_3 level in its blood is normal or above normal for most of its life (45,48). Only at a very early age is a hypothyroid state detectable (45,73-75). It is, however, possible that some tissues of the ob/ob mouse may fail to respond to the T_3 present in its blood. These mice have an exaggerated increase in metabolic rate in response to a dose of thyroid hormone that is without effect in lean mice (35,43,77), suggesting a partial resistance to the effect of endogenous T_3. Moreover, treatment of ob/ob mice with thyroid hormone permits a normal thermogenic response of the mouse to injected NA and of its BAT to cold-exposure (35). Since the only role for T_3 in BAT function and growth appears to be a permissive one that allows the acute thermogenic effect of NA on the tissue (70), the effect of thyroid hormone on BAT of the ob/ob mouse is interpreted as due to improved responsiveness to NA. It follows that the defect in BAT of the ob/ob mouse is most probably in its sensitivity to that action of T_3 ("permissive effect") that controls responsiveness to NA, possibly by control of α- and/or β-adrenergic receptors.

That DIT is also defective in the ob/ob mouse is suggested by the low thermogenic state of its BAT mitochondria despite its hyperphagia (30, 34) and by its refractoriness to NA (67), known to be the mediator of DIT (58,61,81). We have found a normal activation of sympathetic activity in BAT of the cafeteria-fed ob/ob mouse (Zaror-Behrens, Himms-Hagen, unpublished results). It is of interest, however, that prolonged cafeteria feeding of ob/ob mice promotes some thermogenic activation of BAT mitochondria (increase in GDP binding) and growth of BAT (68 and Hogan, Himms-Hagen, unpublished results). It seems likely that this response is due to the change in composition of the diet rather than to overeating, since cafeteria feeding does not increase any further the already elevated food intake of the ob/ob mouse (68). The response appears to be mediated by the increase in T3 level that occurs (Hogan, Himms-Hagen, unpublished results); as noted above, treatment of the ob/ob mouse with thyroid hormone improves the thermogenic responsiveness of its BAT to NA.

BAT of the db/db mouse resembles that of the ob/ob mouse in all respects so far studied (24,65,66). Like the ob/ob mouse, the db/db mouse is extremely cold-sensitive.

The Zucker fa/fa rat is also hyperphagic and hypometabolic and has a very high metabolic efficiency (9,37). Much variability in cold-sensitivity has been reported (2,23,27,41,69,71,79); the variability may be due to variation in the age of the rats, younger rats being more resistant. We have found that BAT of young (7-8 w) fa/fa rats is present in normal amounts and shows a normal thermogenic response (increase in GDP binding) when the rat is exposed to cold (71). In contrast, cafeteria feeding of the young fa/fa rat is without effect on either the thermogenic state of its BAT mitochondria (no increase in GDP binding) or on its size (no increase in DNA, protein or cytochrome oxidase) (71). This finding is in keeping with the recent demonstration that fa/fa rats have a reduced thermic response to a single meal (55).

Thus, the fa/fa rat differs from the ob/ob mouse in that its BAT can respond thermogenically to cold-exposure. Whereas the defect in the ob/ob mouse appears to be at the tissue level (refractoriness of BAT to NA, perhaps secondary to resistance to T3) and thus to impair all responsiveness of BAT to acute stimulation, the defect in the fa/fa rat would appear to be in the hypothalamic response to diet or in the neural connections between the site of this response and the point of conver-gence with the neural route which mediates the activation of the sympathetic innervation of BAT by cold-exposure (71). The fa/fa rat exhibits a slower development of obesity than the ob/ob mouse, possibly because of the partial nature of the defect in its control of BAT thermo-genesis, in contrast to the virtually total defect in the ob/ob mouse.

BAT THERMOGENESIS AND ENERGY BALANCE IN ANIMALS WITH HYPOTHALAMIC OBESITY

BAT has been studied in two types of laboratory animal with hypothalamic obesity, the goldthioglucose [GTG]-obese mouse and the medial hypothalamic [MH]-lesioned rat.

The GTG mouse is hyperphagic initially, during the dynamic phase of its obesity (11,16,25) and exhibits an increased metabolic efficiency (11,16). It is not, however, cold-sensitive (36,78). The hypothalamic lesions are mainly in glucose-sensitive regions and are somewhat variable in size, depending on the dose of GTG (10,42). BAT of the GTG mouse is present in normal amounts and can respond thermogenically in the normal way to cold-exposure of the mouse (increase in GDP binding, see FIG.3).

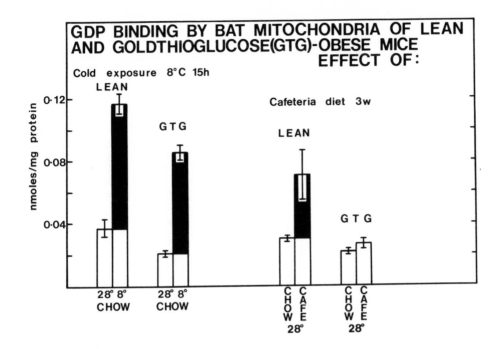

FIG.3.   Effect of cold-exposure or of cafeteria feeding on GDP binding by
          BAT mitochondria of lean and GTG-obese mice. Bars shows means
±SEM for 4 experiments. Black portions of bars denote a significant
(P<0.05) effect of treatment. Mice were studied 3 w after receiving GTG,
i.e., in the dynamic phase of their obesity. GDP binding by BAT mitochondria of GTG mice is significantly lower than that of lean mice; the
unmasking response (increase in GDP binding) occurs in response to cold
but not in response to cafeteria feeding.

Acclimation of the GTG mouse to cold induces a normal growth of BAT
(Hogan, Himms-Hagen, submitted for publication). Thus, there appears to
be no defect inherent in BAT, in the immediate innervation of BAT, in the
control of BAT growth or in the sympathetic control of BAT thermogenesis
in the GTG mouse. In contrast, the GTG mouse that is fed a cafeteria
diet during the dynamic phase of its obesity fails to activate thermogenesis in its BAT (no increase in GDP binding, see FIG.3) although a
normal growth of BAT occurs (Hogan, Himms-Hagen, submitted for
publication).
    The defect in control of BAT thermogenesis in the GTG-obese mouse
would appear to be, as in the fa/fa rat, located in the hypothalamus and
to result in a failure of diet, but not of cold, to activate the
sympathetic innervation of BAT. This suggestion is in keeping with the
demonstrated abnormal responsiveness of the sympathetic nervous system
of the GTG-obese mouse to diet (80).
    The MH-lesioned rat is hyperphagic and exhibits a high metabolic
efficiency; it is not, however, cold-sensitive (1,22,76). BAT is
present in normal amounts in both male and female MH-lesioned rats and is
able to respond thermogenically (increase in mitochondrial GDP binding)
when the rats are exposed to cold (33). BAT of the MH-lesioned rat does

not, however, respond thermogenically to a cafeteria diet, fed during the dynamic phase of the obesity (first 3 w); it also does not grow in response to this treatment (Hogan, Coscina, Himms-Hagen, unpublished results). The defect in the MH-lesioned rat would appear to lie in the hypothalamic mechanisms involved in responsiveness to diet. This defect does not impede cold-induced sympathetic activation of BAT.

CONCLUSIONS: ANIMAL MODELS OF OBESITY

A defect in BAT thermogenesis occurs in all animal models of human obesity so far studied. All these animals are hyperphagic, at least in the dynamic phase of their obesity, and it is obvious that hyperphagia itself contributes to the development of their obesity. All, however, also exhibit an elevated metabolic efficiency and become obese even when pair fed to lean control animals. The elevated metabolic efficiency can be correlated with a reduction in energy expenditure that is accounted for by reduced thermogenesis in BAT. Only for the ob/ob mouse has the deficit in energy expenditure been quantitatively related to reduced BAT functioning (64). However, it appears likely that the same is true of the other animal models.

Study of the nature of the defect in BAT functioning reveals some differences between the animal models (summarized in TABLE 1), not surprising in view of the differing causes of their obesity. The ob/ob mouse has the most severe defect (and the most rapidly developing obesity) since its BAT fails to respond thermogenically to either of the two main environmental stimuli to energy expenditure in this tissue under usual laboratory conditions (temperature below thermoneutrality; chow food). In contrast, in the other three animal models BAT has an unimpaired thermogenic responsiveness to cold and fails to respond only to diet; their obesity develops more slowly, in keeping with the partial nature of the defect in control of energy expenditure in their BAT.

TABLE 1. Summary of BAT Function in Animal Models of Human Obesity

Stimulus	Response of BAT	Genetic obesity		Hypothalamic obesity	
		ob/ob mouse	fa/fa rat	GTG mouse	MH rat
COLD	Thermogenic	No (Yes)[a]	Yes	Yes	Yes
	Growth	Yes	Yes	Yes	Yes
DIET	Thermogenic	No (Yes)[a]	No (No)[a]	No (No)[a]	No (No)[a]
	Growth	Yes	No	Yes	No

[a]Denotes the long-term effect of adaptation to cold or to cafe diet

It is of interest that control of growth of BAT induced by cold-acclimation is normal in all four animal models, even in the ob/ob mouse in which BAT appears to be refractory to the acute thermogenic effect of NA. Since growth of BAT is thought to be mediated, at least in part, by NA, it seems likely that the growth-promoting effect of NA is mediated in a different way from its thermogenic effect.

The failure of cafeteria feeding to promote BAT thermogenesis and growth in two of the types of obesity (the fa/fa rat, the MH-lesioned rat) would be in keeping with a hypothalamic defect in these animals that prevents the transduction and/or transmission of signals derived from the diet to the sympathetic innervation of BAT. However, the nature of the defect in BAT functioning in the GTG-obese mouse is difficult to explain. The failure of diet-induced activation would suggest a defect similar to that in the fa/fa rat and in the MH-lesioned rat, in keeping with the known defective sympathetic responsiveness of the GTG-obese mouse to diet (80). However, the observed growth of BAT in response to diet in the GTG mouse could not then be attributed to increased sympathetic stimulation and another explanation would have to be sought. It may be relevant that the GTG mouse, unlike the other three animal models, is not stunted, and indeed may show increased body growth (12). Moreover, cafeteria feeding of the GTG mouse promotes overall body growth (Hogan, Himms-Hagen, submitted for publication). Although both GTG- and MH lesion-induced obesities are hypothalamic in origin, their etiologies differ, particularly in the involvement of the pituitary, which appears to participate in the obesity induced by GTG but not in that induced by MH lesions (51). Thus, some other factor, possibly of pituitary origin, may be implicated in the growth of BAT induced in the GTG-obese mouse by cafeteria feeding.

Thus there is a correlation between thermogenic functioning of BAT and energy balance. At one extreme is the lean cold-acclimated rat with highly effective BAT thermogenesis as a major component of its energy expenditure; at the other extreme is the massively obese ob/ob mouse with defective BAT thermogenesis leading to reduced energy expenditure. In between is the cafeteria-fed rat with effective BAT thermogenesis as an adaptable component of its overall energy expenditure and lean, or only moderately obese, despite its hyperphagia (there are sex and strain differences in responsiveness of rats to cafeteria feeding, as yet not explored in detail). Three other obesities (the fa/fa rat; the GTG-obese mouse; the MH-lesioned rat) are associated with partial defects in BAT thermogenesis, some deficit in energy expenditure and slowly developing obesity.

The correlation between effectiveness of thermogenesis in BAT and leanness or obesity lends support to the concept that thermogenesis in BAT is normally regulated to buffer energy intake over a fairly wide range so as to minimize changes in body fat content; the effectiveness of caloric buffering by BAT is inversely correlated with the proportion of body fat.

IMPLICATIONS FOR THE FUTURE

The extent to which the concept of BAT thermogenesis as a caloric buffer applies to man is as yet uncertain. There is no doubt that BAT is present in adult man and that thermogenesis can be demonstrated to occur in the areas expected from the distribution of BAT in experimental animals. Sympathetic activity and resting metabolic rate are increased in man by feeding and decreased by fasting, as in experimental animals. It has not, however, so far been possible to quantitate in man either the amount of BAT or the contribution of BAT thermogenesis to overall energy expenditure. It might be noted that the only quantitative technique available for this purpose in animals is the measurement of blood flow using radioactive microspheres (20,21,59,64), a technique obviously not applicable to man.

If, however, it is assumed that the hypothesis that BAT serves as a caloric buffer applies to man, it is clearly of importance to understand in some detail the control mechanisms involved and the nature of the defects in these mechanisms in the animal models of human obesity. An ultimate objective in the treatment of obesity would be to develop means of modifying BAT thermogenesis and thus of modifying energy expenditure and energy balance. One important point which arises from the studies of experimental animals described here is that study of a single animal model would be entirely inadequate for providing a framework on which to base studies of human obesity. In the four animal models studied, at least three different types of defective control of BAT thermogenesis can be identified. It is likely that still other types of defective control will be uncovered if other obese animal strains are studied. In view of the highly heterogeneous nature of human obesity and the strong genetic component it is clear that only a large collection of animal models will suffice to provide a clear understanding of defects which might occur and contribute to obesity in man.

REFERENCES

1. Bernardis, L.L., and Goldman, J.K.(1976): J.Neurosci.Res. 2:91-116.
2. Bray, G.A., and York, D.A. (1972): Am.J.Physiol. 223:176-179.
3. Bray, G.A., and York, D.A. (1979): Physiol. Rev. 59:719-809.
4. Brooks, S.L., Rothwell, N.J., and Stock, M.J. (1982): Quart.J.exp. Physiol. 67:259-268.
5. Bukowiecki, L., Collet, A.J., Follea, N., Guay, G., and Jahjah, L., (1982): Am.J.Physiol. (in press).
6. Bukowiecki, L., Follea, N., Lupien, J., and Paradis, A., (1981): J. biol. Chem. 256:12840-12848.
7. Cannon, B., Nedergaard, J., and Sundin, U. (1981): In: Survival in the Cold: Hibernation and Other Adaptations, edited by X.J.Musacchia and L. Jansky, pp.99-120. Elsevier North Holland, Amsterdam.
8. Cannon, B., Sundin, U., and Romert, L. (1977): FEBS Lett. 74:43-46.
9. Deb, S., Martin, R.J., and Hershberger, T.V.(1976) J.Nutr. 106:191-197.
10. Debons, A.F., Krimsky, I., Maayan, M.J., Fani, K., and Jimenez, F.A. (1977): Fed. Proc. 36:143-147.
11. De Laey, P., Dent, C., Terry, A.C., and Quinn, E.H. (1975): Arch.int. Pharmacodyn. 213:145-162.
12. De Leeuw, I., Van Rooy, P., and D'Hollander, M. (1981): Diabetologia 20:145-147.
13. Desautels, M., and Himms-Hagen, J. (1979): Can.J.Biochem. 57:968-976.
14. Desautels, M., and Himms-Hagen, J. (1980): Can.J.Biochem. 58:1057-1068.
15. Desautels, M., Zaror-Behrens, G., and Himms-Hagen, J. (1978): Can.J.Biochem. 56:378-383.
16. Djazayery, A., Miller, D.S., and Stock, M.J. (1979): Nutr.Metab. 23:357-367.
17. Fellenz, M., Triandafillou, J., Gwilliam, C., and Himms-Hagen, J. (1982): Can.J.Biochem. (in press).
18. Foster, D.O., and Depocas, F. (1981): Can.J.Physiol.Pharmacol. 58:1418-1425.
19. Foster, D.O., and Frydman, M.L. (1978) Can.J.Physiol.Pharmacol. 58:97-109.
20. Foster, D.O., and Frydman, M.L. (1978) Can.J.Physiol.Pharmacol. 56:110-122.

21. Foster, D.O., and Frydman, M.L. (1979): Can.J.Physiol.Pharmacol. 57:257-270.
22. Frohman, L.A. (1978): In: Recent Advances in Obesity Research II, edited by G.A. Bray, pp.133-141. Newman, London.
23. Godbole, V., York, D.A., and Bloxham, D.P. (1978): Diabetologia 15:41-44.
24. Goodbody, A.E., and Trayhurn, P. (1981): Biochem.J. 194:1019-1022.
25. Gray, G.F., and Liebelt, R.A. (1961): Texas Rep.Biol.Med. 19:80-88.
26. Hardeveld, C.Van, Zuidwijk, M.J., and Kassenaar, A.A.H. (1979): Acta Endocrinol. 91:473-483.
27. Harris, R.B.S. (1982): J.Physiol.Lond.) 324:58P-59P.
28. Heick, H.M.C., Vachon, C., Kallai, M.A., Begin-Heick, N., and Leblanc, J. (1973): Can.J.Physiol.Pharmacol. 51:751-758.
29. Himms-Hagen, J. (1981): In: Nutritional Factors: Modulating Effects on Metabolic Processes, edited by R.F.Beers, Jr., and E.G. Bassett, pp.85-99. Raven Press, New York.
30. Himms-Hagen, J., and Desautels, M. (1978):Biochem.Biophys.Res.Commun. 83:628-634.
31. Himms-Hagen, J., Dittmar, E., and Zaror-Behrens, G. (1980): Can.J.Biochem. 58:336-344.
32. Himms-Hagen, J., Triandafillou, J., and Gwilliam, C. (1981): Am.J.Physiol. 241:E116-E120.
33. Hogan, S., Coscina, D.V., and Himms-Hagen, J. (1982): Am.J.Physiol. (in press).
34. Hogan, S., and Himms-Hagen, J. (1980): Am.J.Physiol. 239:E301-E309.
35. Hogan, S., and Himms-Hagen, J. (1981): Am.J.Physiol. 241:E436-E443.
36. Joosten, H.F.P., and Van der Kroon, P.H.W. (1974): Metabolism 23:425-436.
37. Kaplan, M.L. (1979): Metabolism 28:1147-1151.
38. Knehans, A.W., and Romsos, D.R. (1982): Am.J.Physiol. 242:E253-E261.
39. Landsberg, L., and Young, J.B. (1981): Life Sci. 28:1801-1819.
40. Landsberg, L., and Young, J.B. (1981) In: Nutritional Factors: Modulating Effects on Metabolic Processes, edited by R.F. Beers,Jr., and E.G. Bassett, pp.155-174. Raven Press, New York.
41. Levin, B.E., Triscari, J., and Sullivan, A.C. (1980):Pharmacol. Biochem. Behav. 13:107-113.
42. Liebelt, R.A., and Perry, J.H. (1967):Handbook of Physiology 6: sect.1, 271-285. American Physiological Society, Washington.
43. Lin, M.H., Vander Tuig, J.G., Romsos, D.R., Akera, T., and Leveille, G.A. (1979) Am.J.Physiol. 237:E265-E272.
44. Locke, R.M., and Nicholls, D.G. (1981): FEBS Lett. 135:249-252.
45. Mobley, P.W., and Dubuc, P.U. (1979): Horm.Metab.Res.11:37-39.
46. Mory, G., Ricquier, D., and Hemon, P. (1980):J.Physiol.(Paris) 76:859-864.
47. Mory, G., Ricquier, D., Pesquies, P., and Hemon, P. (1981): J.Endocrinol. 91:515-524.
48. Naltchayan, S., Bouhnik, J., and Michel, R. (1981):C.R.Soc.Biol. 174:118-120.
49. Nedergaard, J., and Lindberg, O. (1982): Int.Rev.Cytol.74:187-286.
50. Nicholls, D.G. (1979): Biochim. Biophys. Acta 549:1-29.
51. Powley, T.L., and Plocher, T.A. (1980): Behavioral Neural Biology 28:300-318.
52. Ricquier, D., and Kader, J.-C. (1976): Biochem. Biophys.Res.Commun. 73:577-583.
53. Ricquier, D., Mory, G., and Hemon, P.(1975): FEBS Lett. 53:342-346.

54. Ricquier, D., Mory, G., and Hemon, P. (1979) Can.J.Biochem. 57:1262-1266.
55. Rothwell, N.J., Saville, M.E., and Stock, M.J. (1982): Int.J.Obesity 6:53-59.
56. Rothwell, N.J., and Stock, M.J. (1979): Nature (Lond.) 281:31-35.
57. Rothwell, N.J., and Stock, M.J. (1980): Can.J.Physiol.Pharmacol. 58:842-848.
58. Rothwell, N.J., and Stock, M.J. (1981): Ann.Rev.Nutr. 1:235-256.
59. Rothwell, N.J., and Stock, M.J. (1981): Pfluegers Arch. 389:237-242.
60. Smith, R.E., and Horwitz, B.A. (1969): Physiol.Rev. 49:330-425.
61. Stock, M.J., and Rothwell, N.J. (1981): In: Nutritional Factors: Modulating Effects on Metabolic Processes, edited by R.F. Beers, Jr., and E.G. Bassett, pp.101-113. Raven Press, New York.
62. Suter, E.R. (1969): J.Ultrastruct.Res. 26:216-241.
63. Thomson, J.F., Habeck, D.A., Nance, S.L., and Beetham, K.L. (1969): J. Cell Biol. 41:312-334.
64. Thurlby, P.L., and Trayhurn, P. (1980): Pfluegers Arch. 385:193-201.
65. Trayhurn, P. (1979): Pfluegers Arch. 380:227-232.
66. Trayhurn, P., and Fuller, L. (1980): Diabetologia 19:148-153.
67. Trayhurn, P., and James, W.P.T. (1978): Pfluegers Arch. 373:189-193.
68. Trayhurn, P., Jones, P.M., McGuckin, M.M., and Goodbody, A.E. (1982): Nature (Lond.) 295:323-325.
69. Trayhurn, P., Thurlby, P.L., James, W.P.T. (1976): Proc.Nutr.Soc. 35:133A.
70. Triandafillou, J., Gwilliam, C., and Himms-Hagen, J. (1982): Can.J.Biochem. 60:530-537.
71. Triandafillou, J., and Himms-Hagen, J. (1982):Am.J.Physiol.(in press).
72. Vallin, I. (1970): Acta Zoologica 51:129-139.
73. Van der Kroon, P.H.W., and Boldewijn, H. (1980): IRCS Med.Sci. 8:859.
74. Van der Kroon, P.H.W., Boldewijn, H., and Langeveld-Soeter, N. (1982): Int.J.Obesity 6:83-90.
75. Van der Kroon, P.H.W., Wittgen-Struik, G., and Vermeulen, L. (1981): Int.J.Obesity 5:353-358.
76. Vander Tuig, J.G., Flynn, A.M., Romsos, D.R., and Leveille, G.A. (1980): Fed. Proc. 39:887.
77. Vander Tuig, J.G., Trostler, N., Romsos, D.R., and Leveille, G.A. (1979): Proc. Sco. exp. Biol. Med. 160:266-271.
78. Webb, G.A., Jagot, S.A., Rogers, P.D., and Jakobson, M.E. (1980): IRCS Med.Sci. 8:163-164.
79. York, D.A., Hershman, J.M., Utiger, R.D., and Bray, G.A. (1972): Endocrinology 90:67-72.
80. Young, J.B., and Landsberg, L. (1980): J.clin.Invest. 65:1086-1094.
81. Young, J.B., Saville, E., Rothwell, N.J., and Stock, M.J. (1982): J.clin.Invest. 69:1061-1071.
82. Zaror-Behrens, G., and Himms-Hagen, J. (1982): Am.J.Physiol. (in press).

The Adipocyte and Obesity: Cellular and Molecular Mechanisms, edited by A. Angel, C. H. Hollenberg, and D. A. K. Roncari. Raven Press, New York © 1983.

Thermic Effect of Overfeeding: Role of Thyroid Hormones, Catecholamines, and Insulin Resistance

Elliot Danforth, Jr. and Ethan A. H. Sims

Metabolic Unit, Department of Medicine, College of Medicine, University of Vermont, Burlington, Vermont 05405

Newman: How comes it, my lord, that thou dost engorge thyself and add nere a stone to thy weight, whilst thine peer, under restraint, dost so sadly augment himself?
                    Shakespere Henry VII Part IV, Act II, Scene 1.

Every since Lavoisier demonstrated animal respiration, there has been the tendency to assume that man burns his fuels with a constant even flame and with a constant efficiency. The question has been raised whether individuals utilize energy with the same nutritional efficiency under all dietary conditions. There is now evidence in man as well as in animals of adaptive changes in thermogenesis during overnutrition which may be responsible for changes in the efficiency with which fuels are utilized and which could have important survival value in times of famine, but which could be a liability in times of affluence.

Several potentially thermogenic metabolic processes have been suggested that separately or in concert might explain such a phenomenon (25). These processes are hormonally regulated, with modulation by availability of substrates and also by central nervous control. Most hormones are thermogenic to some degree, but the thyroid hormones and catecholamines in the form of sympathetic nervous system activity appear to carry the principal burden for regulating the thermogenic processes of the body. These two hormonal systems are ideally suited for this purpose, the thyroid hormones contributing to the slow response and catecholamines to the more rapid response of thermogenesis to environmental factors. In addtion, there is recent evidence that the thermogenic response to insulin varies with the degree of insulin resistance. The nutritionally induced alterations in thyroid hormone and catecholamine metabolism and the possible role of insulin resistance will be reviewed, with particular reference to their possible roles in regulating thermogenesis and the thermogenic response to overnutrition.

ENERGY EXPENDITURE: RESPONSE TO OVERNUTRITION

In the Vermont studies of experimental obesity in man, it was clear that there was great individual variation in the ability of lean, prison volunteers to gain weight following long periods of overeating (26). These observations resurrected the old and generally discredited theories that man could adapt to excess intake

271

by expending calories inefficiently. During this century this assumption has been questioned and tested by a number of authors. Neumann (15) was the first to demonstrate in man, by means of three marathon experiments, that his weight could remain at a constant plateau in spite of wide variations of caloric intake. This ability, however, did not prevent him from developing a middle-age spread between experiments. Garrow (9) has recently reviewed the fifteen studies prior to 1977 which were designed to test what Neumann referred to as "luxuskonsumption". The concept probably had its origin in the work of Voit (29), who emphasized that animals utilized only what they needed from available food and who included energy intake in this. His pupil Rubner (6) clearly described the concept of adaptive thermobenesis when he wrote "The stream of food increases, but it does not determine the size of consumption. Apparently the organism does. At first the organism builds reserves, then it deposits additional substance, and finally, with increasing heat production it gets rid of the ample food intake, at least in part." Such an adaptation could have survival value in enabling an animal or person to take an excess of foodstuff of poor quality to obtain an essential nutrient, such as protein or sodium, while being less subject to the development of obesity. It is not always agreed, however, that this increased energy expenditure is in excess of the energy requirements for all the processes required for energy storage and for synthesize of new tissue, as well as for physical activity. The problem then is to determine whether excess calorie intake in the adult individual, who has acheived his or her genetically determined weight and body compostion, results in the predicted storage of energy, or whether individual differences in energy expenditure may exist which might contribute to or perpetuate obesity to a greater extent in one individual than in another. Solving this problem is not an easy task.

Two approaches have generally been used in man in the attempt to demonstrate adaptive thermogenesis during periods of overfeeding. The first, is to determine whether nutritional efficiency is altered following long periods of overfeeding and significant change in body composition. This is no longer practical because of the long-term confinement required for this kind of studies. Our own extended studies (26) with prison inmates as volunteers were consistently successful from a humane point of view, but in the present climate prisoners are no longer eligible to volunteer for such studies. The second method is to overfeed lean and obese volunteers over shorter periods of time and then to estimate whether there are differences in the components of thermogenesis or in the response to thermogenic stimuli. During short-term studies of overfeeding the changes in weight are small. Unfortunately, the methods for estimating the composition of this change in weight, and therefore the energy stored, are not sensitive enough to detect individual differences in energy expenditure (adaptive thermogenesis). A direct approach to this problem would be the simultaneous measurement of energy expenditure and nitrogen balance with overfeeding. Studies of this nature have been performed in man (16) but energy expenditure has only been estimated and not actually measured. These studies have been complicated by including supposedly normal subjects with widely varying metabolic status and response to overeating. It is possible that individuals with differing subtypes of obesity may differ in their response to overfeeding, and inclusion of different types in a single experimental group of obese, such as those with early and late onset obesity, and those with a genetic tendency toward type II diabetes, may mask significant differences. Therefore, there are no studies to date which have convincingly proved or disproven whether individual differences may exist in energy expenditure in response to over-feeding in man.

MEASURING ENERGY EXPENDITURE IN MAN

The formula which expresses the energy stored within the body in response to intake is not complicated.

$$\text{Energy In} = (\text{Energy Stored}) - (\text{Energy Expended})$$

Energy expenditure can only be measured or estimated with difficulty. It can be estimated directly by measuring heat losses in a whole body calorimeter. However, this procedure is too confining for the subjects for the long-periods required for these studies. Fortunately, early in this century, Atwater and Benedict (1) confirmed that the heat released from the body by the oxidation of fuels could be accurately predicted from the oxygen consumed and carbon dioxide produced by measurement of respiratory exchange using an indirect calorimeter, if appropriately adjusted for the protein catabolized. Ideally, an "indirect calorimeter" should be built large enough to allow a subject to live, eat and sleep for several days in it while relatively unencumbered. There are only a few chambers, such as the one in the Physiology Institute at the University of Lausanne, Switzerland, at the Dunn Research Laboratory in Cambridge and the Medical Research Council Laboratories in Harrow, England, which are accurate enough to measure the small individual differences in energy expenditure which may exist. A less satisfactory method is to measure thermogenesis indirectly using a mouth-peice or a ventilated hood for collections of expired gases. Such methods of energy expenditure are limited to relatively short periods of time.

For conceptual reasons, energy expenditure can be divided into several components (Figure 1).

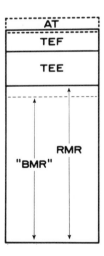

Figure 1.
(See text)

COMPONENTS OF THERMOGENESIS

The most familiar of these components of thermogenesis is the basal metabolic rate (BMR). While at the Mayo Clinic, Boothby defined and popularized the use of the BMR for the diagnosis of disorders of the thyroid. He defined this function as the energy expended by an individual when bodily and mentally at rest 12 to 18 hours after a meal in a thermoneutral environment. Much to the inconvenience of the patient and physician alike, measurements were done during the early morning hours when the circadium rhythm of oxygen consumption was known to be at a low. Because of the increase in metabolism caused by the muscular and mental unrest introduced by this procedure, it is unlikely that the true "basal" metabolism was often measured. Therefore, for practical and conceptual reasons, the BMR is now rarely measured. In its place we now measure what is referred to as the resting metabolic rate (RMR), which may be (but is not always) higher than the BMR as defined by Boothby. Particularly for comparison of the RMR between individuals, relating the RMR to fat free mass, as kcal/kg FFM, when body composition can be measured is more meaningful and hopefully will become accepted practice.

Resting Metabolic Rate

RMR usually accounts for 60 to 75% of our energy expenditure. The RMR varies among individuals. For instance, obese subjects generally have higher RMR (and BMR) than lean people. This was recognized by the early investigators who "normalized" these values. They noted that metabolic rate correlated loosely with surface area and therefore corrected the metabolic rate for the subjects surface areas. This did not account for the usually higher values observed for women and lower values for older subjects. Therefore, correction factors were also applied for sex and age. Today, the fat free mass, sometimes erroneously referred to as lean body mass, is considered the most important determinate of resting metabolism. However, even when related to the fat free mass, there may be as much as a 30% variation in the RMR between and within individuals. Part of this variation can be related to the antecedent diet and nutritional state.

Subjects who have been starving, or who have been given diets restricted in caloric intake just prior to the measurements, have a lowering of the RMR which is out of proportion to any change in fat free mass. However, if a patient has lost weight and a new plateau of body weight has been established, the RMR, corrected for fat free mass, will usually have returned to normal (8). The acute reduction in RMR is a source of frustration to those attempting to lose weight by dieting, since weight loss becomes less than expected as adaptation takes place.

Early in our studies of experimental obesity in man we became aware of a marked variation in the ability to individuals to "augment themselves". Lean dedicated volunteers, earnestly overeating, had an increased requirement of calories relative to size to maintain their added weight. Their intake at each meal and supplemental feeding was closely monitored and the caloric content estimated from tables. Physical activity and initiative tended to diminish as they became overweight, though there was of course the added cost of moving their increased bulk. They gained 14-25% above their ideal starting weight by overeating over a period of several months, and required 50% more calories per square meter of B.S.A. to maintain this heavier weight. In more recent studies we have found an increment of 10% in the RMR accompanying overfeeding (30). Naturally overweight subjects, with some exceptions, also increase their RMR when challenged with excess calories. However, when expressed as a percent of resting metabolism properly corrected for fat free mass, this is usually less than in lean subjects (12). More studies are required to determine whether the increase in RMR in response to overfeeding is blunted in obese subjects.

Thermic Effect of Exercise

The second largest component of thermogenesis is the energy above RMR expended for muscular activity. In a sedentary individual, this does not exceed 15 to 20% while in more active subjects this may amount to 30% of the 24 hour energy expenditure. Except perhaps in lumberjacks and mountain climbers and the like, it is unlikely that the expenditure, even in the most active individuals can average greater than 50% of the individuals 24 hour energy requirements. We have found no convincing evidence for a difference in the caloric costs of exercise between lean and obese subjects, except for that due to the obviously increased energy costs to the obese of moving their increased weight and to a possilbe hobbling effect of the adipose tissue itself. No difference in efficiency of exercise was discovered after overfeeding in our lean or obese volunteers. There, however, remains a question as to whether there may be a synergistic effect on energy expenditure when exercise is performed directly following ingestion of a meal (14,23).

Thermic Effect of Food (TEF)

The third compartment of thermogenesis is the increased thermogenesis that accompanies ingestion of a meal. In the past, this was thought to be a specific effect of the protein in the meal that was metabolized to urea and was referred to as the specific dynamic action (SDA) of protein. It is now recognized that the increased thermogenesis following a meal is not restricted to this, but is related to the caloric content and probably the composition of the meal and other factors as well. It varies with the antecedent state of nutrition and possibly even with the degree of obesity. The thermic response to a meal can be calculated by relating the energy expended above resting to the caloric value of the meal, or more simply, as the increase in oxygen consumption above resting for the several hours following the meal. Most of the thermic effect of food can be accounted for by the digestion, absorption, transport, metabolism, and storage of the ingested food.

Thermic Effect of Insulin

Insulin secretion is a factor in the thermic effect of food. DeFronzo et al. (6) while working in Jequier's laboratory in Lausanne, showed that by combining te euglycemic hyperinsulinemic clamp technique with measurement of the respiratory exchange, hepatic glucose production, and nitrogen excretion it is possible to estimate the routes of disposal of glucose during insulin stimulation as well as the changes in thermogenesis. Ravussin and Bogardus (18) have recently used this combined technique to study the thermic response to insulin of normal subjects. As suggested by Ravussin et al. (19) one component of insulin's action may operate to reduce net thermogenesis by reducing the cost of the gluconeogenic component of hepatic glucose production. The importance of blunting of these effects of insulin in the obese and in the non-insulin-dependent diabetic is discussed below.

The energy costs of these processes may not account for the entire thermogenic response to the meal. Activation of the sympathetic nervous system by carbohydrate or some other component in the meal may be responsible for part of this thermogenic response. We, (4) as well as others, (17) have found a reduced TEF in obese compared to lean subjects. Obese subjects generally have an increase in hepatic glucose production which contributes to their total energy output. As suggested by Ravussin et al. (19), when insulin is given to such subjects or when insulin sensitivity is improved, this component of thermogenesis is decreased, and this may partly explain a lesser net change. We have found no augmentation in the TEF following overfeeding in either lean or obese subjects.

ADAPTIVE THERMOGENESIS

When the rat is exposed to cold, after acclimitization there is an increase in thermogenesis, referred to as non-shivering thermogenesis, which is well established and which is dependent upon increase in thyroid hormone and catecholamine activity and involves stimulation of brown adipose tissue. The question of the presence of this component of thermogenesis in man is still controversial.

Rothwell and Stock (20) have developed a model of overfeeding in rats which in many respects mimics our experiments of overfeeding in man. In this model, the rat overeats in response to an interesting selection of foods. This "cafeteria" overfeeding program is remarkably successful in encouraging gluttony in the rat. The interesting point, is that the rats, like the subjects of our overfeeding experiments in man, do not always gain the weight expected as a result of the increased intake, and they also show increased thermogenesis, both at rest and in response to infusion of norepinephrine. We have recently confirmed these observations in the rat (27,28). In this model there is hyperplasia of brown adipose tissue, which raises the possibility that the mechanisms responsible for the increased thermogenesis in the cafeteria rat are the same as those responsible for the increased thermogenesis in these animals following cold acclimitization (22). In the cold-adapted rat, the increased thermogenesis is regulated by the central nervous system through release of norepinephrine from nerve endings in the brown adipose tissue. This process requires the presence of either intact or increased thyroidal activity. The intriguing similarities between the increased thermogenesis and hormonal responses of the cold-adapted and "cafeteria" overfed rat suggested to us that we should further investigate nutritionally-induced alterations in thyroid hormone and catecholamine (norephinephrine) metabolism.

NUTRITIONALLY-INDUCED ALTERATIONS IN THYROID HORMONE METABOLISM

Under normal conditions, only a small amount of triiodothyronine (T_3) is secreted from the thyroid gland, whereas the remainder is formed through the monodeiodinative pathways which are dependent upon intermediary metabolism. There is evidence that important outer ring deiodinase, 5'-diodinase, which is responsible for the conversion of T_4 to T_3, may be the same enzyme as for the conversion of rT_3 to $3,3'-T_2$ (Figure 2). The highest activity of this enzyme is found in the microsomal membrane fractions of the liver and the kidneys. Accelerated glucose metabolism and a redux state yielding favorable conditions for reduced sufhydryl groups enhance 5'-deiodinase activity (2).

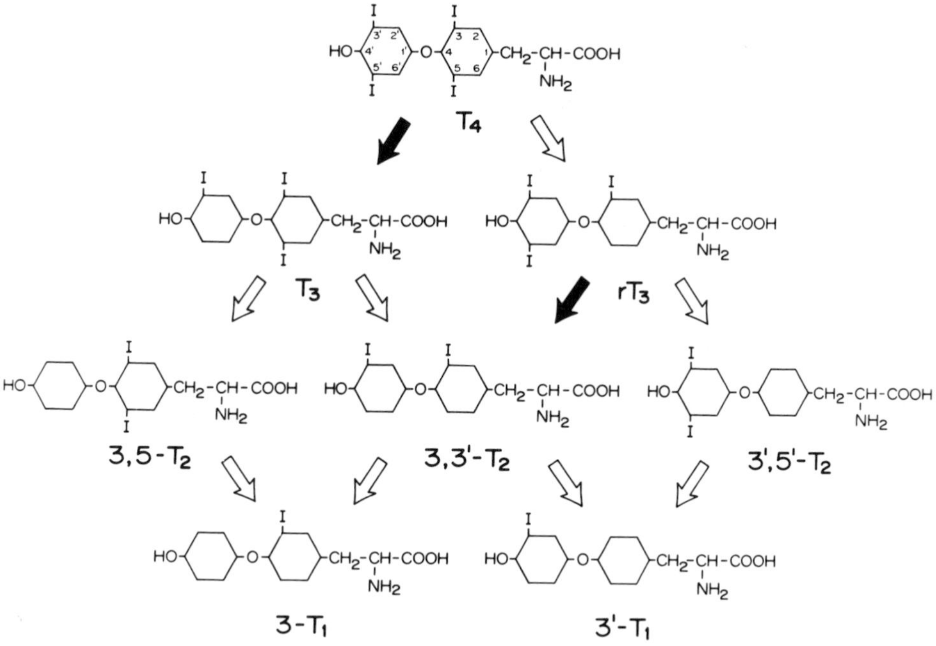

Figure 2. (See text)

Figure 3 summarizes the recognized effects of overnutrition and undernutrition on peripheral thyroid hormone metabolism. Starvation induces a shift of the metabolism of T_4 from outer to inner ring monodeodination, which results in decreased serum concentrations of T_3 and increased concentrations of rT_3. It appears that the caloric restriction alters the conversion of T_3 and rT_3 by reducing the peripheral conversion of T_4 to T_3 and by reducing the metabolic clearance rate of rT_3. Since the metabolic clearance rate of T_4 during starvation remains unchanged or declines slightly, there is a net shunting of T_4 metabolism away from T_3 and toward rT_3. Overnutrition, on the other hand, is associated with increased concentrations of T_3 without a change in the T_4 concentration.

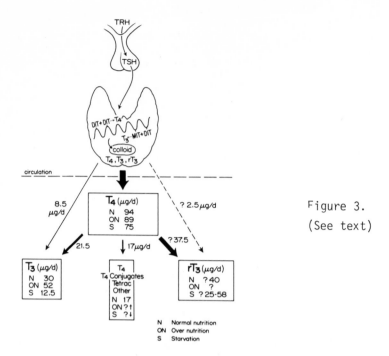

Figure 3.

(See text)

Figure 4 depicts the peripheral kinetics of T_4 and T_3 before and during three weeks of overfeeding of lean caucasians and obese Pima Indians. No alteration was found in the kinetics of T_4 following overfeeding in either group of subjects. As noted, overfeeding caused an increased metabolic clearance and production rate of T_3 in the lean subjects but not in the obese subjects. In another group of overfed obese caucasions, we found no increase in the metabolic clearance rate but a small increase in the production rate of T_3, again without an alteration in the T_4 kinetics following overfeeding. Further studies will be required to determine whether there may be quantitative and/or qualitative differences in peripheral thyroid hormone metabolism in response to overfeeding between lean and obese subjects.

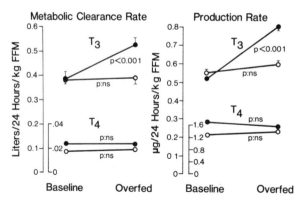

Figure 4. (See text)

NUTRITIONALLY-INDUCED ALTERATIONS IN NOREPHINEPHRINE METABOLISM

The role of the sympathetic nervous system in non-shivering thermo-genesis in rats exposed to cold is well established. As noted earlier, the similarity between the increased thermogenesis accom-paning cold acclimitization and overfeeding in the rat is consistent with a role for the sympathetic nervous system in both conditions. Sympathetic blockade antagonizes the increased oxygen consumption of cold acclimitized (21) and also of overfed rats, (20) and the sympath-omimetic agent, levodopa, prevents in man the decline in oxygen consumption which accompanies caloric restriction (24).

Until recently, it was assumed that sympathetic nervous system activity was increased by acute caloric restriction. In fact, just the opposite appears to be the case. Caloric restriction diminishes plasma catecholamines and decreases urinary catecholamines and cate-cholamine metabolites (7,11). Increased plasma norepinephrine concen-trations and increased oxygen consumption in association with cardio-vascular signs of sympathetic stimulation, follow glucose ingestion in normal man. Changes in sympathetic nervous system activity, therefore appear to accompany changes in dietary intake in man. Further evidence in support of this can be found in the following chapter by Landsberg on diet induced changes in sympathetic nervous system activity.

The effect of short-term overfeeding on sympathetic nervous system activity in man is under active investigation. The important question is whether differences may exist between lean and obese subjects which could lead to difference in energy expenditure in response to overfeeding. In recent studies (13) we have examined the sensitivity of lean and obese caucasian volunteers to graded in-fusions of norepinephrine. No differences in energy expenditure were uncovered either before or after short-term overfeeding in these studies. However, in similar studies in obese Pima Indians (5), there was an increase in the thermogenic response to graded doses of norepinephrine which normalize following overfeeding. This dif-ference in responsiveness from lean caucasians appear to be the result of increased concentrations of norepinephrine achieved following the infusions. This has been interpreted to indicate that there might be a defect in the metabolic clearance rate of norepi-nephrine in these obese subjects. It is too soon to say whether there are other differences in the metabolism of norepinephrine between lean and obese subjects or between lean and obese subjects after overfeeding.

NUTRITIONALLY INDUCED ALTERATIONS IN INSULIN RESPONSE

By combining the euglycemic hyperinsulinemic clamp technique with indirect calorimetry, Ravussin et al. at Vermont (16) found that the obese have an impaired thermogenic response, and the non-insulin-dependent diabetic a further impairment. This takes the form of blunting and a delay in the response. Whether the total thermic response per mole of glucose disposed is reduced is difficult at present to say. This suggests that one component of the reduced thermogenic response to overfeeding of the obese and of the Type IIB diabetic may be this blunted insulin sensitivity. This is given strong support by an important observation of Cummingham et al (30). They found that when mature rat were fed a cafeteria diet they ate 45-60 percent more and gained 40-50 percent in weight. Brown fat increased in all. Forty-three percent of the rats developed slightly inpaired glucose tolerance. Those that did not had the expected increase in adaptive thermogenesis, with only 3.3 gm of body tissue laid down per 100 kcal of intake, as opposed to 3.7 in chow fed rats. Those that developed impaired glucose tolerance, however, had even greater efficiency of weight gain in comparison with the controls, forming 3.9 gm of tissue per 100 kcal of intake, in spite of a 20-30% greater increase in brown fat. This work has the important implication that acquired impairment in glucose tolerance can be associated with increased tendency toward weight gain. We know from the Vermont study that simple overeating can lead to impairment of glucose tolerance, but our subjects promptly gravitated back to their previous normal weight. In this respect they behaved like the rats that showed no impairment of glucose tolerance. Apparently there must be an additional factor or factors to account for the imparied tolerance and inefficiency of weight gain in the glucose intolerant group of rats. In the case of overweight patients with non-insulin dependent diabetes in an inherited factor leading to glucose intolerance may lead to the same efficiency of gain in weight.

CONCLUSIONS

The evidence has been reviewed which suggests that overnutrition alters peripheral thyroid hormone metabolism and sympathetic nervous system activity, both of which changes could have important effects on thermogensis and, either singly or in concert, cause the increase in resting metabolic rate and inefficiency of weight gain when lean and some obese subjects are overfed. Possible differences in the thermogenic adaptation to overfeeding between lean and obese subjects have been discussed. Evidence to date is still inconclusive as to whether impaired adaptation to overfeeding may contribute to the development of obesity in man. The thermogenic response to insulin is decreased in the obese with insulin resistance and further decreased in the overweight non-insulin-dependent diabetic. This may impair an adaptive response in these subjects and may predispose them to further development of obesity.

ACKNOWLEDGEMENTS

Supported in part by U.S. Public Health Service grants GCRC RR-109, AM 18535 (Dr. Danforth) and AM 10254 (Dr. Sims).

REFERENCES

1.   Atwater, W.V., Benedict, F.G. (1905): Carnegie Institution of Washington Publication, 42.

2.   Burger, A.G., Burger, M., Wimpfheimer and Danforth, E., Jr. (1980): Acta. Endocrinologica, 93:322-331.

3. Cunningham, J., Calles, J., Eisikowitz, L., Zawalich, W., and Felig, P. (1982): Clin. Res., 30:699A.

4. Danforth, E., Jr., Daniels, R.J., Katzeff, H.L., Ravussin, E. and Garrow, J.S. (1981): Clin. Res. 29:663A.

5. Daniels, R.J., Katzeff, H.L., Ravussin, E., Garrow, J.S. and Danforth, E., Jr. (1982): Clin. Res. 30:244A.

6. DeFronzo, R.A., Jacot, E., Jequier, E., Maeder, E., Wahren, J. and Felber, J.P. (1981): Diabetes, 30:1000-1007.

7. DeHaven, J., Sherwin, R., Hendler, R. and Felig, P. (1980): N. Engl. J. Med., 302:477-482.

8. Doré, C., Hesp, R., Wilkins, W. and Garrow, J.S. (1982): Human Nutrition: Clinical Nutrition, 36C:41-48.

9. Garrow, J.S. (1977): Recent Advances in Obesity Research II Proceedings of the 2nd International Congress on Obesity edited by G.S. Bray, pp. 200-210.

10. Goldman, R.F., Haisman, M.F., Bynum, G., Salans, L.B., Danforth, E., Jr., Horton, E.S. and Sims, E.A.H. (1976): In: Obesity in Perspective, edited by G.A.Bray, pp. 165-186. Fogarty International Center Series on Preventive Medicine, Washington, D.C. DHEW Publication No. NIH 75-708.

11. Jung, R.T., Shetty, P.S., Barrand, M., Callingham, B.A. and James, W.P.T. (1979): Br. Med. J. 1:12-13.

12. Katzeff, H.L. and Danforth, E., Jr. (1981): Clin. Res. 29: 663A.

13. Katzeff, H.L. and Danforth, E., Jr. (1982); Clin. Res. 30:245A.

14. Miller, D.S., Mumford, P. and Stock, M.J. (1967): Clin. Nut. 20:1223.

15. Neumann, R.O. (1902): Archives of Hygiene 45:1.

16. Norgan, N.G. and Durnin, V.G.A. (1980); Am. J. Clin. Nut. 33: 978-988.

17. Pittet, P., Chappuis, P., Acheson, K., Detechtermann, F. and Jéquier, E. (1976): Brit. J. Nutri. 35:281-292.

18. Ravussin, E. and Bogardus, C. (in press). Life Sciences.

19. Ravussin, E., Bogardus, C., Schwartz, R.S., Robbins, D.C., Wolfe, R.R., Horton, E.S., Danforth, E., Jr. and Sims, E.A.H. (1982): Submitted.

20. Rothwell, N.J., Stock, M.J. (1979): Nature, 281:31-35.

21. Rothwell, N.J., and Stock, M.J. (1980): Can. J. Physiol. Pharm.
     58:842-848.

22. Rubner, M. (1902): Die Gestze des Energie Verbrauchs bei die
     Ernährung. Translated 1968 R.J.T. Joy, U.S. Army Research
     Institute of Environmental Medicine, Natick, Massachusetts.

23. Segal, K. and Gutin, B. (1982): Joint AIN-ASCN-CSNS Meeting,
     July 22-24 in press.

24. Shetty, P.S., Jung, R.T., James, W.P.T. (1979): Lancet, 1:77-79.

25. Sims, E.A.H., (1976): Clin. Endo. Metab. 5:377-393.

26. Sims, E.A.H., Danforth, E., Jr., Horton, E.S., Bray, G.A.,
     Glennon, J.A. and Salans, L.B. (1973): Recent Progress in
     Hormone Research, 29:457-496.

27. Tulp, O.L., Frink, R., and Danforth, E., Jr. (1982): Nutrition,
     in press.

28. Tulp, O.L., Gregory, M.H. and Danforth, E., Jr. (1982): Life
     Sciences, in press.

29. Voit, C. (1881): Handbuch der Physiologie, 6:209.

The Adipocyte and Obesity: Cellular and
Molecular Mechanisms, edited by A. Angel,
C. H. Hollenberg, and D. A. K. Roncari.
Raven Press, New York © 1983.

Diet-Induced Changes in Sympathetic Nervous System Activity

Lewis Landsberg and James B. Young

*Charles A. Dana Research Institute and Thorndike Laboratory, Department of Medicine,
Beth Israel Hospital, Harvard Medical School, Boston, Massachusetts 02215*

The relationship between dietary intake and sympathetic nervous system activity has been studied in our laboratory over the last seven years. Measurements of norepinephrine (NE) turnover in sympathetically innervated organs of the rat have provided evidence that diet exerts an important influence on the functional state of the sympathetic nervous system (SNS). Fasting suppresses, while overfeeding stimulates sympathetic activity. Experiments demonstrating an effect of diet on the SNS are summarized here along with evidence that suggests a role for insulin-mediated glucose metabolism within the central nervous system in the coupling of dietary intake and sympathetic outflow.

The experiments described here were performed on female Sprague-Dawley (SD) rats weighing approximately 180 grams with the exception of the cafeteria fed and cold exposed animals in which 120 gram male SD rats were used and the experiments on fat intake which employed 120 gram female SD rats. NE turnover was determined from the rate of disappearance of a tracer dose of tritiated NE from heart, interscapular brown adipose tissue, or other organs. After administration as an IV bolus, ^{3}H-NE is rapidly cleared from the circulation and taken up by sympathetic nerve endings throughout the body, where it equilibrates with the endogenous NE store. The decline in NE specific activity over time follows first order kinetics and permits computation of a fractional turnover rate or slope, as well as a calculated turnover rate, which is equal to the product of the slope and the steady state endogenous NE level. Since sympathetic activity is the major determinant of NE turnover, the NE turnover rate provides an index of SNS activity.

DIETARY INTAKE AND SYMPATHETIC ACTIVITY

Fasting and Restricted Caloric Intake

As shown in Table 1, fasting and caloric restriction suppress NE turnover in heart (9,17). Suppression of cardiac NE turnover begins promptly during the first day of a fast (10) and is rapidly restored towards normal with refeeding (18). The reduction in cardiac NE turnover is secondary to diminished central sympathetic activity as indicated by

experiments involving ganglionic blocking agents (6,17). Decreased
sympathetic activity is demonstrable in a variety of organs other than
heart (18) and occurs throughout the lifespan of the rat, from six weeks
through two years of age (8).

TABLE 1.   Effect of fasting and caloric restriction on cardiac NE turnover
in the rat

	Fractional NE Turnover (k), %/h	Calculated NE Turnover Rate (NETR) ng/h	% Change NETR vs Control	Reference
Exp 1				
Control fed	5.7 + 0.1	23.1 + 1.5		
Fast 48h	2.7 + 0.2[a]	13.1 + 1.2	-43%	(17)
Exp 2				
Control fed	6.4 + 0.1	42.4 + 8.0		
Fast 15h	3.8 + 1.0[b]	28.3 + 8.4	-29%	(10)
Fast 48h	3.3 + 1.0[b]	27.7 + 8.9	-35%	
Exp 3				
Control fed	6.8 + 0.2	32.5 + 3.1		
Fast 48h	1.8 + 0.2[a]	9.4 + 1.4	-71%	(18)
Refed 1d after 48h fast	3.8 + 0.2[c]	21.2 + 1.7	-35%	
Exp 4				
Control fed	6.4 + 0.7	36.2 + 5.6		
Caloric restriction 35% control intake	3.6 + 0.8[c]	25.0 + 6.2	-61%	(9)

[a]$p<0.001$,   [b]$p<0.05$,   [c]$p<0.01$, vs control

Studies in humans are not as definitive, although the available
evidence is consistent with sympathetic suppression during fasting or
caloric restriction. Plasma NE levels are reduced in obese subjects on
restricted caloric intake (2,5), as well as in patients with anorexia
nervosa (4). Unpublished studies from our laboratory demonstrate a
significant fall in urinary NE excretion during a three day fast in
normal weight human subjects. A recent study utilizing a tracer technique to estimate rate of appearance of NE in the circulation, and rate
of NE clearance, demonstrated significant reduction of NE appearance
after ten days of a 400 kcal per day balanced diet in normal weight human
subjects (7), a finding consistent with diminished sympathetic activity.

Overfeeding

Sucrose.
Overfeeding sucrose increases cardiac NE turnover as shown in Table 2
(16). When ad lib access to dilute solutions of sucrose (in addition to
standard chow diet) is provided, rats increase their caloric intake by
about 30%. Under these circumstances, cardiac NE turnover is increased

within the first day of overfeeding sucrose (10); the increase persists throughout eight days of sucrose overfeeding, and is restored to normal one day after sucrose is withdrawn and normal chow feeding resumed (10). Experiments with ganglionic blocking agents indicate that the increase in NE turnover is secondary to increased central sympathetic activity (6,16). Increased sympathetic activity in response to sucrose occurs throughout the lifespan of the rat (8), and is demonstrable in a variety of organs other than heart (18).

TABLE 2. Effect of overfeeding on cardiac NE turnover in the rat

	Fractional NE Turnover (k), %/h	Calculated NE Turnover Rate (NETR) ng/h	% Change NETR vs Control	Reference
Exp 1				
Control fed	4.8 + 0.2	21.4 + 1.9		
Sucrose fed 3d	8.5 + 0.1[a]	30.6 + 2.3	+43%	(16)
Exp 2				
Control fed	7.7 + 0.9	44.7 + 6		
Sucrose fed 15h	11.4 + 0.9[b]	61.8 + 7.1	+38%	(10)
Sucrose fed 3d	13.2 + 3.0[b]	71.0 + 17.7	+59%	
Exp 3				
Control fed	5.3 + 0.9	33.2 + 6.6		
Sucrose fed 8d	7.9 + 0.9[b]	44.5 + 6.5	+35%	(10)
Exp 4				
Control fed	7.2 + 0.5	48.3 + 5.3		
Cafeteria fed 9d	12.7 + 1.0[b]	80.2 + 9.7	+66%	(22)

[a]$p<0.001$,   [b]$p<0.05$, vs control

In human subjects, the acute administration of glucose increases plasma NE levels (15,21) in association with increased oxygen consumption and evidence of cardiovascular stimulation. These observations are consistent with, but do not prove, sympathetic activation during the immediate postprandial state following glucose administration. Long term effects of overfeeding sucrose in man have not been reported.

Mixed diet.
Rats overfed a mixed, highly palatable (cafeteria) diet increase caloric intake approximately 50-100% (11). After ten days of "cafeteria" feeding, cardiac NE turnover is increased (22) as shown in Table 2. Although only a limited amount of information is available in human subjects, the recent study utilizing ^{3}H-NE mentioned above demonstrates that the NE appearance rate in plasma increases when normal human subjects were fed a mixed diet, 1,000 calories above the level required for weight maintenance, for ten days (7), consistent with increased sympathetic nervous system activity.

Fat.
Recent experiments also demonstrate the effect of fat intake on SNS

activity (14). In the experiments shown in Table 3, chow intake was restricted to the same level in three groups of animals; one group received only the restricted chow (control), another received fat supplements in the form of lard, and the third was supplemented with sucrose, the fat and sucrose supplements being isocaloric. In comparison with the restricted chow control, both sucrose and fat markedly increased cardiac NE turnover. This experiment does not represent fat overfeeding, but does demonstrate that fat, when added to the diet, affects the sympathetic nervous system. Subsequent preliminary studies indicate that the increase in NE turnover is secondary to an increase in sympathetic activity and that organs other than heart are similarly affected.

TABLE 3. Effect of fat intake on cardiac NE turnover

	Fractional NE Turnover (k), %/h	Calculated NE Turnover Rate (NETR) ng/h	% Change NETR vs Control	Reference
Control (restricted chow)	1.8 ± 0.8	6.5 ± 2.9		
Fat (chow + lard)	15.4 ± 2.1^a	50.8 ± 9.1	+780%	(14)
Sucrose (chow + sucrose)	11.6 ± 1.3^a	35.6 ± 5.4	+550%	(14)

[a]$p < 0.001$, vs control

THE SIGNAL THAT COUPLES CHANGES IN DIETARY INTAKE WITH SYMPATHETIC ACTIVITY

Hypoglycemia and 2-Deoxy-Glucose

The stimulatory effect of hypoglycemia on the adrenal medulla has been recognized for over 50 years. Recent studies from our laboratory have demonstrated that hypoglycemia, induced in pregnant rats by fasting (19), or by administration of a glycosuric agent (phlorizin) to fasting rats (6), suppresses SNS activity depsite concomitant stimulation of the adrenal medulla. Similarly, 2-deoxy-glucose, a glucose analog which disrupts intracellular glucose metabolism, when administered to fed rats diminishes sympathetic activity while the adrenal medulla is stimulated (9). The fact that fasting, hypoglycemia, and 2-deoxy-glucose all suppress sympathetic activity suggest that glucose utilization within the central nervous system may be involved in the relationship between dietary intake and sympathetic activity. In fasting normal animals, in whom plasma glucose concentration is maintained above 50 mg/dl, marked stimulation of the adrenal medulla does not occur.

Potential Role of Insulin

Thus, plasma glucose level, by influencing intracellular glucose metabolism within the brain, may affect SNS activity. The plasma glucose level, however, is unlikely to serve as the sole signal in the link between diet and sympathetic activity. Under ordinary circumstances, the plasma glucose level is maintained within rather narrow limits despite wide variations in dietary intake and sympathetic activity. Insulin levels, on the other hand, vary widely throughout the day and reflect caloric intake, particularly intake of carbohydrates. Certain regions of the central nervous system, furthermore, are known to be sensitive to insulin (1). Recent studies from our laboratory have provided evidence that insulin may be involved in the coupling of dietary intake and sympathetic activity. Utilizing insulin and glucose "clamp" techniques, these studies demonstrate that infusion of insulin, with maintenance of the plasma glucose level by simultaneous glucose infusion, is associated with a dose-related increase in plasma NE level (13). Cardiovascular signs of sympathetic stimulation were noted during the insulin infusion. Since insulin infusion was without effect on plasma clearance of NE these data are consistent with an effect of insulin on sympathetic activity. Steady state hyperglycemia, on the other hand, had a negligible effect both on plasma NE level and the cardiovascular system.

Studies in the mouse suggest that the ventromedial portion of the hypothalamus is involved in the initiation of diet-induced changes in sympathetic activity. Gold thioglucose, an agent which destroys portions of the ventromedial hypothalamus, has been shown to block fasting-induced suppression of sympathetic activity in the mouse (20). These findings have been interpreted as indicating an inhibitory pathway from the hypothalamus to the brainstem; during fasting this inhibitory pathway is stimulated resulting in suppression of SNS activity (20). The ventromedial portion of the hypothalamus, furthermore, is sensitive to insulin and glucose (1). Taken as a whole these data are consistent with the hypothesis that insulin mediated glucose metabolism within certain critical hypothalamic neurons, perhaps related to the ventromedial hypothalamus, are involved in the initiation and maintenance of changes in sympathetic activity in response to changes in dietary intake.

Although the insulin hypothesis appears to be a reasonable one, it is unlikely that insulin-mediated glucose metabolism is the sole signal in the relationship between diet and sympathetic activity. The fact that fat affects sympathetic activity (Table 3) suggests that other signals are probably involved as well. Other hormones of enteric origin, as well as afferent neural impulses from the liver and the gut, are probably involved in the relationship between dietary intake and the activity of the sympathetic nervous system.

PHYSIOLOGIC SIGNIFICANCE OF DIET-INDUCED CHANGES IN SYMPATHETIC ACTIVITY

The Sympathetic Nervous System and Diet-Induced Thermogenesis

The sympathetic nervous system plays a critical role in the regulation of adaptive changes in thermogenesis in response to cold exposure. The fact that diet influences sympathetic activity raises the possibility that the sympathetic nervous system may be involved in the regulation of changes in thermogenesis that accompany changes in dietary intake. This hypothesis is supported by recent studies from our laboratory which demonstrate diet-induced changes in SNS activity in brown adipose tissue, the major thermogenic organ in the rat (3).

Sympathetic Activity in Interscapular Brown Adipose Tissue (IBAT) in the Rat

NE turnover techniques have recently been applied to the study of sympathetic outflow to IBAT in the rat (22). As shown in Table 4, these studies demonstrate significant depression of sympathetic activity in IBAT during fasting and significant increase during nine days of "cafeteria" feeding or cold exposure (22). Other studies from our laboratory indicate that overfeeding increases sympathetic activity in IBAT for periods of at least three weeks. These findings are consistent with an important role for the sympathetic nervous system in the regulation of changes in thermogenesis that are known to occur in association with changes in dietary intake in the rat (11,12).

TABLE 4. Effect of diet and cold exposure on IBAT NE turnover in the rat

	Fractional NE Turnover (k), %/h	Calculated NE Turnover Rate (NETR) ng/h	% Change NETR vs Control	Reference
Exp 1				
Control fed	8.6 + 0.8	29.1 + 4.2		
Fast 48h	5.2 + 1.4[a]	18.9 + 5.9	−59%	(22)
Exp 2				
Control	5.8 + 0.8	24.8 + 4.5		
Cafeteria fed 9d	11.0 + 1.1[b]	51.7 + 6.8	+108%	(22)
Cold exposed 9d	11.9 + 1.7[c]	59.5 + 11.0	+138%	

[a] $p < 0.05$,   [b] $p < 0.003$,   [c] $p < 0.001$, vs control

Implications of Diet-Induced Changes in Sympathetic Activity

Famine, starvation and overfeeding.

During periods of famine or starvation suppression of SNS activity would have the useful physiological effect of decreasing metabolic rate and conserving calories. The effect of sympathetic suppression on metabolic rate might be synergistic with the reduced peripheral conversion of T4 to T3 that accompanies fasting or starvation. Alterations in both thyroid hormone metabolism and sympathetic nervous system activity, therefore, may be involved in the metabolic adaptation to the fasting state, an adaptation that reduces energy output and would, therefore, enhance survival.

Conversely, increased sympathetic nervous system activity with overfeeding would increase energy expenditure and aid in the dissipation of calories as heat. Sympathetic stimulation might, in this regard, be synergistic with the increased peripheral conversion of T4 to T3 that occurs during overfeeding. The ability to dissipate excess calories would be of special advantage to organisms on a subsistence diet; by enhancing intake of low quality foodstuffs, the need for essential nutrients, such as protein, could be satisfied without excessive weight gain. The ability to increase energy expenditure with overfeeding would, therefore, insure adequate intake of vital nutrients while preventing storage of excessive calories as fat.

Obesity.

If, in fact, the hypothesis that diet-induced changes in sympathetic activity are important in the regulation of metabolic energy expenditure is correct, important implications for the pathogenesis and treatment of obesity may emerge. An abnormality in either sympathetic activation with feeding or overfeeding, or in the thermogenic response to NE, might be associated with a "thrifty" metabolic trait resulting in efficient utilization of foodstuffs with excessive fuel storage. Such a trait would serve well during periods of semi-starvation and famine; with an abundant food supply, however, individuals with this "thrifty" trait would be predisposed to the development of obesity. Both the sympathetic responses to feeding and the responsiveness to obese individuals to the thermogenic effects of catecholamines require additional study.

Similarly, if suppression of sympathetic activity and decreased peripheral conversion of T4 and T3 contribute to the metabolic adaptation to starvation by reducing energy output, these same metabolic adaptations will be called into play during therapeutic dieting. By decreasing energy output in response to diminished caloric intake, these metabolic adaptations would serve to limit weight loss and imapir the effectiveness of low energy diets.

Finally, diet-induced changes in sympathetic activity may also be involved, at least in part, in the changes in blood pressure that occur when caloric intake is altered. Suppression of sympathetic activity with caloric restriction may contribute to the beneficial effect of diet on blood pressure in hypertensive subjects. Conversely, the relationship between obesity and hypertension may involve, at least in part, diet-induced changes in sympathetic activity. Excessive stimulation of the sympathetic nervous system in response to overfeeding may contribute to the elevated blood pressure that frequently complicates obesity. Increased blood pressure, as well as increased storage of foodstuffs as fat, may be a consequence of overeating in some obese hypertensive individuals.

REFERENCES

1. Debons, A.F., Krimsky, I., From, A., and Cloutier, R.J.(1969): Am. J. Physiol., 217:1114-1118.

2. DeHaven, J., Sherwin, R., Hendler, R., and Felig, P.(1980): N. Engl. J. Med., 302:477-482.

3. Foster, D.O., and Frydman, M.L.(1978): Can. J. Physiol. Pharmacol. 56:110-122.

4. Gross, H.A., Lake, C.R., Ebert, M.H., Ziegler, M.G., and Kopin, I.J. (1979): J. Clin. Endocrinol. Metab., 49:805-809.

5. Jung, R.T., Shetty, P.S., Barrand, M., Callingham, B.A., and James, W.P.T.(1979): Br. Med. J., 1:12-13.

6. Landsberg, L., Greff, L., Gunn, S., and Young, J.B.(1980): Metabolism, 29:1128-1137.

7. O'Dea, K., Esler, M., Leonard, P., Stockigt, J.R., and Nestel, P. Metabolism, In press.

8. Rappaport, E.B., Young, J.B., and Landsberg, L.(1981): <u>J. Gerontology</u>, 36:152–157.

9. Rappaport, E.B., Young, J.B., and Landsberg, L.(1982): <u>Endocrinology</u>, 110:650–656.

10. Rappaport, E.B., Young, J.B., and Landsberg, L.(1982): <u>Metabolism</u>, 31:143–146.

11. Rothwell, N.J., and Stock, M.J.(1979): <u>Nature</u>, 281:31–35.

12. Rothwell, N.J., and Stock, M.J.(1980): <u>Can. J. Physiol. Pharmacol.</u> 58:985–991.

13. Rowe, J.W., Young, J.B., Minaker, K.L., Stevens, A.L., Pallotta, J., and Landsberg, L.(1981): <u>Diabetes</u>, 30:219–225.

14. Schwartz, J., Young, J.B., and Landsberg, L.(1982): <u>Clin. Res.</u>, 30:247A.

15. Welle, S., Lilavivanthana, U., and Campbell, R.G.(1980): <u>Metabolism</u>, 29:806–809.

16. Young, J.B., and Landsberg, L.(1977): <u>Nature</u>, 269:615–617.

17. Young, J.B., and Landsberg, L.(1977): <u>Science</u>, 196:1473–1475.

18. Young, J.B., and Landsberg, L.(1979): <u>Am. J. Physiol.</u>, 236:E524–E533.

19. Young, J.B., and Landsberg, L.(1979): <u>J. Clin. Invest.</u>, 64:109–116.

20. Young, J.B., and Landsberg, L.(1980): <u>J. Clin. Invest.</u>, 65:1086–1094.

21. Young, J.B., Rowe, J.W., Pallotta, J.A., Sparrow, D., and Landsberg, L.(1980): <u>Metabolism</u>, 29:532–539.

22. Young, J.B., Saville, E., Rothwell, N.J., Stock, M.J., and Landsberg, L.(1982): <u>J. Clin. Invest.</u>, 69:1061–1071.

The Adipocyte and Obesity: Cellular and
Molecular Mechanisms, edited by A. Angel,
C. H. Hollenberg, and D. A. K. Roncari.
Raven Press, New York © 1983.

Obesity and the Fat Cell: Future Prospects

C. H. Hollenberg, D. A. K. Roncari, P. Djian

Department of Medicine, Banting and Best Diabetes Centre, Institute of Medical Sciences,
University of Toronto, Toronto, Ontario, M5S 1A1 Canada

During the course of this symposium, information has been
presented in a number of areas that link adipose tissue function and
obesity. I would like to conclude this review by focusing on three
areas that may be of particular importance in furthering our understanding of the tissue and the disease. These areas include energy
balance, the adaptation of adipose tissue to positive energy balance
and the cellular biology of adipose tissue. In discussing each area,
I will attempt to highlight certain problems that require solution
if we are to advance significantly our understanding of the cellular
and molecular mechanisms that accompany obesity. Obviously this
approach is highly personal and prejudiced but as long as it is not
taken too seriously, it might lead to useful argument.

The Genesis of Obesity

Our present understanding of the genesis of human obesity can be
simply stated. For reasons that may be obscure, an individual enters
into positive caloric balance. This perturbation is signalled to
adipose tissue by alterations in the plasma concentration of certain
hormones and nutrients. White adipose tissue responds to these
signals by changes in the activity of key enzyme systems which result
in an increase in both nutrient removal from the circulation and in
storage of this nutrient as neutral fat. Expansion of adipose tissue
results, and if the state of positive caloric balance is maintained
over a long enough period, clinical obesity ensues. In this concept,
adipose tissue is seen as a passive accomplice to the crime of positive
caloric balance. Unexpended calories are pushed into the tissue
which, while capable of being adapted to receive extra nutrient, plays

no role at all in the fundamental abnormality of caloric balance that initiates the problem.

Examination of each step of this process reveals major gaps in our knowledge. Our understanding of energy balance in obesity is at best fragmentary and while we have a much better comprehension of the processes that allow adipose tissue to adapt to positive caloric balance, we can describe this adaptation in general rather than in quantitative terms. Finally, although we are just beginning to explore the cellular biology of adipose tissue, there are already hints that adipose tissue may not simply be a passive recipient of calories but may play a more active and genetically determined role in the genesis of obesity. I would like to examine each of these areas in more detail.

III Energy Balance and Obesity

Earlier in this symposium, Dr. Himms-Hagen reviewed the evidence linking the development of obesity in some rodents to a defect in energy expenditure. In some animals with inherited obese syndromes, an abnormality in brown fat metabolism leads to a reduced capacity for thermogenesis when the animals are exposed to stimuli such as cold or catecholamine administration (28,29). These data, plus the common clinical observation that some obese patients fail to lose weight with normal energy intakes, have suggested to many that some forms of human obesity may mimic animal models and may be due to a constitutional abnormality in energy expenditure. Search for this abnormality represents one of the central themes of contemporary obesity research. The role, if any, of brown fat in energy balance in adult man remains a subject of debate and the applicability of the animal models to man cannot even be approached until this role and indeed the presence of brown fat in adult man is established. Further, although provocative data have been produced suggesting that obese humans have a blunted thermogenic response to food and norepinephrine (11,21), other studies have produced either equivocal results or have failed to demonstrate any abnormality (4,5,13). Another approach to this problem is based on the observation that sodium-potassium pump activity is an important contributor to total energy expenditure and that sodium-potassium ATPase is the enzymatic basis of pump activity. Hence a search has been made for differences between normal and obese individuals in the activity of this enzyme in several tissues. While provocative data have emerged from one laboratory, consistent differences have not been observed; indeed some of the results are totally contradictory (2,6,18). Thus, the question of whether a constitutional abnormality of energy balance exists in the obese remains unanswered despite two entirely different approaches to the problem. It is quite possible that the present techniques are not sufficiently sensitive or reproducible to detect the very small change in energy expenditure that will, over time, lead to excessive fatness. Further, it is very likely that the obese population is comprised of groups of different etiologies and that only some patients have a genetically determined abnormality of energy balance. If the obese group were to be stratified according to genetic markers, a sub-group might be identified in which a genetic abnormality would be more likely and hence more easily identified.

Selection on the basis of family history is unlikely by itself to be
satisfactory and a more rigorous genetic analysis will be required.
A possible approach to this analysis involves HLA typing of obese
patients with a strong family history of the disease. Another
approach is to study massively obese patients who display accelerated
replication of adipocyte precursors, an abnormality very likely to be
genetically determined (24).

The entire concept of a constitutional abnormality in energy
expenditure in obesity rests on the supposition that genetic factors
are important in the regulation of thermogenesis. As likely as this
proposition is, it has never, to my knowledge, been proven. Hence
it would be of great interest to determine whether resting metabolism
and the thermogenic response to physiological stimuli such as food
and exercise are genetically controlled. This question can be
explored in man using mono and dizygotic twins provided that attention
is paid to assuring equal similarities in body composition between
the two groups of twins. This would appear to be an important and
feasible study. A positive result would clearly establish the genetic
control of energy metabolism and would place on a firm footing those
concepts that explain inter-individual variation in energy output on
the basis of genetic variability.

IV   The Adaptation of Adipose Tissue to Positive Energy Balance

I would now like to leave the rather unsatisfactory field of
energy balance and move into an area where we have considerably more
knowledge, the adaptation of adipose tissue to positive energy
balance. This adaptation involves the generation of signals
indicating assumption of positive caloric balance, receipt of these
signals by adipose tissue and translation of these signals in this
tissue so that fat storage rather than fat mobilization becomes its
predominant function. In adipose tissue, the translation process
involves alterations in the activity of those enzyme systems involved
in assimilation of circulating lipoprotein triglyceride, in the
synthesis of new adipose triglyceride and in the regulation of
lipolysis. While we have considerable knowledge about the regulation
of each of these enzyme systems, we still lack essential information
about some crucial steps in enzyme control, the quantitative significance of some changes in enzyme activity, and the mechanisms that
integrate the entire process.

It has long been established that circulating lipoprotein triglyceride is the main precursor of adipose lipid and that assimilation of
this lipid by fat cells requires its prior hydrolysis by lipoprotein
lipase (9,10). It is also well established that the activity of this
enzyme in fat tissue is high in fed, non-diabetic animals and
decreases with fasting and insulin deficiency. These changes are
considered to represent an important adaptation of the organism to an
altered nutritional state and to facilitate assimilation of plasma
triglyceride by fat tissue when calories are abundant. Gastric
inhibitory polypeptide (GIP), a hormone secreted after either glucose
or fat feeding, also increases adipocyte lipoprotein lipase activity
(7) and may be of importance in signalling the tissue that a fat meal
has been ingested. It is known that the effect of both insulin and

GIP on enzyme activity in adipocytes can be blocked by inhibitors of protein synthesis (7,20), and this fact together with the known rapid turnover of the enzyme leads to the reasonable assumption that these hormones influence enzyme activity in fat cells by enhancing enzyme synthesis. It is also assumed that enzyme synthesized in adipocytes is released by the cell, migrates to the vascular tree and binds to heparan sulphate on the surface of capillary endothelial cells where it exerts its lipolytic action.

Despite the fact that this enzyme has received an extraordinary amount of attention, there is surprisingly little more known about its regulation. It is unclear whether the effect of insulin on lipo-protein lipase represents a specific effect of the hormone on the enzyme or whether it is a manifestation of the overall stimulation of adipocyte protein synthesis produced by insulin. Further, it is not known whether insulin influences the transcriptional, translational or post-translational steps in enzyme synthesis. While it is con-sidered likely that in adipose tissue the enzyme exists in two forms, one less active and possibly the precursor of the other, differences in the molecular structure of the two forms have not been elucidated nor have the factors governing their interconversion been established. Further, it is not as yet known whether regulation of enzyme activity occurs at any of the steps involving release of enzyme from the fat cell, transport to capillary endothelium, binding to endothelium, and turnover of bound enzyme. It would be of particular interest to determine if turnover of enzyme bound to capillary endothelium is related to the flux of lipoprotein triglyceride through the capillary bed. It is also important to obtain more quantitative information on the effect of diurnal variations in adipocyte lipoprotein lipase activity on the distribution of lipoprotein triglyceride amongst tissues such as heart and adipose tissue. Changes in the quantity of enzyme in adipose tissue will only affect plasma triglyceride uptake by this tissue when the enzyme is rate limiting. There are as yet insufficient data to determine whether, at normal plasma triglyceride concentrations, the adipose enzyme ever becomes rate limiting even after overnight fasting. If it does not, then the redistribution of plasma triglyceride away from fat tissue and towards cardiac muscle produced by fasting may not be due to a reduction in the quantity of adipose enzyme but may be more a reflection of differences between the heart and adipose enzymes in substrate affinity.

A second component of the adaptation of adipose tissue to positive caloric balance involves the transfer of fatty acids, produced by hydrolysis of lipoprotein triglyceride, from the capillary endothelium into fat tissue and the formation within the tissue of new adipose triglyceride. If the tissue is not to be poisoned with fatty acids, these adjustments must occur in a highly co-ordinated fashion. At first glance, the problem seems simple; fatty acids diffuse into fat cells along a concentration gradient and are esterified with glycero-phosphate which is generated in increased amounts because of the enhanced metabolism of glucose that occurs in the tissue during feeding. However, it is likely that this co-ordination is a far more complex process. There is recent evidence indicating that entry of fatty acids into fat cells involves a saturable transport system and that diffusion comes into play only at high concentrations of unbound fatty acid (1). The possibility that the capacity of this transport system is sensitive to hormonal and nutritional alterations deserves early exploration. Further, some of the crucial enzymes involved in triglyceride synthesis are subject to metabolic regulation by processes including phosphorylation - de-phosphorylation and induction by insulin (22,23). Obviously the entire function of adipose tissue as a lipid storage site depends upon the co-ordinated regulation of lipoprotein lipase, the adipocyte fatty acid transport system and the key enzymes involved in triglyceride synthesis, and yet little is known about how this co-ordination is produced. It is very likely that insulin plays an important role in this process and the availability of adipocyte cell culture systems should open the way to a careful study of the effect of this hormone on these catalytic and transport proteins at various stages of fat cell development. It is also conceivable that the cell culture approach, when combined with the availability of purified enzymes, will allow localization of the genes coding for these proteins. Indeed localization and sequencing of the lipoprotein lipase gene should be approachable given present knowledge and would be of immense benefit in furthering our understanding of the control of this key enzyme.

A third adaptation of the fat cell to positive caloric balance involves changes in the lipolytic system and hence in the rate of fat mobilization. The elucidation of the mechanism of activation of hormone sensitive lipase has been a matter of intense and successful study over the past 25 years. It is known that the enzyme is activated by phosphorylation, a reaction catalyzed by a cyclic AMP-dependent protein kinase, while inactivation results from dephosphorylation catalyzed by a protein phosphatase. Hormonal control of the lipase usually, but not invariably, involves hormonal regulation of the intracellular concentration of cyclic AMP which in turn results from hormonal effects on adenylate cyclase or cyclic AMP phosphodiesterase. It has recently become clear that the cyclase is part of a three component complex including hormone-specific receptors, a GTP sensitive coupling subunit and the catalytic component of the cyclase. New information concerning the functioning of the complex is accumulating very rapidly with attention being focused particularly on the mobility, molecular structure and ligand-induced chemical change of receptors, on the coupling activity of the GTP-binding subunit and on the mechanism of activation of the cyclase. There is no doubt but that this area of research will continue to be one of the most fruitful in modern biology.

Obviously the physiological control of lipolysis is exerted not only by agents that activate hormone-sensitive lipase but also by those that reduce the activity of this enzyme. Three hormones or groups of hormones exhibit anti-lipolytic properties, insulin, E-prostaglandins and those catecholamines that occupy alpha-2 receptors. Of these, there is general agreement only about the physiological importance of the anti-lipolytic effect of insulin. This is a most sensitive effect of the hormone; indeed insulin is probably the most important factor regulating the mobilization of fat on a moment-to-moment basis. Despite much work, the precise mechanism by which insulin inhibits lipolysis remains unclear. Three effects of insulin in adipocytes have been reported, each of which could influence the lipolytic process. These effects include inhibition of adenylate cyclase (8), activation of low Km phosphodiesterase (16,30), and production of a series of mediators from the plasma membrane when the membrane is exposed to insulin (14,26). One of the mediators inhibits cyclic AMP-dependent protein kinase, activates a phosphoprotein phosphatase and is likely responsible for the effect of insulin on both adenylate cyclase and phosphodiesterase. It is not as yet clear whether this mediator is also responsible for the inhibitory effect of insulin on the lipase and, if so, whether the mediator acts via altering cyclic AMP levels or through activation of a phosphatase. Given the poor correlation between effects of insulin on lipolysis and on adipocyte cyclic AMP values, the latter possibility is perhaps the more likely. The entire problem of the mechanism of regulation of lipolysis by insulin is intimately bound up with elucidation of the fundamental mode of action of the hormone and currently extraordinary progress is being made in this area.

The inhibition of lipolysis produced by alpha-2 agonists is a well recognized phenomenon that is mediated via inhibition of adenylate cyclase by mechanisms that are as yet unclear. This response is most evident, both in vivo and in vitro, when the stimulatory beta adrenergic receptors are blocked. Data attempting to explain the alterations in lipolysis seen in hypo and hyperthyroidism, diabetes and fasting on alterations in the balance of adipocyte alpha-2 and beta receptors are confusing and contradictory. Indeed it is unlikely that the effect of thyroid hormone on altering the sensitivity of the lipase system to catecholamines is due to changes in catecholamine receptor balance; this action is more probably a result of an influence of the hormone on the coupling subunit of the cyclase complex (17). Nonetheless, there are interesting regional variations in catecholamine receptor balance that correlate with regional variations in propensity to fat storage (12,19). These differences in receptor ratio are of interest from another viewpoint since they may be indicative of a distinct genetic origin of fat cells in different depots.

The E class of prostaglandins is another group of substances that have anti-lipolytic properties. Adipose tissue possesses the enzymatic machinery to convert free arachadonic acid to prostaglandins and hence prostaglandin synthesis in fat tissue proceeds most rapidly during lipolysis. This fact suggests that prostaglandins may act as effectors of a negative feed-back loop that limits the lipolytic response to lipolytic agents. Prostaglandins alter lipolysis by inhibition of adenylate cyclase and it will be interesting to determine whether the cyclase inhibition produced by alpha-2 agonists, prostaglandins and insulin have any common features. At present, it is uncertain whether alpha-2 agonists and prostaglandins are of physiological importance in the control of lipolysis. This is an important area for future study and deserves more attention than it has heretofore received.

In looking ahead to other research in this area, it is of importance to remember that adipose tissue is frequently exposed to a mixture of signals that often carry contradictory messages. For example, feeding produces both insulin and catecholamine release while exposure of the tissue to lipolytic agents produces both lipolysis and

production of prostaglandins. Hence in addition to exploring the
separate molecular mechanisms that subserve the action of each hormone,
it is important to study these mechanisms in the presence of
physiological combinations of hormones and over concentration ranges
that apply in intact man. Further, it might be expected that the
integrated responses to several hormones will change as cells enlarge
and that this change will vary depot to depot. Indeed the exploration
of differences due to region and cell size may be one of the most
fruitful areas for future research.

V   Cellular Biology of Adipose Tissue

Finally, I would like to turn to the cellular biology of adipose
tissue, a field which in my opinion holds the greatest promise for
fundamental advances in our understanding of the role of adipose tissue
in the genesis of obesity. The development of techniques of estimation
of fat cell number, of adipocyte DNA synthesis in intact animals and of
procedures for cell culture of primordial fat cells of animal and human
origin have provided powerful tools for the study of the genesis and
differentiation of fat cells and of fat cell turnover at various times
of life. Of the various new concepts that have emerged from these
approaches, there are several that are of particular interest.

Earlier in this symposium, Roncari elaborated on his observation
that primordial fat cells derived from massively obese patients and
propogated in tissue culture replicate more rapidly than cells from
normal weight individuals (25). This is, of course, a most important
observation since it is one of the few indications that a fraction of
the obese population may harbour a genetic abnormality of adipocyte
reproduction. More recent work from this laboratory has demonstrated
that mature human fat cells, when placed in a medium deficient in
factors necessary to promote fat cell maturation, will de-differentiate,
a process which involves loss of lipid, elongation of cells and the
return of a capacity for cell replication. New observations indicate
that the replication rate of de-differentiated cells derived from
massively obese patients is at least as rapid as that of primordial
cells obtained from the same biopsy. Hence as fat cells from the
massively obese mature, they retain the mechanism responsible for
accelerated replication and this mechanism is again expressed when
mature cells de-differentiate. The process that allows this mechanism
to be turned off and on as the cell gains and loses lipid is of
fundamental interest and will be the subject of much future research.
Further, the de-differentiated cell may well prove to be an important
new tool for studies of the regulation of fat cell division and differentiation since the origin of this cell is known precisely. This is,
of course, not the case in working with primordial fat cells derived
from a mixed stromal population.

There is yet another, even more highly speculative aspect of the
cellular biology of adipose tissue that requires exploration. This
concerns the possibility that the adipocyte precursor pool consists of
multiple clones of genetically distinct cells rather than a single,
genetically homogeneous family. This concept is, of course, not unique
to adipose tissue for it is considered likely that many normal adult
tissues are polyclonal in origin. A very striking example of this

phenomenon can be seen in the thyroid when autoradiography is performed shortly after injection of l^{125}. Nearly all follicles contain at least two families of cells, one which rapidly iodinates intracellular thyroglobulin and another which has little capacity for iodination (27).

While the polyclonal nature of adipose tissue has not been as definitively established, it is strongly suggested by the differing properties displayed by fat tissue obtained from different anatomic regions. For example, in man, alpha-1 receptors are detectable on omental adipose tissue and are entirely lacking in subcutaneous fat (3). Further, recent studies in our laboratory indicate that adipocyte precursors obtained from perirenal fat replicate more rapidly than those from the epididymal region. These results are independent of the age of the animal and are obtained with precursors grown in secondary culture and hence many generations removed from the animal. This fundamental difference in behaviour of tissue derived from the two sites may explain why high fat feeding produces a much greater increase in fat cell number of perirenal than in epididymal fat (15).

Recently, Djian, working in Roncari's laboratory, has obtained very preliminary data suggesting that precursors obtained from a single tissue sample may be polyclonal. In this study, preadipocytes derived from rat perirenal fat were grown in a tissue culture system in which colonies of preadipocytes were produced, each colony being derived from a single parent preadipocyte. During tissue culture, there was marked variation between colonies in the rate at which constituent cells accumulated lipid. These results strongly suggest that there were marked differences amongst parent cells in the programme of differentiation and hence in genomic regulation.

The possibility that adipocyte precursors are a polyclonal mixture raises some interesting questions as to the contribution of adipose tissue to the genesis of obesity. It is conceivable that there is inter-individual variation in the mixture of cell families that make up the adipocyte precursor pool. Hence an individual could be predisposed to obesity because of the presence within this adipocyte precursor pool of an unusual proportion of cells programmed for rapid differentiation. Exposure of this individual to positive caloric balance would result in more rapid and more extensive recruitment of mature fat cells from the precursor pool than in an individual not so predisposed. If this inter-individual difference is great enough, the same caloric input could result in a greater accumulation of fat in the one with the genetic predisposition. Hence it is conceivable that in some of the obese, adipose tissue may not be simply a passive recipient of extra calories that are pushed into it. This tissue may actively assist in its own growth by pulling into its primordial cell pool an unusual fraction of circulating energy due to the presence within this pool of an unusual number of cells programmed for rapid differentiation.

Obviously this "push-pull" theory of obesity is highly speculative but perhaps is no more so than others we have all been testing over the past few years. In any event, this hypothesis is sufficiently fanciful to serve as a fitting conclusion to one of the most hazardous of enterprises, an attempt to forecast the future of research in a complex and rapidly moving area.

1. Abumrad, N.A., Perkins, R.C., Park, J.H., and Park, C.R. (1981): J. Biol. Chem., 256:9183-9191.

2. Bray, G., Kral, J.G., and Björntorp, P. (1981): N. Engl. J. Med., 304:1580-1582.

3. Burns, T.W., Langley, P.E., Terry, B.E., Bylund, D.B., Hoffman, B.B., Tharp, M.D., Lefkowitz, R.J., Garcia-Sainz, J.A., and Fain, J.N. (1981): J. Clin. Invest., 67:467-475.

4. Cunningham, J., Levitt, M., Hendler, R., Nadel, E., and Felig, P. (1982): Clin. Res., 30:244A.

5. Daniels, R., Katzeff, H., Ravussin, E., Garrow, J., and Danforth, E. (1982): Clin. Res., 30:244A.

6. De Luise, M., Blackburn, G., and Flier, J.S. (1980): N. Engl. J. Med., 303:1017-1022.

7. Eckel, R.H., Fujimoto, W.Y., and Brunzell, J.D. (1979): Diabetes, 28:1141-1142.

8. Hepp, K.D. (1971): Fed. Eur. Biochem. Soc. Lett., 12:263-266.

9. Hollenberg, C.H. (1959): Am. J. Physiol., 197:667-670.

10. Hollenberg, C.H. (1966): J. Clin. Invest., 45:205-216.

11. Jung, R.T., Shetty, P.S., James, W.P.T., Barrand, M.A., and Callingham, B.A. (1979): Nature, 279:322-323.

12. Kather, H. (1981): Triangle, 20:131-143.

13. Katzeff, H. and Danforth, E. (1982): Clin. Res., 30:245A.

14. Larner, J., Galasko, G., Cheng, K., DePaoli-Roach, A.A., Huang, L., Daggy, P., and Kellogg, J. (1979): Science, 206: 1408-1410.

15. Lemonnier, D. (1972): J. Clin. Invest., 51:2907-2915.

16. Loten, E.G. and Sneyd, J.G.T. (1970): Biochem. J., 120:187-193.

17. Malbon, C.C., Moreno, F.J., Cabelli, R.J., and Fain, J.N. (1978): J. Biol. Chem., 253:671-677.

18. Mir, M.A., Charalambous, B.H., Morgan, K., and Evans, P.J. (1981): N. Engl. J. Med., 305:1264-1267.

19. Östman, J., Arner, P., Engfeldt, P., and Kager, L. (1979): Metabolism, 28:1198-1205.

20. Patten, R.L. (1970): J. Biol. Chem., 245:5577-5584.

21. Pittet, P., Chappuis, P., Acheson, K., de Techtermann, F., and Jequier, E. (1976): Br. J. Nutr., 35:281-292.

22. Roncari, D.A.K., Mack, E.Y.W., and Yip, D.K. (1979): Can. J. Biochem., 57:573-577.

23. Roncari, D.A.K. and Mack, E.Y.W. (1981): Can. J. Biochem., 59: 944-950.

24. Roncari, D.A.K., Lau, D.C.W., and Kindler, S. (1981): Metabolism, 30:425-427.

25. Roncari, D.A.K., Lau, D.C.W., Djian, Ph., Kindler, S., and Yip, D.K. (1982): In: The Adipocyte and Obesity: Cellular and Molecular Mechanisms, edited by A. Angel, C.H. Hollenberg, and D.A.K. Roncari, pp. . Raven Press, New York.

26. Seals, J.R., McDonald, J.M., and Jarett, L. (1979): J. Biol. Chem., 254:6997-7001.

27. Studer, H. and Ramelli, F. (1982): Endocrine Reviews, 3:40-61.

28. Thurlby, P.L. and Trayhurn, P. (1978): Br. J. Nutr., 39:397-402.

29. Thurlby, P.L. and Trayhurn, P. (1980): Pflugers Arch., 385: 193-201.

30. Zinman, B. and Hollenberg, C.H. (1974): J. Biol. Chem., 249: 2182-2187.

Subject Index